Pediatric Endocrinology and Diabetes

Editors

DENIS DANEMAN
MARK R. PALMERT

PEDIATRIC CLINICS
OF NORTH AMERICA

www.pediatric.theclinics.com

Consulting Editor
BONITA F. STANTON

August 2015 • Volume 62 • Number 4

ELSEVIER

1600 John F. Kennedy Boulevard • Suite 1800 • Philadelphia, Pennsylvania, 19103-2899

http://www.theclinics.com

THE PEDIATRIC CLINICS OF NORTH AMERICA Volume 62, Number 4
August 2015 ISSN 0031-3955, ISBN-13: 978-0-323-39350-8

Editor: Kerry Holland
Developmental Editor: Casey Jackson

The Pediatric Clinics of North America (ISSN 0031-3955) is published bimonthly by Elsevier Inc., 360 Park Avenue South, New York, NY 10010-1710. Months of issue are February, April, June, August, October, and December. Periodicals postage paid at New York, NY and additional mailing offices. Subscription prices are $200.00 per year (US individuals), $493.00 per year (US institutions), $270.00 per year (Canadian individuals), $657.00 per year (Canadian institutions), $325.00 per year (international individuals), $657.00 per year (international institutions), $100.00 per year (US students and residents), and $165.00 per year (international and Canadian residents and students). To receive students/resident rare, orders must be accompanied by name of affiliated institution, date of term, and the signature of program/residency coordinator on institution letterhead. Orders will be billed at individual rate until proof of status is received. Foreign air speed delivery is included in all *Clinics* subscription prices. All prices are subject to change without notice. **POSTMASTER:** Send address changes to *The Pediatric Clinics of North America*, Elsevier Health Sciences Division, Subscription Customer Service, 3251 Riverport Lane, Maryland Heights, MO 63043. **Customer Service: 1-800-654-2452 (US and Canada). From outside of the US and Canada: 1-314-447-8871. Fax: 1-314-447-8029. For print support, E-mail: JournalsCustomerService-usa@elsevier.com. For online support, E-mail: JournalsOnlineSupport-usa@elsevier.com**.

Reprints. For copies of 100 or more, of articles in this publication, please contact the Commercial Reprints Department, Elsevier Inc., 360 Park Avenue South, New York, NY 10010-1710. Tel.: 212-633-3874; Fax: 212-633-3820; E-mail: reprints@elsevier.com.

The Pediatric Clinics of North America is also published in Spanish by McGraw-Hill Inter-americana Editores S.A., Mexico City, Mexico; in Portuguese by Riechmann and Affonso Editores, Rua Comandante Coelho 1085, CEP 21250, Rio de Janeiro, Brazil; and in Greek by Althayia SA, Athens, Greece.

The Pediatric Clinics of North America is covered in *MEDLINE/PubMed (Index Medicus), Excerpta Medica, Current Contents, Current Contents/Clinical Medicine, Science Citation Index, ASCA, ISI/BIOMED,* and *BIOSIS*.

PROGRAM OBJECTIVE

The goal of the *Pediatric Clinics of North America* is to keep practicing physicians and residents up to date with current clinical practice in pediatrics by providing timely articles reviewing the state-of-the-art in patient care.

TARGET AUDIENCE

All practicing pediatricians, physicians and healthcare professionals who provide patient care to pediatric patients.

LEARNING OBJECTIVES

Upon completion of this activity, participants will be able to:
1. Review the consequences and long term outcomes of childhood diabetes.
2. Discuss disorders in sex development in the infant and gender identity in the child.
3. Recognize the impact of novel technology on diabetes diagnosis and management.

ACCREDITATION

The Elsevier Office of Continuing Medical Education (EOCME) is accredited by the Accreditation Council for Continuing Medical Education (ACCME) to provide continuing medical education for physicians.

The EOCME designates this enduring material for a maximum of 15 *AMA PRA Category 1 Credit*(s)™. Physicians should claim only the credit commensurate with the extent of their participation in the activity.

All other health care professionals requesting continuing education credit for this enduring material will be issued a certificate of participation.

DISCLOSURE OF CONFLICTS OF INTEREST

The EOCME assesses conflict of interest with its instructors, faculty, planners, and other individuals who are in a position to control the content of CME activities. All relevant conflicts of interest that are identified are thoroughly vetted by EOCME for fair balance, scientific objectivity, and patient care recommendations. EOCME is committed to providing its learners with CME activities that promote improvements or quality in healthcare and not a specific proprietary business or a commercial interest.

The planning committee, staff, authors and editors listed below have identified no financial relationships or relationships to products or devices they or their spouse/life partner have with commercial interest related to the content of this CME activity:
Catherine Birken, MD, FRCPC; Herbert J. Bonifacio, MD, MSc, MPH, MA; Fergus J. Cameron, BMedSci, MBBS, DipRACOG, FRACP, MD; Wayne S. Cutfield, MBChB, MD; Denis Daneman, MBBCh, DSc (Med), FRCPC; Elisa De Franco, PhD; Johnny Deladoëy, MD, PhD; José G.B. Derraik, PhD; Sian Ellard, PhD, FRCPath; Anjali Fortna; Melissa Gardner, MA; Katharine Garvey, MD, MPH; Maria Güemes, MD; Alistair J. Gunn, MBChB, PhD; Muskaan Gurnani, BHSc; Jennifer Harrington, MBBS, FRACP, PhD; Kerry Holland; Khalid Hussain, MD, PhD; Mary Anne Jamieson, MD; Craig A. Jefferies, MBChB, MD; Indu Kumari; Meranda Nakhla, MSc, MD, FRCPC; Mark R. Palmert, MD, PhD; Stephen M. Rosenthal, MD; David E. Sandberg, PhD; Etienne Sochett, MB ChB, FRCPC; Bonita F. Stanton, MD; Megan Suermann; Guy Van Vliet, MD; Diane K. Wherrett, MD, FRCPC; Neil H. White, MD, CDE; Joseph I. Wolfsdorf, MB, BCh.

The planning committee, staff, authors and editors listed below have identified financial relationships or relationships to products or devices they or their spouse/life partner have with commercial interest related to the content of this CME activity:
Jill Hamilton, MD, FRCPC has research support from Mead Johnson & Company, LLC.

UNAPPROVED/OFF-LABEL USE DISCLOSURE

The EOCME requires CME faculty to disclose to the participants:
1. When products or procedures being discussed are off-label, unlabelled, experimental, and/or investigational (not US Food and Drug Administration [FDA] approved); and
2. Any limitations on the information presented, such as data that are preliminary or that represent ongoing research, interim analyses, and/or unsupported opinions. Faculty may discuss information about pharmaceutical agents that is outside of FDA-approved labelling. This information is intended solely for CME and is not intended to promote off-label use of these medications. If you have any questions, contact the medical affairs department of the manufacturer for the most recent prescribing information.

TO ENROLL

To enroll in the *Pediatric Clinics of North America* Continuing Medical Education program, call customer service at 1-800-654-2452 or sign up online at http://www.theclinics.com/home/cme. The CME program is available to subscribers for an additional annual fee of USD 290.

METHOD OF PARTICIPATION

In order to claim credit, participants must complete the following:

1. Complete enrollment as indicated above.
2. Read the activity.
3. Complete the CME Test and Evaluation. Participants must achieve a score of 70% on the test. All CME Tests and Evaluations must be completed online.

CME INQUIRIES/SPECIAL NEEDS

For all CME inquiries or special needs, please contact elsevierCME@elsevier.com.

Contributors

CONSULTING EDITOR

BONITA F. STANTON, MD
Vice Dean for Research and Professor of Pediatrics, School of Medicine, Wayne State University, Detroit, Michigan

EDITORS

DENIS DANEMAN, MBBCh, FRCPC, DSc (Med)
R.S. McLaughlin Foundation Chair in Paediatrics; Professor and Chair, Department of Paediatrics, Paediatrician-in-Chief, The Hospital for Sick Children, University of Toronto, Toronto, Canada

MARK R. PALMERT, MD, PhD
Head, Division of Endocrinology, The Hospital for Sick Children; Professor, Departments of Paediatrics and Physiology, University of Toronto, Toronto, Ontario, Canada

AUTHORS

CATHERINE BIRKEN, MD, FRCPC
Division of Paediatric Medicine, Department of Paediatrics, The Hospital for Sick Children, University of Toronto, Toronto, Ontario, Canada

HERBERT J. BONIFACIO, MD, MSc, MPH, MA
Division of Adolescent Medicine, Lecturer, Department of Pediatrics; Clinical Lead, Transgender Youth Clinic, The Hospital for Sick Children, University of Toronto, Toronto, Ontario, Canada

FERGUS J. CAMERON, BMedSci, MBBS, DipRACOG, FRACP, MD
Professor, Department of Endocrinology and Diabetes, Royal Children's Hospital, Murdoch Childrens Research Institute; Department of Paediatrics, University of Melbourne, Melbourne, Australia

WAYNE S. CUTFIELD, MBChB, FRACP, MD
Paediatric Endocrinology Service, Starship Children's Hospital, Auckland District Health Board; Liggins Institute, University of Auckland, Auckland, New Zealand

DENIS DANEMAN, MBBCh, FRCPC, DSc (Med)
R.S. McLaughlin Foundation Chair in Paediatrics; Professor and Chair, Department of Paediatrics, Paediatrician-in-Chief, The Hospital for Sick Children, University of Toronto, Toronto, Canada

ELISA DE FRANCO, PhD
Postdoctoral Fellow, Institute of Biomedical and Clinical Science, University of Exeter Medical School, Exeter, United Kingdom

JOHNNY DELADOËY, MD, PhD
Associate Clinical Professor, Department of Pediatrics, Endocrinology Service and Research Center, Centre Hospitalier Universitaire Sainte-Justine; Department of Biochemistry, University of Montreal, Montreal, Quebec, Canada

JOSÉ G.B. DERRAIK, PhD
Liggins Institute, University of Auckland, Auckland, New Zealand

SIAN ELLARD, PhD, FRCPath
Professor of Human Molecular Genetics, Institute of Biomedical and Clinical Science, University of Exeter Medical School, Exeter, United Kingdom

MARIA GÜEMES, MD
Developmental Endocrinology Research Group, Molecular Genetics Unit, Institute of Child Health, University College London, United Kingdom

MELISSA GARDNER, MA
Child Health Evaluation & Research (CHEAR) Unit and Division of Child Behavioral Health, Department of Pediatrics, University of Michigan, Ann Arbor, Michigan

KATHARINE GARVEY, MD, MPH
Attending in Endocrinology, Division of Endocrinology, Department of Medicine, Boston Children's Hospital; Instructor in Pediatrics, Department of Pediatrics, Harvard Medical School, Boston, Massachusetts

ALISTAIR J. GUNN, MBChB, FRACP, PhD
Paediatric Endocrinology Service, Starship Children's Hospital, Auckland District Health Board; Department of Physiology, University of Auckland, Auckland, New Zealand

MUSKAAN GURNANI, BHSc
Division of Endocrinology, Department of Paediatrics, The Hospital for Sick Children, University of Toronto, Toronto, Ontario, Canada

JILL HAMILTON, MD, FRCPC
Division of Endocrinology, Department of Paediatrics, The Hospital for Sick Children, University of Toronto, Toronto, Ontario, Canada

JENNIFER HARRINGTON, MBBS, FRACP, PhD
Division of Endocrinology, Department of Pediatrics, The Hospital for Sick Children, University of Toronto, Toronto, Ontario, Canada

KHALID HUSSAIN, MD, PhD
Developmental Endocrinology Research Group, Molecular Genetics Unit, Institute of Child Health, University College London, London, United Kingdom

MARY ANNE JAMIESON, MD
Associate Professor, Department of Obstetrics and Gynecology, Queen's University, Kingston, Ontario, Canada

CRAIG A. JEFFERIES, MBChB, FRACP, MD
Paediatric Endocrinology Service, Starship Children's Hospital, Auckland District Health Board; Liggins Institute, University of Auckland, Auckland, New Zealand

MERANDA NAKHLA, MSc, MD, FRCPC
Department of Paediatrics, Montreal Children's Hospital, McGill University, Montreal, Canada

STEPHEN M. ROSENTHAL, MD
Professor of Pediatrics, Director, Pediatric Endocrine Outpatient Services; Program
Director, Pediatric Endocrinology; Medical Director, Child and Adolescent Gender Center,
University of California, San Francisco, San Francisco, California

DAVID E. SANDBERG, PhD
Child Health Evaluation and Research (CHEAR) Unit and Division of Child Behavioral
Health, Department of Pediatrics, University of Michigan, Ann Arbor, Michigan

ETIENNE SOCHETT, MB ChB, FRCPC
Division of Endocrinology, Department of Pediatrics, Hospital for Sick Children, University
of Toronto, Toronto, Ontario, Canada

GUY VAN VLIET, MD
Professor, Department of Pediatrics, Endocrinology Service and Research Center, Centre
Hospitalier Universitaire Sainte-Justine, Montreal, Quebec, Canada

DIANE K. WHERRETT, MD, FRCPC
Associate Professor, Division of Endocrinology, Department of Pediatrics, Hospital for
Sick Children, University of Toronto, Toronto, Ontario, Canada

NEIL H. WHITE, MD, CDE
Professor of Pediatrics, Department of Pediatrics, Washington University School of
Medicine, St Louis, Missouri

JOSEPH I. WOLFSDORF, MB, BCh
Clinical Director and Associate Chief, Division of Endocrinology, Department of Medicine,
Boston Children's Hospital; Professor, Department of Pediatrics, Harvard Medical
School, Boston, Massachusetts

Contents

> One-third of North American children are overweight or obese. Pathologic obesity accounts for only a small percentage of these cases. The vast majority are the result of a complex interaction of genetic and hormonal, nutritional, physical activity, and physical and social environmental factors. Obesity increases the risk for various cardiometabolic, pulmonary, and psychosocial complications for children, which often continues into adulthood. Multidisciplinary care, focusing on family-centered behavior change, is an evidence-based, essential part of the treatment, along with pharmacologic and surgical options for more complex cases. Prevention and early intervention strategies are key to reversing the obesity epidemic.

> Fractures are common during childhood; however, they can also be the presenting symptom of primary or secondary causes of bone fragility. The challenge is to identify those children who warrant further investigation. In children who present with multiple fractures that are not commonly associated with mild to moderate trauma or whose fracture count is greater than what is typically seen for their age, an initial evaluation, including history, physical examination, biochemistry, and spinal radiography, should be performed. In children with bone pain or evidence of more significant bone fragility, referral for specialist evaluation and consideration of pharmacologic treatment may be warranted.

> Diabetic ketoacidosis (DKA) is a major cause of morbidity and mortality in children with type 1 diabetes mellitus (T1DM). This article examines the factors associated with DKA in children with T1DM, both at first presentation and in recurrent cases. The challenge for future research is to find effective ways to improve primary care physician and general community awareness of T1DM to reduce DKA at presentation and develop practical, cost-effective programs to reduce recurrent DKA.

Technological innovations have revolutionized the treatment of type 1 diabetes. Although technological advances can potentially improve diabetes outcomes, maintenance of target glycemic control, at the present time, remains largely dependent on patient and family motivation, competence, and adherence to daily diabetes care requirements. Trials of closed loop or "artificial pancreas" technology show great promise to automate insulin delivery and achieve near normal glucose control and reduced hypoglycemia with minimal patient intervention.

In this article, the author reviews the long-term outcomes and their precursors of type 1 diabetes starting in youth. The author also contrasts the changing incidence of these long-term complications as we have moved from the pre–Diabetes Control and Complications Trial (DCCT) to the post-DCCT standard of care and reviews the emerging data related to complications in youths with type 2 diabetes. Finally, the author reviews the recent understanding related to the effects of diabetes on the brain and cognition.

A constant supply of glucose to the brain is critical for normal cerebral metabolism. The dysglycemia of type 1 diabetes (T1D) can affect activity, survival, and function of neural cells. Clinical studies in T1D have shown impairments in brain morphology and function. The most neurotoxic milieu seems to be young age and/or diabetic ketoacidosis at onset, severe hypoglycemia under the age of 6 years followed by chronic hyperglycemia. Adverse cognitive outcomes seem to be associated with poorer mental health outcomes. It is imperative to improve outcomes by investigating the mechanisms of injury so that neuroprotective strategies independent of glycemia can be identified.

Overt thyroid dysfunction is documented by serum thyrotropin or T4 concentrations are often ordered for nonspecific complaints and will by definition fall outside of the 95% reference range 5% of the time. In addition, most laboratories quote adult ranges, which are not necessarily applicable to young children, and regression toward the mean is common, justifying that the test be repeated before embarking on treatment. On the other hand, neck ultrasounds are frequently performed for diffuse goiter or non-thyroid conditions. Yet, an ultrasound is not required to make a diagnosis of Hashimoto thyroiditis and small cysts and nodules discovered incidentally often lead to unjustified concerns about neoplasia.

associated with a high risk of brain injury because insulin inhibits lipolysis and ketogenesis thus preventing the generation of alternative brain substrates (such as ketone bodies). Hence HH must be diagnosed as soon as possible and the management instituted appropriately to prevent brain damage. This article reviews the mechanisms of glucose physiology in the newborn, the mechanisms of insulin secretion, the etiologic types of HH, and its management.

The use of targeted gene panels now allows the analysis of all the genes known to cause a disease in a single test. For neonatal diabetes, this has resulted in a paradigm shift with patients receiving a genetic diagnosis early and the genetic results guiding their clinical management. Exome and genome sequencing are powerful tools to identify novel genetic causes of known diseases. For neonatal diabetes, the use of these technologies has resulted in the identification of 2 novel disease genes (*GATA6* and *STAT3*) and a novel regulatory element of *PTF1A*, in which mutations cause pancreatic agenesis.

PEDIATRIC CLINICS OF NORTH AMERICA

THE CLINICS ARE AVAILABLE ONLINE!
Access your subscription at:
www.theclinics.com

Foreword

Pediatric Endocrinology and Diabetes

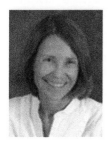

Bonita F. Stanton, MD
Consulting Editor

Dear colleagues,

In May 2015, the world learned that the National Aeronautics and Space Administration (NASA) believes that Antarctica's Larsen B Ice Shelf will disappear by 2020. This Ice Shelf is estimated to have existed for over 10,000 years. As recently as 1995, it was 4445 square miles; by February 2002, it was only 2573 square miles. Then, after another major disintegration a month later, Larsen B was down to 1337 square miles. Currently, it is thought to be about 618 square miles. This Antarctic Ice Shelf is expected to be gone by the year 2020 (http://www.cnn.com/2015/05/16/us/antarctica-larsen-b-ice-shelf-to-disappear/index.html).

This news is distressing for sure, but, you might be wondering, what does it have to do with an issue on pediatric endocrine disorders?

Well, actually, quite a lot. Please note that half of the articles in this fascinating and extremely well-written issue deal with diabetes. There are several reasons for this focus. One reason represents a "good thing": there have been many advances in our understanding of the causes and treatments of diabetes.

Another reason is neither a "good thing" nor a "bad thing"—but is glacierlike. Like glaciers, diabetes has been recognized as a disorder of mankind for thousands of years. In fact, even the term "diabetes" was used by the Greeks over two thousand years ago (http://www.diabetescausestreatments.com/history-of-diabetes.html). In 1936, the two types of diabetes were recognized. Since that time, until recently, diabetes type II has been described as very rare in children.

The third reason is a "bad thing": this long-recognized disorder has been increasing dramatically among children and adults in recent years. Since the year 2000, accompanying the greatly increased rate of obesity among children around the globe, the rate of diabetes mellitus type II has also been increasing dramatically.[1] Diabetes mellitus II is expected to exceed 5% of the global population within the next decade; it already afflicts an estimated 4% of the population. It is expected that by 2050, diabetes may

Pediatr Clin N Am 62 (2015) xv–xvi
http://dx.doi.org/10.1016/j.pcl.2015.05.007
0031-3955/15/$ – see front matter © 2015 Published by Elsevier Inc.

pediatric.theclinics.com

impact one in three US adults. Nearly all of this increase reflects dietary changes, and the global burden will disproportionately impact emerging nations.[2]

Moreover, as is the case with glaciers, much of this increase is a result of things that we are doing, that potentially we could change—if society had the will to do so.

Bonita F. Stanton, MD
School of Medicine
Wayne State University
1261 Scott Hall
540 East Canfield, Suite 1261
Detroit, MI 48201, USA

E-mail address:
bstanton@med.wayne.edu

REFERENCES

1. Springer SC, Silverstein J, Copeland K, et al. Management of type 2 diabetes mellitus in children and adolescents. Pediatrics 2013;131(2):e648–64. http://dx.doi.org/10.1542/peds.2012-3496.
2. Zarshenas MM, Khademian S, Moein M. Diabetes and related remedies in medieval Persian medicine. Indian J Endocrinol Metab 2014;18(2):142–9. http://dx.doi.org/10.4103/2230-8210.129103.

Preface

Pediatric Diabetes and Endocrinology

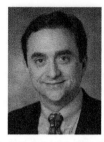
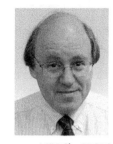

Mark R. Palmert, MD, PhD   Denis Daneman, MBBCh, FRCPC, DSc (Med)
Editors

As guest editors of this issue of *Pediatric Clinics of North America*, "Pediatric Diabetes and Endocrinology," we were tasked with assembling an issue of about a dozen or so articles of direct relevance to the practicing pediatrician. This meant that, rather than dealing with an exhaustive list of topics, we had to be highly selective in ensuring relevance to the target audience. We also had to consider the balance between important updates versus coverage of new topics since the last issues on "Diabetes Mellitus in Children" (December 2005) and general "Pediatric Endocrinology" (December 2011). Our final choices for subject matter span the spectrum from prevention to recognition to cutting-edge clinical translation of recent research findings to outcomes.

Some topics were obvious as they represent the "frontiers" in pediatric endocrinology, namely, childhood obesity and its myriad consequences, and the child with repeated fractures. The vast majority of these children will remain in the care of generalists. Knowing who to investigate and who and when to refer for subspecialty opinion is important both in providing their care and in planning for specialized services.

Preventing diabetic ketoacidosis (DKA) is feasible and the only sure way to prevent the sometimes dire complications of DKA. The remaining three articles in the diabetes section explore, first, the use of technology in achieving goals: the use of pumps and sensors is steadily increasing and, when used optimally, can greatly improve outcomes, but rigorous assessment of cost-effectiveness is still needed. A second article highlights success as current approaches to therapy in type 1 diabetes have begun to show major reductions in the classical diabetes-related complications. The final article highlights that the brain ought to be added to the list of organs needing protection.

We chose to highlight two common reasons for referral to pediatric endocrinologists, namely, minor abnormalities in thyroid function or structure and menstrual irregularities, because most represent normal variations and can be easily separated into the majority that do not require referral from the minority that do. The article on height

Pediatr Clin N Am 62 (2015) xvii–xviii
http://dx.doi.org/10.1016/j.pcl.2015.05.006
0031-3955/15/$ – see front matter © 2015 Published by Elsevier Inc.

enhancement provides reason for pause in the ever-increasing use of growth hormones.

The articles on disorders of sexual differentiation (DSD) and gender dysphoria were included to highlight changing philosophies in these fields: in the indications and timing of surgery for the management of common and uncommon DSDs, and in the approach to and management of gender nonconforming youth. Our patients have taught us enormously in the past 10 years or so.

Finally, the articles on hyperinsulinemic hypoglycemia of infancy and early-onset diabetes (neonatal to about 6 months) highlight the need for molecular genetic diagnosis and the value of next-generation sequencing in informing not only diagnosis but also, perhaps even more importantly, management of these rare conditions.

Much has been left out of this issue, work to do for the next guest editors in pediatric endocrinology and diabetes. We are indebted to an international group of authors and coauthors for their excellent contributions. They all very willingly agreed to participate in this issue of *Pediatric Clinics of North America*.

Mark R. Palmert, MD, PhD
Division of Endocrinology
The Hospital for Sick Children
University of Toronto
555 University Avenue
Toronto, Ontario, Canada M5G 1X8

Denis Daneman, MBBCh, FRCPC, DSc (Med)
Department of Paediatrics
The Hospital for Sick Children
University of Toronto
555 University Avenue
Toronto, Canada M5G 1X8

E-mail addresses:
mark.palmert@sickkids.ca (M.R. Palmert)
denis.daneman@sickkids.ca (D. Daneman)

Childhood Obesity

Causes, Consequences, and Management

Muskaan Gurnani, BHSc[a], Catherine Birken, MD, FRCPC[b], Jill Hamilton, MD, FRCPC[a],*

KEYWORDS

- Childhood • Adolescent • Obesity • Cardiometabolic risk • Lifestyle interventions
- Prevention

KEY POINTS

- Routine body mass index (BMI) screening of children on age-appropriate growth charts is necessary to identify those requiring further assessment.
- Central adiposity is associated with increased risk for type 2 diabetes (T2DM), dyslipidemia, hypertension, sleep-disordered breathing, nonalcoholic fatty liver disease, and polycystic ovarian syndrome (PCOS).
- Family-centered behavior therapy should focus on small goals to improve nutritional intake and physical activity and reduce sedentary behaviors.
- Studies demonstrate modest weight loss of 5% to 10% with improvement in cardiometabolic parameters.
- Psychosocial stressors and comorbidities may make behavior change difficult; empathetic counseling using techniques such as motivational interviewing may be useful adjuncts to therapy.
- Prevention strategies must be implemented across various domains, as children are influenced in the context of their families, cultures, communities, and on a broader population level.

BACKGROUND

Obesity prevalence has increased during the past decades in children and adolescents, leading to a significant current and future health burden.[1] In North America, approximately one-third of children are either overweight or obese.[2,3] Although the overall proportion of children with obesity may be plateauing, the rates of severe obesity in children continue to rise, particularly in very young children.[2–5] Furthermore,

Disclosure Statement: The authors have nothing to disclose.
[a] Division of Endocrinology, Department of Paediatrics, The Hospital for Sick Children, University of Toronto, 555 University Avenue, Toronto, Ontario M5G 1X8, Canada; [b] Division of Paediatric Medicine, Department of Paediatrics, The Hospital for Sick Children, University of Toronto, 555 University Avenue, Toronto, Ontario M5G 1X8, Canada
* Corresponding author.
E-mail address: jill.hamilton@sickkids.ca

the incidence of overweight/obesity for children younger than 5 years in low- and middle-income countries is higher than the rates of wasting.[6] As obesity tends to track into adulthood, especially for those with the most severe degrees of obesity and in older age groups, prevention and intervention strategies should begin at the earliest age possible.[7]

Overweight and obesity in children are assessed clinically by calculation of BMI, obtained by dividing weight (in kilograms) by height squared (square meters). BMI values can be plotted on age- and sex-specific growth charts. Several definitions of pediatric obesity exist, as defined by growth charts compiled by the Centers for Disease Control (CDC), the World Health Organization (WHO), and the International Obesity Task Force.[8] Most commonly, overweight is defined as BMI 85th to 95th percentile (CDC) or 85th to 97th percentile (WHO) and obesity as greater than or equal to 95th percentile (CDC) or greater than or equal to 97th percentile (WHO).[9,10]

ETIOLOGY/RISK FACTORS

Childhood obesity is a complex condition, influenced by genetics, nutritional intake, level of physical activity, and social and physical environment factors.[11,12] Rare pathologic causes may also lead to rapid weight gain; however, in most children, there is no single underlying cause. Red flags for pathologic obesity that may warrant further investigation include rapid onset of weight gain, very early age of onset, obesity discordant with parent weights, hypogonadism, short stature/poor linear growth, and association of dysmorphic features or developmental delay.[13,14]

Environmental Factors

Intrauterine and postnatal factors
Substantial evidence from epidemiologic and experimental animal studies suggest that fetal and early postnatal environmental exposures impact significantly on the development of obesity, diabetes, and heart disease.[15] The "developmental origins of health and disease (DOHaD)" hypothesis posits a stimulus or insult to an organism during a critical period of development can alter gene expression via epigenetic modifications. For example, being either small or large for gestational age is associated with an increased risk of developing childhood obesity.[12] Prenatal exposure to gestational diabetes mellitus (hyperglycemia, hyperinsulinemia), maternal smoking, and high maternal adiposity are correlated with increased incidence of childhood obesity, independent of birth size.[12,16] A systematic review found a strong increased risk of overweight and obesity in individuals delivered by cesarean section.[17] Outcomes related to mode of delivery and obesity may be due to accumulation of differing bacteria in the gut (the microbiome), which influences inflammation, nutrient ingestion, and immune system development in the infant.[18]

Exclusive breast-feeding in the first 6 months correlates with a lower incidence of childhood obesity in cohort studies, although a large randomized clinical trial promoting breast-feeding failed to show a protective effect at age 6.5 years.[19,20] Rapid weight gain in the first few months of life, in addition to an earlier age of BMI rebound (the physiologic increase in slope of the BMI curve normally occurring at age 5–7 years), is also associated with higher rates of childhood obesity and adult cardiometabolic risk.[21,22]

Nutrition/Feeding behaviors
Several dietary factors including higher caloric food intake during infancy, introduction of solid foods before 6 months of age, higher consumption of sweetened drinks (juice, soda), increased fast food consumption, eating while watching television (TV), skipping breakfast, reduced family meal times eating together, and lower daily milk, fruit,

and vegetable intake have all been associated with increased rates of childhood obesity.[12,13,23,24]

Most guidelines recommend 60 minutes of moderate to vigorous daily physical activity for children and adolescents. In Canada, approximately 93% and 96% of Canadian children aged 5 to 11 and 12 to 17 years, respectively, fail to meet these guidelines.[20,25] Low habitual levels of physical activity are associated with higher obesity incidence in multiple studies.[12,16,20] Sedentary behavior, in particular time spent at the TV or computer screen, is associated with higher BMIs,[20] although systematic reviews examining reduced screen time showed no effect on BMI in children.[26]

Obesity and sociodemographic influences

Cross-sectional studies have shown that members of certain ethnic groups (eg, Aboriginal, Hispanic, and South Asian) are more prone to obesity during childhood. Children from low-income countries with greater food security are more prone to becoming obese, as are those in urban areas as compared with children in rural areas. In high-income countries, children in the lowest socioeconomic classes have higher obesity rates in comparison to children from a more affluent socioeconomic position.[12]

Pathologic Causes of Obesity

Endocrine causes

Endocrine disorders, such as hypothyroidism, Cushing syndrome, growth hormone deficiency, and pseudohypoparathyroidism, can present with weight gain and slowed growth. Of these, only Cushing syndrome typically presents with severe obesity; however, all disorders may lead to a more central pattern of weight deposition. Endocrine causes of obesity are rare and are found in less than 1% of children and adolescents with obesity, with hypothyroidism being the most common cause of endocrine-related weight gain.[27] The level of leptin, a hormone produced by adipocytes that acts at the level of the hypothalamus to regulate weight and induce satiety, is elevated in obesity. However, similar to the insulin resistance that develops with increased adiposity, leptin resistance also occurs, and both of these may contribute to reduced satiety and subsequent weight gain.[27,28]

Genetic causes

Rare single gene defects, which specifically result in obesity, are those that affect the leptin-melanocortin regulating pathway.[12,13,29] The genes identified thus far include leptin, the leptin receptor, proopiomelanocortin, prohormone convertase 1, melanocortin receptors (MCR) 3 and 4, and the transcription factor single-minded 1. Of these, only MCR4 mutations are common, accounting for approximately 4% of early-onset and childhood cases of severe obesity.[29,30] There are also several genetic syndromes associated with obesity, including Prader-Willi, Bardet-Biedl, Alström, and WAGR (Wilms tumor, aniridia, genitourinary anomaly, mental retardation) syndromes, which generally exhibit some degree of neurocognitive delay and characteristic dysmorphic features.[12,30]

Common genetic variants associated with high adiposity and weight gain, but having weak individual effects, have been identified through genome-wide association studies, although no single variant contributes in a large way to predict obesity.[12]

Other causes

Central nervous system tumors such as craniopharyngioma located in the hypothalamic region and the subsequent surgery to debulk these tumors can result in reduced satiety, resistance to insulin and leptin, and enhanced insulin secretion due to auto-nomic dysregulation.[31] The net result of these physiologic changes leads to rapid and unrelenting weight gain.[12,16,28] Lastly, medication-induced obesity can occur from the use of atypical antipsychotics and high-dose glucocorticoids.[12,16]

COMORBIDITIES/CONSEQUENCES OF CHILDHOOD OBESITY

There are multiple potential comorbidities associated with obesity, many of which track into adulthood.[11] However, not all overweight or obese children exhibit medical or psychological sequelae; a subset of individuals may exhibit no clinical complica-tions or health risks related to their weight.[32]

In adults, the metabolic syndrome is defined as a clustering of features including in-sulin resistance/elevated glucose, hypertension, abdominal obesity and dyslipidemia that portends risk for T2DM, and cardiovascular disease.[33] The metabolic syndrome is also prevalent in other conditions linked to insulin resistance, such as PCOS and nonalcoholic fatty liver disease (NAFLD).[13,16] In children and adolescents, features of the metabolic syndrome cluster in a similar fashion, although there is no single accepted definition.[34] A systematic review of studies performed in the pediatric age range indicates a prevalence of metabolic syndrome in population-based studies of 3.3%, 11.9%, and 29.2% of normal-weight, overweight, and obese children, respectively.[35]

There is compelling evidence that the obesity-associated dyslipidemia tracks from early life into adulthood.[36,37] In a report from the Bogalusa Heart Study, pathology studies of children and young adults aged 2 to 39 years who died primarily from trau-matic injuries, fatty streaks in the aorta and coronary arteries were documented early in life, and these atherosclerotic changes were associated with elevated cholesterol and higher BMI.[38] In the large population-based US study, the National Health and Nutrition Examination Survey (NHANES) reported that the overall prevalence of dysli-pidemia in children and adolescents is 20.3% and increases to 42.9% in obese youth.[39] Recommendations supporting the use of non–high-density lipoprotein (HDL) cholesterol (calculated as total cholesterol − HDL cholesterol) have been pub-lished, with further evaluation with fasting lipid profile if non-HDL cholesterol is abnormal.[40]

Hypertension is defined as elevated systolic or diastolic blood pressure (BP) greater than or equal to 95th percentile for age, sex, and height-based tables.[41] Studies in American children indicate a prevalence estimate of 10% with prehypertension (95th percentile > BP ≥90th percentile) and 3.7% with hypertension, increasing with increasing BMI and waist circumference.[42] Recognition of elevated BP in the office setting is unrecognized in approximately 25% of cases.[43]

Rates of T2DM in children have increased in parallel with increases in obesity. In 2009, the total prevalence of T2DM in a representative sample of youth younger than 20 years in the United States was 0.24 cases per 1000 individuals, with increasing prevalence with age, whereas the incidence of T2DM in Canada was 11.3 cases per 100,000 children (<18 years) per year, similar to American incidence statistics.[44–46] Impaired glucose tolerance is particularly common in severely obese adolescents, with up to 25% exhibiting this finding.[47] Of great concern are an increasing number of reports indicating that youth diagnosed with T2DM go on to develop significant microvascular and macrovascular complications of diabetes early in adulthood.[48]

Fat deposition in the liver visualized by ultrasonography or elevated levels of hepatic alanine aminotransferase are distinctive for NAFLD, which can progress to more serious liver dysfunction and is a common consequence of obesity in all ages.[13,16]

In addition, gallstones are found to be more prevalent in obese adolescents (2%) as compared with nonobese teens (0.6%), although the mechanisms leading to this have not been completely elucidated.[13,16]

PCOS is one of the most common endocrine disorders affecting 4% to 6% of young women and is the leading cause of infertility.[49] PCOS is characterized by chronic oligo-ovulation or anovulation, hyperandrogenism, and the appearance of polycystic ovaries on ultrasound imaging. Challenges in diagnosing youth with PCOS include physiologic anovulation in the first year postmenarche, presence of acne during puberty, and multifollicular (but not polycystic) appearance of the ovaries during adolescence.[50] Insulin resistance is a core feature of PCOS and leads to stimulation of increased androgen, as well as increased risk for the metabolic syndrome. These features, along with the presence of PCOS symptoms 1 to 2 years after menarche, should prompt further assessment.

Obstructive sleep apnea is 4 to 6 times higher in obese children and adolescents than in nonobese peers.[13,16] Sleep-disordered breathing has been associated with insulin resistance and cardiometabolic risk, as has poor sleep quality in children and adolescents.[51,52] The causal association between obesity and asthma is debatable. However, the apparent association may be due to the difficulty in subjectively distinguishing between shortness of breath related to obesity and increased work effort and wheezing-related symptoms due to asthma.[12,13]

Excessive weight can lead to injury of the developing epiphyseal growth plates, resulting in pain and limited mobility. Blount disease (tibia vara), flatfoot, scoliosis, osteoarthritis, slipped capital femoral epiphysis, and spondylolisthesis leading to low back pain have all been associated with overweight/obesity.[12,13,53,54]

Obese children and adolescents are susceptible to dermatologic conditions such as acanthosis nigricans (hyperpigmented, hyperkeratotic plaques) and intertriginous irritation or infection.[13] Neurologic conditions include an increased risk for intracranial hypertension.[13] Renal pathologies such as hyperfiltration and microalbuminuria may also be seen.[12] Lastly, both vitamin D and iron deficiencies are shown to be increased in overweight and obese children.[12,55]

Psychosocial Comorbidities

Anxiety, depression, stress, low self-esteem and body image, bullying, social withdrawal, and lower quality of life have all been reported to be more common in obese adolescents.[16] Poor school performance, including difficulty with concentration, homework completion, and missed school days, are 4 times more likely in an adolescent obese population when compared with a healthy control sample.[56] Clinical populations of overweight/obese adolescents also show higher lifetime rates of eating disorders, especially bulimia nervosa, than population-based samples.[57] Binge eating disorder (BED), defined as repetitive loss of control of eating of large quantities of food over discrete time frames, without compensatory weight-reduction activity, is common. About 20% to 40% of adolescents seeking treatment of overweight/obesity report symptoms of BED.[57]

ASSESSMENT/SCREENING

Calculation of BMI and plotting on age- and sex-appropriate growth charts for children older than 6 years are recommended by the US Obesity Task Force as routine screening approach for use in clinical practice. There is insufficient evidence to provide a similar recommendation for children younger than 6 years,[58] although this recommendation will likely change over time given increasing obesity incidence in this age group. Although BMI is correlated with percent body fat, it is also correlated with lean tissue mass and height and represents an indirect measure of adiposity.[59] Measurement of skinfold thickness, waist to height ratio, waist circumference, and bioelectrical impedance analysis, which have been shown to predict cardiometabolic risk, have been used as physical measures of adiposity in pediatric research populations, as BMI may not always be accurate in judging adiposity.[13] However, as no reference standards for these measures have been developed for children, from a practical clinical standpoint, they are not recommended for clinical screening.

Tables 1 and 2 outline specific points to consider when gathering history and conducting a physical examination and list suggested investigations to screen for common obesity-related comorbidities. Additional laboratory tests that could be performed if history indicates risk factors include thyroid function, abdominal ultrasonography to assess fatty liver, renal function, albumin to creatinine ratio, and clinical screening for PCOS.[13,60]

In adults, severity of BMI has historically been described as class I–III and is based solely on BMI level; however, this classification does not take into account comorbidities. The Edmonton Obesity Staging System incorporates the presence and severity of comorbidities in adults, divided into 3 major categories, metabolic, mechanical, and mental health.[61] This system has been shown to better predict mortality in NHANES adult data sets.[62] Development of a similar staging system for the pediatric population, to function as part of the clinical care guidelines and risk assessment procedures for children and adolescents with overweight/obesity, would be beneficial to better target assessment and intervention strategies.

TREATMENT

The goals of weight management are to prevent and reduce the risk of obesity-related sequelae, with a focus on healthy behavioral change. For growing children, weight maintenance may be a goal, and for those who have a more significantly elevated BMI, a steady, gradual weight loss (ie, not more than 0.5 kg/wk) is recommended.[63]

A key message is that improvement of health outcomes, with reduced focus on weight loss, is the primary goal of treatment. The American Academy of Pediatrics Expert Committee established a 4-tiered approach to the management of obesity, outlined in **Fig. 1**.[64] Motivational interviewing approaches to communication are also recommended.[65] The Canadian Obesity Network has developed an office approach for clinicians to use with children with obesity: the 5A's of Obesity Management—Ask, Assess, Advice, Agree, and Arrange (**Box 1**).[66,67] This 5A approach has been used previously to address numerous other health interventions, including smoking cessation.[67]

Nonpharmacologic Approaches

Family-based interventions centered on changing dietary habits, physical activity, and thinking/behavior can lead to improvements in weight-related comorbidities, even with modest weight loss of 5% to 10%.[59] A 2009 Cochrane systematic review of lifestyle management for pediatric obesity demonstrated an overall reduction of −0.06 BMI-standard deviation score (SDS) (95% confidence interval [CI], −0.12 to −0.01) in children younger than 12 years compared with standard care or controls at 6 months and an overall reduction of −0.14 BMI-SDS (95% CI, −0.17 to −0.12) in children older than 12 years.[68] A 2014 systematic review showed an overall reduction of −0.47 BMI-SDS (95% CI, −0.58 to −0.36) in studies of comprehensive lifestyle family

Table 1
Information to consider during assessment of the obese child/adolescent

Checklist	Rationale
History	
Past attempts at weight loss; recent weight gain/loss	Methods used in weight loss attempts; rate of weight changes
Developmental delay, stunted linear growth, pattern of weight gain (age of onset)	Genetic syndromes, endocrine disorders
Headaches, blurred vision	Hypertension, intracranial hypertension
Breathing difficulty while sleeping, snoring, daytime drowsiness	Obstructive sleep apnea
Joint pain	Slipped femoral capital epiphysis, Blount disease, spondylolisthesis
Menstrual history, hirsutism	Hyperandrogenism, PCOS
Polyuria, nocturia	T2DM
Increased fatigue, cold intolerance, constipation, dry skin	Hypothyroidism
Medications	Drug-induced obesity
Fetal/infant history	
Maternal BMI, maternal gestational diabetes, maternal nutrition	To identify prenatal/postnatal exposure that may have contributed to the development of overweight/obesity
Birth weight	
Breast-feeding, introduction of complementary food	
Nutrition, physical activity, and sedentary behaviors	
Food choices, daily caloric intake, eating behaviors—snacking, family meals, eating disorders	To elucidate modifiable unhealthy sedentary and dietary behaviors
Time spent in physical activity, intensity	
Screen time and other sedentary behaviors	
Environmental factors	
Access to fresh produce, grocery stores, food security	To gather information about potential environmental barriers
Access to parks and recreational community centers	
Access to primary health care providers	
Psychosocial factors	
Negative affect (depression, anxiety, stress)	To identify psychosocial issues and need for intervention
Body image, self-esteem	
Peer influence (bullying, support, teasing)	
Readiness to change, motivation, confidence	
School functioning	
Family history	
Obesity, T2DM, hypertension, dyslipidemia, coronary artery disease, sleep apnea	Genetic inheritance of risk factors and risk for comorbidities

Data from Refs.[11,13,64,76]

interventions.[69] Less than 5% of people undertaking diet or activity interventions maintain weight loss unless psychological interventions ensure behavior change support for these individuals.[27] **Box 2** highlights some specific recommendations and key messages for the clinician to use when working with families.

Table 2
Laboratory tests for comorbidity screening

Test	Age Group/Criteria	Outcomes/Thresholds
Dyslipidemia		
FLP If nonfasting, calculate non-HDL (total cholesterol −HDL), and repeat with FLP if non-HDL cholesterol is high or HDL-cholesterol is low Repeat every 2 y	Children >2 y of age if BMI ≥85th percentile[a]	Total cholesterol >5.2 mmol/L (200 mg/dL), high Triglycerides >1.7 mmol/L (150 mg/dL), high HDL cholesterol <0.9 mmol/L (35 mg/dL), low Non-HDL >3.8 mmol/L (145 mg/dL), high Low-density lipoprotein >3.4 mmol/L (130 mg/dL), high[a]
IGT & T2DM		
FPG 2-h OGTT, 1.75 mg/kg up to max 75 g. HbA1c Repeat every 3 y	Overweight (BMI >85th percentile for age and sex and one or more of the following[b]: 1. Family history of T2DM or 2. High-risk race/ethnicity or 3. Signs of IR or conditions associated with IR or 4. Exposed to GDM in utero	Prediabetes: IFG 5.6–6.9 mmol/L (100–125 mg/dL) IGT OGTT 2-h glucose 7.8–11.0 mmol/L (140–199 mg/dL) A1C 5.7%–6.4% Diabetes: FPG >7.0 mmol/L (126 mg/dL) or OGTT 2-h glucose >11.0 mmol/L (200 mg/dL) Requires second confirmatory test if patient is asymptomatic
NAFLD		
ALT/AST Repeat every 2 y	Children >10 y, with BMI 85th–94th percentile and metabolic risk factors, or BMI ≥95th percentile[c]	ALT/AST 2 × normal levels Upper limit of normal: ALT = 22–25 U/L
Sleep-disordered breathing		
Sleep study (polysomnography or nocturnal pulse oximetry) Repeat if symptoms arise.	All, if symptoms to suggest OSA are documented	Detection of hypopneas, apneas, sleep disruption and fragmentation, or cyclic desaturations

Abbreviations: ALT, alanine aminotransferase; AST, aspartate aminotransferase; FLP, fasting lipid profile; FPG, fasting plasma glucose; HDL, high-density lipoprotein; IFG, impaired fasting glucose; IGT, impaired glucose tolerance; IR, insulin resistance; OGTT, oral glucose tolerance test; OSA, obstructive sleep apnea.

[a] Lipid threshold cutoffs may vary depending on number of individual risk factors.

[b] Guidelines for diabetes screening are those recommended by the American Diabetes Association, which differ slightly from those suggested by the Canadian Diabetes Association.

[c] Recommendations from the American Academy of Pediatrics expert committee on child obesity. The American Association for the Study of Liver Diseases does not support screening because of a lack of evidence and specific management guidelines of NAFLD in children.

Data from Refs.[64,77–83]

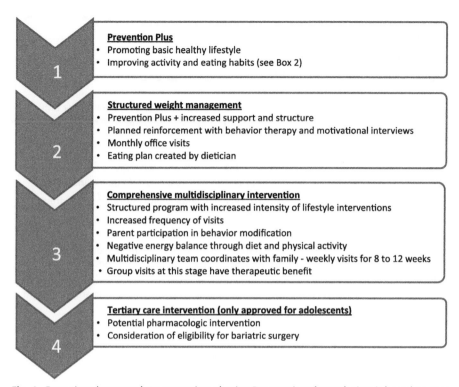

Fig. 1. Four-tiered approach to managing obesity. Progression through tiers is based on case severity and lack of improvement in health outcomes. (*Data from* Barlow SE, Expert C. Expert committee recommendations regarding the prevention, assessment, and treatment of child and adolescent overweight and obesity: summary report. Pediatrics 2007;120 Suppl 4:S164–92.)

Pharmacologic Approaches

Adjunctive pharmacotherapy to enhance weight loss may accrue additional weight loss of 4 to 7 kg in studies of 6 months duration, but there are limited options available.[70] Orlistat, an enteric lipase inhibitor, prevents breakdown and absorption of fat during digestive process and is approved for use in children older than 10 years.[20] In the authors' experience, undesired side effects, including gas and oily stools, lead to high rates of discontinuation. Off-label use of metformin has been studied for weight loss in adolescents, and one trial lasting 6 months showed significant BMI reduction (-0.5 kg/m^2, 1.3% from baseline; $P<.02$) with use of metformin compared with placebo[70]; however, some do experience side effects including nausea, vomiting, and diarrhea. Sibutramine, a serotonin reuptake inhibitor, has shown similar to slightly higher degrees of weight loss compared with placebo[20] but has been withdrawn from the market because of significant central nervous system side effects and is no longer used in children and adolescents.

Bariatric Surgery

Adolescent bariatric surgery is an effective method to reduce weight, with reduction of BMI by about one-third 2 years after surgery.[71] Studies have also demonstrated

---

Box 1
The 5A's of pediatric obesity management

The 5A's of Pediatric Obesity Management	Approach
Ask	
	• Ask for permission to discuss the child's weight and/or BMI
	• Be nonjudgmental while gauging readiness to change
Assess	
	• Underlying cause and contributing factors
	• Inquire about enablers and barriers in weight management
	• Conduct physical and mental health assessment to address any complications
Advise	
	• Ask for permission to provide information about obesity-related risks, investigations, and treatment options
	• Stress the importance of achieving behavioral and health-related improvements rather than focusing primarily on weight loss
Agree	
	• Aim to have child and family choose behavioral goals themselves, with physician assistance
	• Assess confidence in achieving the goals, use motivational interviewing techniques
	• Agree on a small number of SMART (specific, measurable, achievable, relevant, timely) goals (1–2)
Assist	
	• Summarize management plan and address potential solutions to barriers
	• Provide additional available resources
	• Arrange for follow-up within a short time frame

Data from Canadian Obesity Network. CON. 5As for pediatrics. Available at: http://www.obesitynetwork.ca/5As. Accessed August 1, 2014.

---

postsurgical improvements in metabolic and psychosocial outcomes.[71–73] Despite these encouraging results, adverse consequences of surgery may be significant, including those related to the surgical procedure, significant vitamin deficiencies with the malabsorptive procedures, and the potential for weight regain.[71] As long-term data are not available in adolescents undergoing surgery, predicting who will benefit most from the procedures remains to be determined. As such, consensus criteria for patient selection have been established, including achievement of 95% of growth before surgery, BMI greater than or equal to 40 kg/m² or BMI greater than or equal to 35 kg/m² with a significant obesity-related comorbidity, previous weight loss attempts, a stable and supportive home environment, and stable mental

Box 2	
Recommendations for nonpharmacologic interventions in obesity management	
Intervention	**Recommendations**
Nutrition therapy	
	• Engage dietician support if possible
	• Limit sugar-sweetened beverages
	• Increase fruit and vegetable intake
	• Decrease snacks and portion sizes
	• Diets should be lower energy intake to promote weight loss of ~0.5 kg/wk, but maintain nutritional balance for growth and development
PA and sedentary time	
	• For the young child, increase duration of unstructured free play
	• Older children should be encouraged to pursue PA that they enjoy
	• Limit screen time to <2 h/d
	• 5 y+: 60 min of moderate to vigorous PA daily
	• 0–4 y: 180 min of any intensity PA daily
Behavioral approach	
	• Increase support around PA and healthy nutrition
	• Decrease frequency of eating in restaurants
	• Increase frequency of family meals eaten together at home
	• Encourage SMART goal setting
	• Promote self-monitoring
	• Discourage the use of food as a reward
	• Use problem solving and motivational interview techniques to identify priorities and barriers, and create a sense of family involvement in decision making

Abbreviations: PA, physical activity; SMART, specific, measurable, achievable, relevant, timely.

Data from Refs.[64,84–86]

health status.[71–73] Surgery is contraindicated in patients with cognitive disabilities that would interfere with postoperative treatment, those with active substance use, pregnant/breast-feeding adolescents or those intending to become pregnant within the next year, and those who do not fully understand or acknowledge the risks associated with bariatric surgery. The 3 most studied types of bariatric surgery are detailed in **Table 3** and **Fig. 2**.

PREVENTION

Prevention is a public health priority worldwide. In a 2011 Cochrane review, 37 studies of obesity prevention in 27,946 children aged 6 to 12 years demonstrated that programs were effective at reducing adiposity, although there was a high level of

Table 3
Bariatric surgery procedures

Roux-en-Y Bypass	Gastric Banding	Sleeve Gastrectomy
Procedure		
• Restrictive and malabsorptive • Proximal pouch of stomach attached to jejunum	• Restrictive • Adjustable gastric band around proximal stomach • Band inflated with saline from subcutaneous port	• Restrictive • Stomach resected along greater curvature
Late complications		
• Protein-calorie malnutrition and micronutrient deficiency • Gastric ulceration, stomal stenosis, gastric dilatation, internal/incisional hernias • Dumping syndrome, postprandial hypoglycemia	• Band slippage or erosion • Stomal obstruction • Esophagitis	• Gastric ulceration • Gastric remnant dilatation • Reflux
Adolescent outcomes		
Average BMI loss at 12 mo of -17.2 kg/m^2, with 8 identified studies	Average BMI loss at 12 mo of -10.5 kg/m^2, with 11 identified studies	Average BMI loss was intermediate at -14.5 kg/m^2, with 3 identified studies

Data from Refs.[71–73,87–90]

observed heterogeneity.[74] Overall, children in the intervention groups had a small but significant difference in mean BMI compared with the control groups (-0.15 kg/m^2 [95% CI, -0.21 to -0.09]). Intervention seemed to demonstrate larger effects in younger age groups. Only 8 studies reported on adverse effects, and no evidence of adverse outcomes, such as unhealthy dieting practices, increased prevalence of underweight, or body image sensitivities, was found. The researchers concluded that there was strong evidence to support the beneficial effects of child obesity prevention programs on BMI.[74] Although obesity prevention in young children seemed to demonstrate the largest effect, there have been fewer studies in this age group. Promising strategies from the Cochrane review, recommendations by the American Academy of Pediatrics, and the "No Time to Wait" strategies from the Ministry of Health Ontario Healthy Kids Panel have been summarized in **Box 3** as evidence-based recommendations for practices that can be undertaken at each of the levels of interaction with the child to promote healthy growth and development and protect from the early onset of overweight or obesity.[13,74,75]

FUTURE DIRECTIONS

It is evident that there is no magic pill or one-size-fits-all approach to the prevention or treatment of obesity, and rarely can the cause of obesity be pinpointed to a single, modifiable cause. The underlying pathways leading to the development of the condition are unique for each patient, and a more targeted approach to treatment, based on underlying factors, including physiologic and psychosocial, at the level of the individual, family, community, and society is warranted. Research to develop approaches based on the underlying cause and severity of comorbidities will assist in making

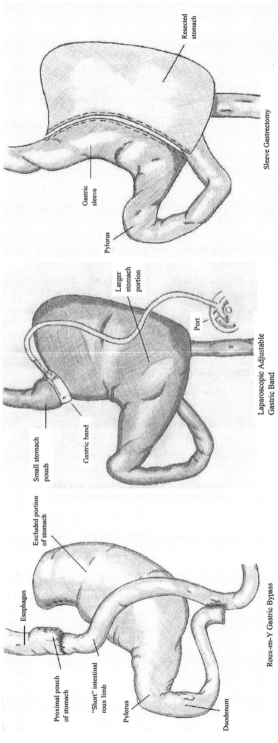

Fig. 2. Surgical alterations in (1) Roux-en-Y bypass, (2) gastric banding, and (3) sleeve gastrectomy. (*Courtesy of Phillip Fournier, BA, Toronto, Canada.*)

Box 3
Obesity prevention recommendations

Structure/Institution	Recommendations
Individual/family	
	• 1 h of physical activity (PA), <2 h of screen time per day
	• Eat breakfast daily
	• Engage in meals and PA together as a family
	• Reduced portion sizes, lower frequency of snacks, low consumption of sugar-sweetened drinks
	• Optimize weight gain during pregnancy, exclusive breast-feeding during first 6 mo of life
Primary care	
	• Monitoring BMI at regular intervals—facilitate early intervention and prevent comorbidities
	• Counsel pregnant mothers regarding adequate maternal nutrition, recommended weight gain in pregnancy, and benefits of breast-feeding
	• Advocate for community and policy action supporting healthy growth of children
	• Support social marketing to promote healthy foods to growing children
School/community	
	• Ensure adequate PA, development of fundamental movement skills, and recess periods at school
	• Mandate nutritional standards for food provided at schools and in vending machines, including in Aboriginal communities
	• Provide nutritional education curriculum to stress importance of healthy eating and positive body image
	• Expand accessibility of play spaces, recreational parks, and safe walking and biking routes in residential areas
	• Implement health promotion strategies (eg, professional development, capacity building activities)
	• Improve mental health services and access
	• Establish comprehensive community programs to promote healthy child development and support those from lower socioeconomic status
Public policy	
	• Ensure adequate funding for treatment of obesity and obesity-related comorbidities
	• Encourage social marketing of healthy food options and legislate bans/restrictions of marketing unhealthy foods to young children
	• Provide incentives to ensure retailers to provide quality, affordable fruits and vegetables

Data from Refs.[64,77,84]

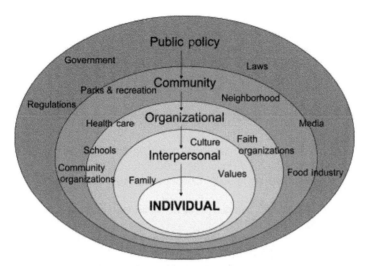

Fig. 3. A socioecological framework depicting various levels of organization involved in promoting and implementing healthy lifestyles. (*From* Caprio S, Daniels SR, Drewnowski A, et al. Influence of race, ethnicity, and culture on childhood obesity: implications for prevention and treatment. Obesity 2008;16(12):2572; with permission.)

the most effective use of limited clinical resources. Prevention will remain the most effective method of reducing the societal burden of obesity and will necessitate attention to the social determinants of health, a focus on the developing child from in utero through to adulthood, and collaboration between multiple organizations at the micro and macro level (**Fig. 3**).

REFERENCES

1. Ng M, Fleming T, Robinson M, et al. Global, regional, and national prevalence of overweight and obesity in children and adults during 1980–2013: a systematic analysis for the Global Burden of Disease Study 2013. Lancet 2014;384(9945): 766–81.
2. Ogden CL, Carroll MD, Kit BK, et al. Prevalence of childhood and adult obesity in the United States, 2011–2012. JAMA 2014;311(8):806–14.
3. Roberts KC, Shields M, de Groh M, et al. Overweight and obesity in children and adolescents: results from the 2009 to 2011 Canadian Health Measures Survey. Health Rep 2012;23(3):37–41.
4. Ogden CL, Carroll MD, Kit BK, et al. Prevalence of obesity and trends in body mass index among US children and adolescents, 1999–2010. JAMA 2012; 307(5):483–90.
5. Skinner AC, Skelton JA. Prevalence and trends in obesity and severe obesity among children in the United States, 1999–2012. JAMA Pediatr 2014;168(6): 561–6.
6. UNICEF, WHO, The World Bank. Levels and trends in child malnutrition. UNICEF-WHO-World Bank Joint Child Malnutrition Estimates. 2012. Available at: http://www.who.int/nutgrowthdb/estimates/en/. Accessed July 11, 2014.
7. Serdula MK, Ivery D, Coates RJ, et al. Do obese children become obese adults? A review of the literature. Prev Med 1993;22(2):167–77.

8. Dinsdale H, Ridler C, Ells LJ. A simple guide to classifying body mass index in children. Oxford (United Kingdom): National Obesity Observatory; 2011. Available at: http://www.noo.org.uk/NOO_about_obesity/measurement.

9. Shields M, Tremblay MS. Canadian childhood obesity estimates based on WHO, IOTF and CDC cut-points. Int J Pediatr Obes 2010;5(3):265–73.

10. Dietitians of Canada, Canadian Paediatric Society, The College of Family Physicians of Canada, Community Health Nurses of Canada. Promoting optimal monitoring of child growth in Canada: using the new WHO growth charts. Can J Diet Pract Res 2010;71(1):e1–3.

11. Plourde G. Preventing and managing pediatric obesity. Recommendations for family physicians. Can Fam Physician 2006;52(3):322–8.

12. Han JC, Lawlor DA, Kimm SY. Childhood obesity. Lancet 2010;375(9727): 1737–48.

13. Speiser PW, Rudolf MC, Anhalt H, et al. Childhood obesity. J Clin Endocrinol Metab 2005;90(3):1871–87.

14. Dietz WH, Robinson TN. Clinical practice. Overweight children and adolescents. N Engl J Med 2005;352(20):2100–9.

15. Reynolds RM, Jacobsen GH, Drake AJ. What is the evidence in humans that DNA methylation changes link events in utero and later life disease? Clin Endocrinol 2013;78(6):814–22.

16. Luca P, Birken C, Grewal P, et al. Complex obesity. Curr Pediatr Rev 2012;8: 179–87.

17. Darmasseelane K, Hyde MJ, Santhakumaran S, et al. Mode of delivery and offspring body mass index, overweight and obesity in adult life: a systematic review and meta-analysis. PLoS One 2014;9(2):e87896.

18. Neu J, Rushing J. Cesarean versus vaginal delivery: long-term infant outcomes and the hygiene hypothesis. Clin Perinatol 2011;38(2):321–31.

19. Kramer MS, Matush L, Vanilovich I, et al. A randomized breast-feeding promotion intervention did not reduce child obesity in Belarus. J Nutr 2009;139(2): 417S–21S.

20. Bagchi D. Global perspectives on childhood obesity: current status, consequences and prevention. Burlington (MA): Academic Press; 2010.

21. Leunissen RW, Kerkhof GF, Stijnen T, et al. Timing and tempo of first-year rapid growth in relation to cardiovascular and metabolic risk profile in early adulthood. JAMA 2009;301(21):2234–42.

22. Whitaker RC, Pepe MS, Wright JA, et al. Early adiposity rebound and the risk of adult obesity. Pediatrics 1998;101(3):E5.

23. Timlin MT, Pereira MA, Story M, et al. Breakfast eating and weight change in a 5-year prospective analysis of adolescents: project EAT (Eating Among Teens). Pediatrics 2008;121(3):e638–45.

24. Wansink B, van Kleef E. Dinner rituals that correlate with child and adult BMI. Obesity 2014;22(5):E91–5.

25. Active Healthy Kids Canada. Is Canada in the running? The 2014 Active Healthy Kids Canada Report Card on Physical Activity for Children and Youth. Toronto: Active Healthy Kids Canada; 2014. Available at: http://www.activehealthykids.ca/ReportCard/2014ReportCard.aspx.

26. Wahi G, Parkin PC, Beyene J, et al. Effectiveness of interventions aimed at reducing screen time in children: a systematic review and meta-analysis of randomized controlled trials. Arch Pediatr Adolesc Med 2011;165(11):979–86.

27. Miller J, Rosenbloom A, Silverstein J. Childhood obesity. J Clin Endocrinol Metab 2004;89(9):4211–8.

28. Lustig RH. Autonomic dysfunction of the beta-cell and the pathogenesis of obesity. Rev Endocr Metab Disord 2003;4(1):23–32.
29. Vaisse C, Clement K, Durand E, et al. Melanocortin-4 receptor mutations are a frequent and heterogeneous cause of morbid obesity. J Clin Invest 2000;106: 253–62.
30. Farooqi S, O'Rahilly S. Genetics of obesity in humans. Endocr Rev 2006;27: 710–8.
31. Hamilton JK, Conwell LS, Syme C, et al. Hypothalamic obesity following craniopharyngioma surgery: results of a pilot trial of combined diazoxide and metformin therapy. Int J Pediatr Endocrinol 2011;2011:417949.
32. Prince RL, Kuk JL, Ambler KA, et al. Predictors of metabolically healthy obesity in children. Diabetes Care 2014;37(5):1462–8.
33. Alberti KG, Eckel RH, Grundy SM, et al. Harmonizing the metabolic syndrome: a joint interim statement of the International Diabetes Federation Task Force on Epidemiology and Prevention; National Heart, Lung, and Blood Institute; American Heart Association; World Heart Federation; International Atherosclerosis Society; and International Association for the Study of Obesity. Circulation 2009; 120(16):1640–5.
34. Ford ES, Li C. Defining the metabolic syndrome in children and adolescents: will the real definition please stand up? J Pediatr 2008;152(2):160–4.
35. Friend A, Craig L, Turner S. The prevalence of metabolic syndrome in children: a systematic review of the literature. Metab Syndr Relat Disord 2013;11(2):71–80.
36. Nicklas TA, von Duvillard SP, Berenson GS. Tracking of serum lipids and lipoproteins from childhood to dyslipidemia in adults: the Bogalusa Heart Study. Int J Sports Med 2002;23(Suppl 1):S39–43.
37. Juhola J, Magnussen CG, Viikari JS, et al. Tracking of serum lipid levels, blood pressure, and body mass index from childhood to adulthood: the Cardiovascular Risk in Young Finns Study. J Pediatr 2011;159(4):584–90.
38. Urbina EM, Gidding SS, Bao W, et al. Association of fasting blood sugar level, insulin level, and obesity with left ventricular mass in healthy children and adolescents: the Bogalusa Heart Study. Am Heart J 1999;138:122–7.
39. US Department of Health and Human Services. Centers for Disease Control and Prevention. Prevalence of abnormal lipid levels among youths: United States, 1999–2006. MMWR Morb Mortal Wkly Rep 2010;59:2.
40. Expert Panel on Integrated Guidelines for Cardiovascular Health and Risk Reduction in Children and Adolescents, National Heart, Lung, and Blood Institute. Expert panel on integrated guidelines for cardiovascular health and risk reduction in children and adolescents: summary report. Pediatrics 2011;128(Suppl 5):S213–56.
41. National High Blood Pressure Education Program Working Group on High Blood Pressure in Children and Adolescents. The fourth report on the diagnosis, evaluation, and treatment of high blood pressure in children and adolescents. Pediatrics 2004;114:555–76.
42. Din-Dzietham R, Liu Y, Bielo MV, et al. High blood pressure trends in children and adolescents in national surveys, 1963 to 2002. Circulation 2007;116(13):1488–96.
43. Hansen ML, Gunn PW, Kaelber DC. Underdiagnosis of hypertension in children and adolescents. JAMA 2007;298:874–9.
44. Pettitt DJ, Talton J, Dabelea D, et al. Prevalence of diabetes in U.S. youth in 2009: the SEARCH for diabetes in youth study. Diabetes Care 2014;37(2):402–8.
45. Amed S, Dean HJ, Panagiotopoulos C, et al. Type 2 diabetes, medication-induced diabetes, and monogenic diabetes in Canadian children: a prospective national surveillance study. Diabetes Care 2010;33(4):786–91.

46. Writing Group for the SEARCH for Diabetes in Youth Study Group, Dabelea D, Bell RA, et al. Incidence of diabetes in youth in the United States. JAMA 2007; 297(24):2716–24.

47. Sinha R, Fisch G, Teague B, et al. Prevalence of impaired glucose tolerance among children and adolescents with marked obesity. N Engl J Med 2002;346: 802–10.

48. Hannon TS, Rao G, Arslanian SA. Childhood obesity and type 2 diabetes mellitus. Pediatrics Aug 2005;116(2):473–80.

49. Legro RS, Arslanian SA, Ehrmann DA, et al. Diagnosis and treatment of polycystic ovary syndrome: an Endocrine Society clinical practice guideline. J Clin Endocrinol Metab 2013;98(12):4565–92.

50. Dokras A, Witchel SF. Are young adult women with polycystic ovary syndrome slipping through the healthcare cracks? J Clin Endocrinol Metab 2014;99(5): 1583–5.

51. Shahar E, Whitney CW, Redline S, et al. Sleep-disordered breathing and cardiovascular disease: cross-sectional results of the Sleep Heart Health Study. Am J Respir Crit Care Med 2001;163(1):19–25.

52. Narang I, Manlhiot C, Davies-Shaw J, et al. Sleep disturbance and cardiovascular risk in adolescents. CMAJ 2012;184(17):E913–20.

53. Gordon JE, Hughes MS, Shepherd K, et al. Obstructive sleep apnoea syndrome in morbidly obese children with tibia vara. J Bone Joint Surg Br 2006;88:100–3.

54. Murray AW, Wilson NI. Changing incidence of slipped capital femoral epiphysis: a relationship with obesity? J Bone Joint Surg Br 2008;90:92–4.

55. Nead KG, Halterman JS, Kaczorowski JM, et al. Overweight children and adolescents: a risk group for iron deficiency. Pediatrics 2004;114:104–8.

56. Schwimmer JB, Burwinkle TM, Varni JW. Health-related quality of life of severely obese children and adolescents. JAMA 2003;289:1813–9.

57. Latzer Y, Stein D. A review of the psychological and familial perspectives of childhood obesity. J Eat Disord 2013;1:7.

58. US Preventive Services Task Force, Barton M. Screening for obesity in children and adolescents: US Preventive Services Task Force recommendation statement. Pediatrics 2010;125(2):361–7.

59. Freedman DS, Sherry B. The validity of BMI as an indicator of body fatness and risk among children. Pediatrics 2009;124(Suppl 1):S23–34.

60. August GP, Caprio S, Fennoy I, et al. Prevention and treatment of pediatric obesity: an endocrine society clinical practice guideline based on expert opinion. J Clin Endocrinol Metab 2008;93:4576–99.

61. Sharma AM, Kushner RF. A proposed clinical staging system for obesity. Int J Obes 2009;33(3):289–95.

62. Padwal RS, Pajewski NM, Allison DB, et al. Using the Edmonton obesity staging system to predict mortality in a population-representative cohort of people with overweight and obesity. CMAJ 2011;183(14):E1059–66.

63. Singhal V, Schwenk WF, Kumar S. Evaluation and management of childhood and adolescent obesity. Mayo Clin Proc 2007;82(10):1258–64.

64. Barlow SE, Expert C. Expert committee recommendations regarding the prevention, assessment, and treatment of child and adolescent overweight and obesity: summary report. Pediatrics 2007;120(Suppl 4):S164–92.

65. Woolford SJ, Sallinen BJ, Clark SJ, et al. Results from a clinical multidisciplinary weight management program. Clin Pediatr 2011;50(3):187–91.

66. Canadian Obesity Network. CON. 5As for Pediatrics. Available at: http://www.obesitynetwork.ca/5As. Accessed August 1, 2014.

67. Rueda-Clausen CF, Benterud E, Bond T, et al. Effect of implementing the 5As of Obesity Management framework on provider–patient interactions in primary care. Clin Obes 2014;4(1):39–44.
68. Oude Luttikhuis H, Baur L, Jansen H, et al. Interventions for treating obesity in children. Cochrane Database Syst Rev 2009;(1):CD001872.
69. Janicke DM, Steele RG, Gayes LA, et al. Systematic review and meta-analysis of comprehensive behavioral family lifestyle interventions addressing pediatric obesity. J Pediatr Psychol 2014;39(8):809–25.
70. Dunican KC, Desilets AR, Montalbano JK. Pharmacotherapeutic options for overweight adolescents. Ann Pharmacother 2007;41(9):1445–55.
71. Hsia DS, Fallon SC, Brandt ML. Adolescent bariatric surgery. Arch Pediatr Adolesc Med 2012;166(8):757–66.
72. Austin H, Smith K, Ward WL. Psychological assessment of the adolescent bariatric surgery candidate. Surg Obes Relat Dis 2013;9(3):474–80.
73. Behrens C, Tang BQ, Amson BJ. Early results of a Canadian laparoscopic sleeve gastrectomy experience. Can J Surg 2011;54(2):138–43.
74. Waters E, de Silva-Sanigorski A, Hall BJ, et al. Interventions for preventing obesity in children. Cochrane Database Syst Rev 2011;(12):CD001871.
75. Ontario Healthy Kids Panel. No time to wait: the healthy kids strategy. Ontario Ministry of Health and Long-Term Care Reports. 2013. Available at: http://www.health.gov.on.ca/en/common/ministry/publications/reports/healthy_kids/healthy_kids.aspx. Accessed July 23, 2014.
76. Krebs NF, Jacobson MS, American Academy of Pediatrics Committee on Nutrition. Prevention of pediatric overweight and obesity. Pediatrics 2003;112:424–30.
77. Daniels SR, Pratt CA, Hayman LL. Reduction of risk for cardiovascular disease in children and adolescents. Circulation 2011;124(15):1673–86.
78. Strauss RS, Barlow SE, Dietz WH. Prevalence of abnormal serum aminotransferase values in overweight and obese adolescents. J Pediatr 2000;136:727–33.
79. Schwimmer JB, Dunn W, Norman GJ, et al. SAFETY study: alanine aminotransferase cutoff values are set too high for reliable detection of pediatric chronic liver disease. Gastroenterology 2010;138(4):1357–64 e1352.
80. Chalasani N, Younossi Z, Lavine JE, et al. The diagnosis and management of non-alcoholic fatty liver disease: practice guideline by the American Association for the Study of Liver Diseases, American College of Gastroenterology, and the American Gastroenterological Association. Hepatology 2012;55(6):2005–23.
81. Marcus CL, Brooks LJ, Ward SD, et al. Diagnosis and management of childhood obstructive sleep apnea syndrome. Pediatrics 2012;130(3):e714–55.
82. Narang I, Mathew JL. Childhood obesity and obstructive sleep apnea. J Nutr Metab 2012;2012:134202.
83. American Diabetes Association. Standards of medical care in diabetes—2014. Diabetes Care 2014;37(Suppl 1):S14–80.
84. Lau DCW, Douketis JD, Morrison KM, et al. 2006 Canadian clinical practice guidelines on the management and prevention of obesity in adults and children [summary]. CMAJ 2007;176(8):S1–13.
85. Birken C, Hamilton J. Obesity in a young child. CMAJ 2014;186(6):443.
86. Tremblay MS, Warburton DE, Janssen I, et al. New Canadian physical activity guidelines. Appl Physiol Nutr Metab 2011;36(1):36–46.
87. O'Brien PE, Sawyer SM, Laurie C, et al. Laparoscopic adjustable gastric banding in severely obese adolescents: a randomized trial. JAMA 2010;303(6):519–26.
88. Black JA, White B, Viner RM, et al. Bariatric surgery for obese children and adolescents: a systematic review and meta-analysis. Obes Rev 2013;14(8):634–44.

89. Alqahtani AR, Antonisamy B, Alamri H, et al. Laparoscopic sleeve gastrectomy in 108 obese children and adolescents aged 5 to 21 years. Ann Surg 2012;256(2): 266–73.
90. Zeller MH, Reiter-Purtill J, Ratcliff MB, et al. Two-year trends in psychosocial functioning after adolescent Roux-en-Y gastric bypass. Surg Obes Relat Dis 2011; 7(6):727–32.

The Child with Multiple Fractures, What Next?

Jennifer Harrington, MBBS, FRACP, PhD*, Etienne Sochett, MB ChB, FRCPC

KEYWORDS

- Fractures • Children • Osteoporosis • Bone mineral density
- Osteogenesis imperfecta

KEY POINTS

- Fractures in children are common; 16% to 25% of children sustain more than 1 fracture by adulthood.
- In the absence of severe trauma, the presence of at least 1 vertebral compression fracture, 2 or more long bone fractures by 10 years of age, or 3 or more long bone fractures by 19 years is an indication for further bone health evaluation.
- Bone fragility in children can arise either from a primary bone disorder (such as osteogenesis imperfecta [OI]) or secondary to an underlying medical condition.
- Ensuring adequate calcium and vitamin D intake, weight-bearing exercise, and minimizing exposure to adverse bone factors are important interventions.
- In children with bone pain or significant bone fragility (vertebral compression fractures or bone mineral density [BMD] z score less than −2), referral for specialist evaluation is indicated.

Fractures are a common occurrence in the pediatric population. With a prevalence that is increasing over time,[1,2] up to 25% to 40% of girls and 30% to 50% of boys sustain a single fracture by adulthood.[3–5] Between 16% and 25% of children have more than 1 fracture.[6–8] Multiple fractures can, however, be an indicator of underlying bone fragility. The dilemma, therefore, when evaluating an otherwise apparently healthy child with a history of multiple fractures, is to distinguish between the child with intact bone health and the child who warrants further detailed investigation.

In adults, BMD as measured by dual-energy x-ray absorptiometry (DXA) is used to help diagnose and define individuals with osteoporosis who have an increased future risk for fractures.[9] In contrast, for children, the diagnosis of osteoporosis cannot be

No external funding was secured for this study. The authors have no financial relationships or conflict of interests relevant to this article to disclose.
Division of Endocrinology, Department of Pediatrics, Hospital for Sick Children, University of Toronto, 555 University Avenue, Toronto, Ontario M5G1X8, Canada
* Corresponding author.
E-mail address: jennifer.harrington@sickkids.ca

made using bone densitometric criteria alone. The 2013 guidelines of the International Society for Clinical Densitometry (ISCD) outlined that bone fragility in children should be defined by a clinical significant fracture history, with, but not mandating, a low BMD or bone mineral content (BMC) below a z score of −2 for age and gender.[10] Understanding the determinants of fracture risk is important to identify children who clinically have a significant fracture history and, therefore, need further assessment.

THE PATTERN OF FRACTURES IN CHILDHOOD

Fractures occur more commonly in boys, with a peak incidence at 11 to 12 years in girls and 13 to 14 years in boys,[2–4] corresponding to periods of increased growth velocity. The rapidly growing adolescent skeleton undergoes a period of relative thinning of the bone cortices[11,12] due to a delay between maximal longitudinal bone growth and peak bone mineral accrual (**Fig. 1**).[13–15]

The site of a fracture often depends on the mechanism of injury and the age of the child. Fractures of the distal forearm constitute the most common site of injury in all ages, accounting for 20% to 25% of fractures.[3,16] Hand fractures, including the phalanges, carpals, and metacarpals, are the second most common fracture occurring in childhood but are seen usually as a result of crush injuries. In comparison, vertebral compression fractures are uncommon, accounting for only 1% to 5% of all fractures in childhood.[3,17] The presence of vertebral body height loss should alert the clinician to the possibility of a bone fragility disorder.[18]

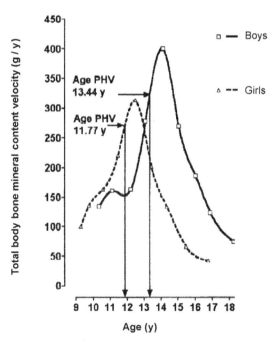

Fig. 1. Peak height velocity (PHV) precedes peak BMC accrual velocity by approximately 0.7 years. (*From* Bailey D, McKay H, Mirwald R, et al. A six-year longitudinal study of the relationship of physical activity to bone mineral accrual in growing children: The University of Saskatchewan Bone Mineral Accrual Study. J Bone Miner Res 1999;14(10):1675; with permission.)

DETERMINANTS OF FRACTURE RISK

A child's risk for having a fracture depends on 3 main factors: the severity of the trauma, the exposure to potential trauma, and the underlying bone strength, including bone density, size, and quality. In a child who undertakes regular vigorous activity and who is frequently exposed to episodes of moderate trauma, a history of multiple fractures may not be unexpected. In contrast, for a child who is exposed to infrequent minor episodes of trauma, fractures may be attributable to an underlying deficit in bone strength.

Severity of Trauma

Given enough force, any bone will break; however, the degree of trauma associated with a fracture relates to the underlying bone quality. Using high-resolution peripheral quantitative CT, children with fractures as a result of mild trauma have been shown to have reduced bone strength and cortical thickness compared with nonfracture controls.[19] In comparison, the presence of a moderate trauma fracture is not associated with bone quality deficits. Thus, the presence of a low trauma fracture should alert clinicians to the potential of underlying bone fragility. This relationship seems to carry through to adulthood, with reduced bone strength, density, and cortical thickness seen in adult men and women with a history of mild but not moderate trauma fractures in childhood.[20] Obtaining an accurate history of the mechanism and circumstances that led to a fracture is, therefore, important to ascertain whether the force associated with the injury seems plausible.

Potential Exposure to Trauma

Exercise and physical activity are associated with increased BMD.[21,22] However, 50% of fractures in children are related to sporting activities.[23] Higher bone mass associated with exercise does not seem to compensate for the increased injury exposure in children who participate in regular vigorous physical activity. Children who undertake daily vigorous physical activity have double the fracture risk of those who do fewer than 4 episodes per week, independent of their bone mass.[24]

Bone Strength: Bone Density, Size, and Quality

Bone strength and its ability to resist fracture depend on bone density, size, and quality. BMD is clearly associated with future fracture risk in adults.[25] Although in children this relationship is not as strong, lower BMD does seem to correlate with increased fracture risk. In a meta-analysis of 8 case-control studies, children with a recent fracture had a standardized mean BMD z score -0.32 lower than children without a history of fractures.[26] A prospective study in children aged 9.9 years also demonstrated that for every 1 SD decrease in volumetric BMD there was an associated 12% increased risk for a subsequent fracture in the following 2 years.[27] A normal BMD z score does not, however, preclude a diagnosis of underlying bone fragility. In a cohort of 66 children with low-trauma vertebral or multiple peripheral fractures, only 8% were found to have a BMD z score less than -2.[8]

Genetic factors play a critical role in peak bone mass determination, with up to 80% of the variance in BMD attributable to heritability.[28] Large genome-wide studies have identified more than 55 different loci associated with attainment of peak BMD.[29] To date, however, these genomic regions and polymorphisms explain only 4% to 5 % of the phenotypic variation seen in adult BMD.[30]

Bone strength is determined not only by BMD but also by bone size and quality. Although the evidence in pediatric cohorts is limited, in adults, nontraumatic vertebral compression fractures have been demonstrated to relate to bone size and trabecular bone microarchitecture independent of the bone density.[31]

CONDITIONS ASSOCIATED WITH BONE FRAGILITY

When a child's history of multiple fractures seems discordant with the severity of or exposure to trauma, further investigation is indicated to assess for potential underlying bone fragility.

Bone fragility can result either as a result of a primary bone condition or as a consequence of a secondary contributing factor or chronic condition (**Box 1**). In all children, particularly infants, nonaccidental injury (NAI) should be excluded as a cause for multiple fractures. Although the pattern of fractures (such as posterior rib and metaphyseal fractures) and associated clinical signs of injury (such as retinal hemorrhage or bruises) may be contributory, differentiating NAI from OI in infants can be difficult.

Primary Osteoporosis

OI is the most common genetic form of primary osteoporosis in children. The majority of cases are associated with mutations in 1 of 2 genes that encode the alpha chains of collagen type I (COL1A1 and COL1A2), although an increasing number of new genes involved in post-translational collagen modification have been described over the past 10 years.[32] OI has a broad clinical phenotype, ranging in severity from perinatal lethality to mild clinical forms without fractures. Typical clinical findings, including blue sclera, gray opalescent primary teeth (dentinogenesis imperfecta), short stature, and joint laxity, can aid in the diagnosis. Radiographic features commonly include vertebral fractures, generalized osteopenia, and gracile long bones with evidence of bowing (**Fig. 2**).[33]

Children with connective tissue disorders, such as Ehlers-Danlos syndrome, can also present with joint laxity in addition to skin hyperelasticity, easy bruising, and recurrent joint dislocations. Connective tissue disorders can be associated with bone fragility, reduced BMD, and increased risk for fractures.[34,35]

Idiopathic juvenile osteoporosis (IJO) is a condition that characteristically presents with bone pain and vertebral fractures prior to the onset of puberty. It is an important differential diagnosis to OI, particularly in the absence of typical OI clinical features or a positive family history. The underlying cause of IJO is unknown, but transiliac histomorphometry studies in patients with IJO demonstrate decreased trabecular bone volume, number, and thickness.[36] Although many children with IJO seem to have spontaneous improvement in symptoms and BMD after the onset of puberty,[37,38] in a subset of patients with more severe symptoms, ongoing bone pain, increased fracture risk, and vertebral deformities can persist into young adulthood.[37]

Several rare genetic conditions involving defects in bone cell signaling and function or bone matrix homeostasis have also been implicated as causes of primary osteoporosis (see **Box 1**).

Secondary Osteoporosis

The presence of impaired bone health as a result of secondary chronic conditions is increasingly recognized in the pediatric population (see **Box 1**). Bone fragility can arise from a combination of factors, including the use of glucocorticoids,[39] increased inflammatory cytokines, diminished nutrition, physical activity, and muscle bulk.[40,41] Although in some children the secondary cause of the fractures may be clearly evident, a history of multiple fractures can be the presenting symptom for an otherwise clinically silent disease. Fractures and decreased BMD are not uncommon

Box 1
Examples of primary and secondary conditions associated with bone fragility and increased risk for fractures in children (not all inclusive). Although some secondary conditions may be evident at the time of the presentation with fractures, a history of frequent fractures can be the presenting symptom

Primary conditions

  Impaired collagen gene expression or collagen post-translational modification

    OI

  Impaired collagen cross-link formation

    Bruck syndrome

  Connective tissue defects

    Ehlers-Danlos syndrome

    Marfan syndrome

    Homocystinuria

  Defective bone mineralization from low alkaline phosphatase activity

    Hypophosphatasia

  Impaired cell signaling and osteoblast function

    Osteoporosis pseudoglioma syndrome

  IJO (cause unknown)

Secondary conditions

  Medication induced

    Glucocorticoids

    Antiepileptic medication

    Anticoagulants

  Reduced weight-bearing activity or muscle bulk

    Duchenne muscular dystrophy

    Cerebral palsy

  Infiltrative conditions

    Leukemia

    Thalassemia

  Chronic inflammatory conditions

    Juvenile idiopathic arthritis

    Inflammatory bowel disease

  Endocrine abnormalities

    Hypogonadism

    Growth hormone deficiency

    Hyperparathryoidism

    Hypercortisolism

  Vitamin and nutritional deficiencies

    Vitamin D deficiency

    Celiac disease

Anorexia nervosa

Cystic fibrosis

Renal disease

Chronic renal failure with secondary hyperparathyroidism

Idiopathic hypercalciuria

presentations for individuals with celiac disease.[42] Acute lymphoblastic leukemia can present with fractures, even with a normal peripheral blood count.[43] Secondary bone fragility can also occur early in the disease process, with 16% of children with acute lymphoblastic leukemia and 7% of children with a rheumatological condition having evidence of vertebral compression fractures within 30 days of diagnosis.[44,45]

Nutritional deficiencies, in particular involving vitamin D, are an important contributor to bone fragility due to decreased bone mineralization. Vitamin D deficiency can arise from inadequate intake as a result of reduced sunlight exposure or decreased absorption from gut malabsorption, or from increased catabolism as seen with some of the antiepileptic medications.[46]

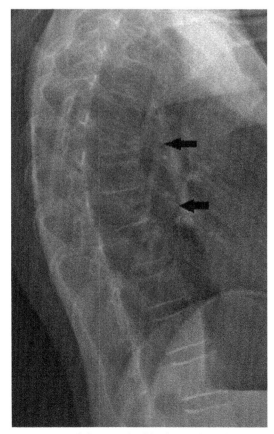

Fig. 2. Osteopenic appearance of the vertebral bodies with multiple vertebral compression fractures as indicated by the black arrows.

APPROACH TO THE CHILD WITH MULTIPLE FRACTURES
Identifying the Child with a Clinically Significant Fracture History

The first step in the evaluation of an otherwise apparently healthy child who presents with multiple fractures is to assess whether the fracture history varies from the normal pattern of fractures seen in childhood and, as such, is clinically significant (**Fig. 3**). Fractures as a result of severe trauma (falling from a height >3 m or as a result of a motor vehicle accident) are not unexpected and, therefore, should not contribute to a child's fracture count. Similarly, crush fractures of fingers, toes, or nose are not classified as fragility fractures.

When a fracture count exceeds what is expected for the age of a child (taking into account the increase in fracture rate in adolescence), or when there are fractures that are not typically seen as a result of mild to moderate trauma (ie, vertebral fractures), then a child is suspected of having a clinically significant fracture history. Based on data from 1412 Finnish children who presented with a new fracture, the definition provided in **Box 2** of a clinically significant fracture history has been proposed by Mayranpaa and colleagues[8] and has been endorsed by the 2013 ISCD guidelines.[10] Data regarding the predictive value of this definition to identify children at increased risk for future fractures are still lacking.

First-Line Evaluation

The aim of the evaluation is to identify potential risk factors leading to the bone fragility, establishing baseline data (eg, BMD and lateral radiograph of the spine) to be able compare subsequent progress with and initiate appropriate supportive treatment to reduce the risk for future fragility fractures (see **Fig. 3**).

History and clinical examination
A detailed history establishes whether there is a family history of multiple fractures (indicating a potential diagnosis of primary osteoporosis) or symptoms of an underlying medical condition. Nutritional assessment of calcium, vitamin D, and other macronutrients can identify potential underlying deficiencies. Physical examination includes the evaluation for features of an underlying collagen or connective tissue disorder and examining for evidence of spinal tenderness or deformity. Evaluation of growth and pubertal stage is critical, because growth and sex hormones are important for normal bone mass accrual. These clinical features also need to be taken into account in the interpretation of BMD measurements.

Biochemistry
Assessment of calcium and phosphate homeostasis includes measurement of serum calcium, phosphate, creatinine, parathyroid hormone, and urinary calcium excretion. Alkaline phosphatase can be elevated in mineralization problems of the bone, such as rickets. Elevated urinary calcium excretion, as seen in idiopathic hypercalciuria, has been associated with decreased BMD and increased fracture risk.[47] Bone turnover markers, such as bone-specific alkaline phosphatase and cross-linked telopeptides, have little diagnostic discrimination but are used more in the monitoring of response to treatment.[48] Evaluation of vitamin D stores should be done by measurement of 25-hydroxyvitamin D (25[OH]D). Although there remains controversy around the optimal 25(OH)D concentration to target, levels at least above 50 nmol/L are optimal in a child with a history of multiple fractures.[49] Measurement of tissue transglutaminase antibody should be undertaken to screen for the possibility of celiac disease. Further investigations, such as of hormone assessments, should be performed if clinically indicated.

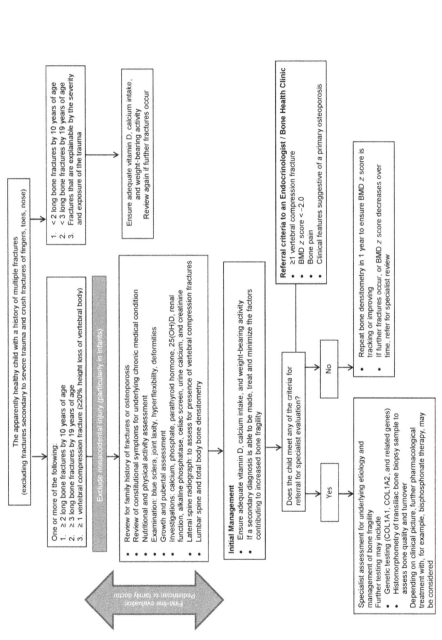

Fig. 3. An algorithm for the management of a child presenting with a clinically significant fracture history, outlining the initial evaluation, management, and when to consider referral for specialist review. (*Data from* Mayranpaa MK, Viljakainen HT, Toiviainen-Salo S, et al. Impaired bone health and asymptomatic vertebral compressions in fracture-prone children: a case-control study. J Bone Miner Res 2012;27(6):1413–24; and Bishop N, Arundel P, Clark E, et al. Fracture prediction and the definition of osteoporosis in children and adolescents: the ISCD 2013 pediatric official positions. J Clin Densitom 2014;17(2):275–80.)

Box 2
Definition of a clinically significant fracture history

One or more of the following in the absence of high-energy trauma

- 2 or more long bone fractures by 10 years of age
- 3 or more long bone fractures at any age up to 19 years
- 1 or more vertebral compression fractures (with a loss of >20% of the vertebral body height at any point)

Lateral spine radiograph

Many children who have underlying bone fragility may also have vertebral height loss.[50] Significant vertebral compression is defined as a vertebral body height loss greater than 20%.[51] Vertebral height loss can lead to deformity, such as kyphosis. In children with secondary osteoporosis, up to 50% of vertebral compression fractures are asymptomatic and can, therefore, be easily overlooked.[44,52] This underlies the importance of including a lateral standing spine radiograph in the evaluation of a child with a significant fracture history.

Bone mineral density

As described previously, lower BMD in children is associated with an increased risk for fractures.[26] Tracking BMD over time is also important in assessing a child's response to treatment. BMD should be routinely measured at the lumbar spine and total body, because hip BMD measurements can be unreliable in younger children.[10]

It is important that clinicians are aware of the potential limitations in the use of DXA to measure bone density in pediatrics. BMD in children should always be reported as a z score compared with age- and gender-matched normative data. There are few normative data for DXA in children less than 5 years of age.[53] DXA does not measure true volumetric BMD (BMC/volume) but provides an areal bone density (BMC/projection area).[54] As a result it underestimates the true density of smaller bones (for example, in children with short stature).[55] Various adjustments to correct for height, pubertal stage, bone age, and lean body mass have been proposed,[56] although the practical application of these corrections is limited.

Initial Management

The key principles in management of children with underlying bone fragility are to minimize the exposure to potential bone adverse factors, encourage weight-bearing physical activity, and ensure adequate nutritional intake, particularly of calcium and vitamin D.

Weight-bearing physical activity

Weight-bearing physical activity improves both bone mass and bone strength in children,[57] although it may not change fracture rate.[58] Mechanical bone loading stimulates osteoblast activity. It seems to be the intensity rather than duration of physical activity that is important in improving bone health. A brief jumping program performed 4 times a week during school hours elicited a significant osteogenic response in 9- to 11-year-old children.[59] Further research is still needed to determine the optimal type of physical activity. If adequate weight-bearing exercise is not possible due to limited mobility, physiotherapy[60] or high-frequency, low-magnitude vibration therapy[61] can increase bone mass.

Calcium and vitamin D

The recommended daily intake of calcium and vitamin D based on 2011 Institute of Medicine guidelines is detailed in **Table 1**.[62] Vitamin D deficiency if present should be corrected, because serum 25(OH)D concentrations less than 50 nmol/L in children have been associated with impairments in bone quality on histomorphometry as well as decreased BMD.[48] In children with chronic diseases, particularly those with malabsorption, significantly higher doses of vitamin D than the recommended daily intake may be needed. Similarly, if a dietary calcium deficit is identified, increasing dietary calcium or, if needed, commencing a calcium supplement, should occur. Although the treatment of calcium deficiency has been demonstrated to improve BMD,[63] the addition of extra calcium supplements in children with sufficient dietary intake does not seem to have significant protective effects on bone health.[64] Given this and the concern about the potential association of calcium supplementation to increased cardiovascular events in adults,[65] calcium supplementation in an otherwise calcium replete child is not recommended.

Second-Line Specialist Evaluation and Management

In children who have symptomatic bone pain or clinical features suggestive of a primary osteoporosis or in whom the severity of the underlying bone fragility is significant, as seen by the presence of vertebral fractures or BMD z score less than -2, referral to an endocrinologist or bone health clinic for further evaluation and consideration for pharmacologic treatment is warranted.

Genetic testing

A provisional clinical diagnosis of OI is based on the presence of characteristic physical and radiological findings. Genetic testing can, however, help confirm the diagnosis. Given that more than 1500 dominant mutations in COL1A1 or COL1A2 have been identified to date, genetic sequencing of either peripheral blood or cultured fibroblasts is required. Additional testing for other dominant and recessive collagen genes can be undertaken if clinically indicated. With the increased availability of whole-exome sequencing, this may provide a valuable tool in the near future to test for rare known and new mutations associated with primary osteoporotic conditions.

Bone biopsy

Histomorphometric analysis of transiliac bone biopsy samples can provide useful information regarding bone quality and turnover. Given its invasive nature and the need to have the appropriate expertise in performing and interpreting the results, however, its use should be reserved for complicated cases in centers where bone biopsies are done regularly.

Table 1
Recommended daily intake of calcium and vitamin D based on the 2011 guidelines from the Institute of Medicine

Age	Calcium	Vitamin D
0–12 mo	250 mg	400 IU
1–3 y	700 mg	600 IU
4–9 y	1000 mg	600 IU
9–18 y	1300 mg	600 IU

Pharmacologic treatments

Depending on the underling bone fragility condition, the presence of bone pain, and the severity of the bone phenotype, pharmacologic intervention may be warranted. Bisphosphonates are the most widely used treatment in the management of bone fragility in children. They decrease osteoclast function and number and inhibit bone resorption,[66] leading to increased cortical bone thickness and BMD.[67] Bisphosphonate treatment is associated with flulike symptoms in up to 85% of children after the first dose and can lead to transient hypocalcemia.[68] Osteonecrosis of the jaw has been described in adult patients on bisphosphonate therapy[69] but has not been reported in pediatric patients to date.

Bisphosphonate therapy is used most commonly in the treatment of moderate to severe OI. Observational trials of bisphosphonate use in children with OI have documented reductions in long bone fracture rate and bone pain as well as improved strength and activities of daily living.[70–72] The improvement in fracture rate has not always been supported with results from randomized control trials.[73,74] In children with secondary osteoporosis from conditions, such as cerebral palsy and juvenile idiopathic arthritis, bisphosphonates have also been demonstrated to improve BMD and reduce bone pain.[75,76] There remains uncertainty about the optimal dose, mode of administration (oral vs cyclic intravenous infusions), duration, and frequency of bisphosphonate treatment. Given that current evidence precludes the ability to make definite recommendations for the routine use of bisphosphonate therapy and that there is a paucity of long-term pediatric safety data, bisphosphonate treatment in children should be limited to centers with the appropriate experience in its use.

SUMMARY

Given that 90% of bone mass is accrued in the first 2 decades of life, bone fragility in childhood and adolescence can have long-term implications through adulthood. In children presenting with multiple fractures, being able to identify those individuals who warrant further evaluation is critical to providing active preventative care to minimize further bone loss and fractures.

REFERENCES

1. Sinikumpu JJ, Lautamo A, Pokka T, et al. The increasing incidence of paediatric diaphyseal both-bone forearm fractures and their internal fixation during the last decade. Injury 2012;43(3):362–6.
2. Khosla S, Melton LJ 3rd, Dekutoski MB, et al. Incidence of childhood distal forearm fractures over 30 years: a population-based study. JAMA 2003;290(11):1479–85.
3. Hedstrom EM, Svensson O, Bergstrom U, et al. Epidemiology of fractures in children and adolescents. Acta Orthop 2010;81(1):148–53.
4. Cooper C, Dennison EM, Leufkens HG, et al. Epidemiology of childhood fractures in Britain: a study using the general practice research database. J Bone Miner Res 2004;19(12):1976–81.
5. Thandrayen K, Norris SA, Pettifor JM. Fracture rates in urban South African children of different ethnic origins: the Birth to Twenty cohort. Osteoporos Int 2009;20(1):47–52.
6. Valerio G, Galle F, Mancusi C, et al. Pattern of fractures across pediatric age groups: analysis of individual and lifestyle factors. BMC Public Health 2010;10:656.

7. Jones IE, Williams SM, Dow N, et al. How many children remain fracture-free during growth? a longitudinal study of children and adolescents participating in the Dunedin Multidisciplinary Health and Development Study. Osteoporos Int 2002; 13(12):990–5.

8. Mayranpaa MK, Viljakainen HT, Toiviainen-Salo S, et al. Impaired bone health and asymptomatic vertebral compressions in fracture-prone children: a case-control study. J Bone Miner Res 2012;27(6):1413–24.

9. Siris ES, Adler R, Bilezikian J, et al. The clinical diagnosis of osteoporosis: a position statement from the National Bone Health Alliance Working Group. Osteoporos Int 2014;25(5):1439–43.

10. Bishop N, Arundel P, Clark E, et al. Fracture prediction and the definition of osteoporosis in children and adolescents: the ISCD 2013 Pediatric Official Positions. J Clin Densitom 2014;17(2):275–80.

11. Kirmani S, Christen D, van Lenthe GH, et al. Bone structure at the distal radius during adolescent growth. J Bone Miner Res 2009;24(6):1033–42.

12. Wang Q, Wang XF, Iuliano-Burns S, et al. Rapid growth produces transient cortical weakness: a risk factor for metaphyseal fractures during puberty. J Bone Miner Res 2010;25(7):1521–6.

13. Fournier PE, Rizzoli R, Slosman DO, et al. Asynchrony between the rates of standing height gain and bone mass accumulation during puberty. Osteoporos Int 1997;7(6):525–32.

14. Faulkner RA, Davison KS, Bailey DA, et al. Size-corrected BMD decreases during peak linear growth: implications for fracture incidence during adolescence. J Bone Miner Res 2006;21(12):1864–70.

15. Bailey DA, McKay HA, Mirwald RL, et al. A six-year longitudinal study of the relationship of physical activity to bone mineral accrual in growing children: the University of Saskatchewan bone mineral accrual study. J Bone Miner Res 1999;14(10):1672–9.

16. Landin LA. Epidemiology of children's fractures. J Pediatr Orthop B 1997;6(2): 79–83.

17. Clark P, Letts M. Trauma to the thoracic and lumbar spine in the adolescent. Can J Surg 2001;44(5):337–45.

18. Tinkle BT, Wenstrup RJ. A genetic approach to fracture epidemiology in childhood. Am J Med Genet C Semin Med Genet 2005;139C(1):38–54.

19. Farr JN, Amin S, Melton LJ 3rd, et al. Bone strength and structural deficits in children and adolescents with a distal forearm fracture resulting from mild trauma. J Bone Miner Res 2014;29(3):590–9.

20. Farr JN, Khosla S, Achenbach SJ, et al. Diminished bone strength is observed in adult women and men who sustained a mild trauma distal forearm fracture during childhood. J Bone Miner Res 2014;29:2193–202.

21. Johannsen N, Binkley T, Englert V, et al. Bone response to jumping is site-specific in children: a randomized trial. Bone 2003;33(4):533–9.

22. Hasselstrom HA, Karlsson MK, Hansen SE, et al. A 3-year physical activity intervention program increases the gain in bone mineral and bone width in prepubertal girls but not boys: the prospective copenhagen school child interventions study (CoSCIS). Calcif Tissue Int 2008;83(4):243–50.

23. Houshian S, Mehdi B, Larsen MS. The epidemiology of elbow fracture in children: analysis of 355 fractures, with special reference to supracondylar humerus fractures. J Orthop Sci 2001;6(4):312–5.

24. Clark EM, Ness AR, Tobias JH. Vigorous physical activity increases fracture risk in children irrespective of bone mass: a prospective study of the independent risk factors for fractures in healthy children. J Bone Miner Res 2008;23(7):1012–22.

25. Kanis JA, Hans D, Cooper C, et al. Interpretation and use of FRAX in clinical practice. Osteoporos Int 2011;22(9):2395–411.
26. Clark EM, Tobias JH, Ness AR. Association between bone density and fractures in children: a systematic review and meta-analysis. Pediatrics 2006;117(2): e291–7.
27. Clark EM, Ness AR, Bishop NJ, et al. Association between bone mass and fractures in children: a prospective cohort study. J Bone Miner Res 2006;21(9): 1489–95.
28. Peacock M, Turner CH, Econs MJ, et al. Genetics of osteoporosis. Endocr Rev 2002;23(3):303–26.
29. Hsu YH, Kiel DP. Clinical review: genome-wide association studies of skeletal phenotypes: what we have learned and where we are headed. J Clin Endocrinol Metab 2012;97(10):E1958–77.
30. Kemp JP, Medina-Gomez C, Estrada K, et al. Phenotypic dissection of bone mineral density reveals skeletal site specificity and facilitates the identification of novel loci in the genetic regulation of bone mass attainment. PLoS Genet 2014; 10:e1004423.
31. Legrand E, Chappard D, Pascaretti C, et al. Trabecular bone microarchitecture, bone mineral density, and vertebral fractures in male osteoporosis. J Bone Miner Res 2000;15(1):13–9.
32. Marini JC, Reich A, Smith SM. Osteogenesis imperfecta due to mutations in noncollagenous genes: lessons in the biology of bone formation. Curr Opin Pediatr 2014;26(4):500–7.
33. Ben Amor IM, Roughley P, Glorieux FH, et al. Skeletal clinical characteristics of osteogenesis imperfecta caused by haploinsufficiency mutations in COL1A1. J Bone Miner Res 2013;28(9):2001–7.
34. Yen JL, Lin SP, Chen MR, et al. Clinical features of Ehlers-Danlos syndrome. J Formos Med Assoc 2006;105(6):475–80.
35. Dolan AL, Arden NK, Grahame R, et al. Assessment of bone in Ehlers Danlos syndrome by ultrasound and densitometry. Ann Rheum Dis 1998;57(10):630–3.
36. Rauch F, Travers R, Norman ME, et al. Deficient bone formation in idiopathic juvenile osteoporosis: a histomorphometric study of cancellous iliac bone. J Bone Miner Res 2000;15(5):957–63.
37. Smith R. Idiopathic juvenile osteoporosis: experience of twenty-one patients. Br J Rheumatol 1995;34(1):68–77.
38. Lorenc RS. Idiopathic juvenile osteoporosis. Calcif Tissue Int 2002;70(5):395–7.
39. van Staa TP, Cooper C, Leufkens HG, et al. Children and the risk of fractures caused by oral corticosteroids. J Bone Miner Res 2003;18(5):913–8.
40. Alsufyani KA, Ortiz-Alvarez O, Cabral DA, et al. Bone mineral density in children and adolescents with systemic lupus erythematosus, juvenile dermatomyositis, and systemic vasculitis: relationship to disease duration, cumulative corticosteroid dose, calcium intake, and exercise. J Rheumatol 2005;32(4): 729–33.
41. Li Y, Li A, Strait K, et al. Endogenous TNFalpha lowers maximum peak bone mass and inhibits osteoblastic Smad activation through NF-kappaB. J Bone Miner Res 2007;22(5):646–55.
42. Bianchi ML, Bardella MT. Bone in celiac disease. Osteoporos Int 2008;19(12): 1705–16.
43. Kayser R, Mahlfeld K, Nebelung W, et al. Vertebral collapse and normal peripheral blood cell count at the onset of acute lymphatic leukemia in childhood. J Pediatr Orthop B 2000;9(1):55–7.

44. Halton J, Gaboury I, Grant R, et al. Advanced vertebral fracture among newly diagnosed children with acute lymphoblastic leukemia: results of the Canadian Steroid-Associated Osteoporosis in the Pediatric Population (STOPP) research program. J Bone Miner Res 2009;24(7):1326–34.

45. Huber AM, Gaboury I, Cabral DA, et al. Prevalent vertebral fractures among children initiating glucocorticoid therapy for the treatment of rheumatic disorders. Arthritis Care Res (Hoboken) 2010;62(4):516–26.

46. Borusiak P, Langer T, Heruth M, et al. Antiepileptic drugs and bone metabolism in children: data from 128 patients. J Child Neurol 2013;28(2):176–83.

47. Moreira Guimaraes Penido MG, de Sousa Tavares M. Bone disease in pediatric idiopathic hypercalciuria. World J Nephrol 2012;1(2):54–62.

48. Mayranpaa MK, Tamminen IS, Kroger H, et al. Bone biopsy findings and correlation with clinical, radiological, and biochemical parameters in children with fractures. J Bone Miner Res 2011;26(8):1748–58.

49. Misra M, Pacaud D, Petryk A, et al. Vitamin D deficiency in children and its management: review of current knowledge and recommendations. Pediatrics 2008; 122(2):398–417.

50. Markula-Patjas KP, Valta HL, Kerttula LI, et al. Prevalence of vertebral compression fractures and associated factors in children and adolescents with severe juvenile idiopathic arthritis. J Rheumatol 2012;39(2):365–73.

51. Genant HK, Wu CY, van Kuijk C, et al. Vertebral fracture assessment using a semiquantitative technique. J Bone Miner Res 1993;8(9):1137–48.

52. Helenius I, Remes V, Salminen S, et al. Incidence and predictors of fractures in children after solid organ transplantation: a 5-year prospective, population-based study. J Bone Miner Res 2006;21(3):380–7.

53. Crabtree NJ, Arabi A, Bachrach LK, et al. Dual-energy X-ray absorptiometry interpretation and reporting in children and adolescents: the revised 2013 ISCD Pediatric Official Positions. J Clin Densitom 2014;17(2):225–42.

54. Bianchi ML. Osteoporosis in children and adolescents. Bone 2007;41(4):486–95.

55. Wren TA, Liu X, Pitukcheewanont P, et al. Bone densitometry in pediatric populations: discrepancies in the diagnosis of osteoporosis by DXA and CT. J Pediatr 2005;146(6):776–9.

56. Zemel BS, Leonard MB, Kelly A, et al. Height adjustment in assessing dual energy x-ray absorptiometry measurements of bone mass and density in children. J Clin Endocrinol Metab 2010;95(3):1265–73.

57. Tan VP, Macdonald HM, Kim S, et al. Influence of physical activity on bone strength in children and adolescents: a systematic review and narrative synthesis. J Bone Miner Res 2014;29:2161–81.

58. Detter F, Rosengren BE, Dencker M, et al. A 6-year exercise program improves skeletal traits without affecting fracture risk: a prospective controlled study in 2621 children. J Bone Miner Res 2014;29(6):1325–36.

59. Macdonald HM, Kontulainen SA, Khan KM, et al. Is a school-based physical activity intervention effective for increasing tibial bone strength in boys and girls? J Bone Miner Res 2007;22(3):434–46.

60. Stark C, Nikopoulou-Smyrni P, Stabrey A, et al. Effect of a new physiotherapy concept on bone mineral density, muscle force and gross motor function in children with bilateral cerebral palsy. J Musculoskelet Neuronal Interact 2010;10(2): 151–8.

61. Reyes GF, Dickin DC, Crusat NJ, et al. Whole-body vibration effects on the muscle activity of upper and lower body muscles during the baseball swing in recreational baseball hitters. Sports Biomech 2011;10(4):280–93.

62. Ross AC, Manson JE, Abrams SA, et al. The 2011 report on dietary reference intakes for calcium and vitamin D from the Institute of Medicine: what clinicians need to know. J Clin Endocrinol Metab 2011;96(1):53–8.
63. Dibba B, Prentice A, Ceesay M, et al. Effect of calcium supplementation on bone mineral accretion in gambian children accustomed to a low-calcium diet. Am J Clin Nutr 2000;71(2):544–9.
64. Winzenberg T, Shaw K, Fryer J, et al. Effects of calcium supplementation on bone density in healthy children: meta-analysis of randomised controlled trials. BMJ 2006;333(7572):775.
65. Bolland MJ, Barber PA, Doughty RN, et al. Vascular events in healthy older women receiving calcium supplementation: randomised controlled trial. BMJ 2008;336(7638):262–6.
66. Russell RG. Bisphosphonates: mode of action and pharmacology. Pediatrics 2007;119(Suppl 2):S150–62.
67. Rauch F, Travers R, Plotkin H, et al. The effects of intravenous pamidronate on the bone tissue of children and adolescents with osteogenesis imperfecta. J Clin Invest 2002;110(9):1293–9.
68. Munns CF, Rajab MH, Hong J, et al. Acute phase response and mineral status following low dose intravenous zoledronic acid in children. Bone 2007;41(3): 366–70.
69. Migliorati CA, Siegel MA, Elting LS. Bisphosphonate-associated osteonecrosis: a long-term complication of bisphosphonate treatment. Lancet Oncol 2006;7(6): 508–14.
70. Glorieux FH, Bishop NJ, Plotkin H, et al. Cyclic administration of pamidronate in children with severe osteogenesis imperfecta. N Engl J Med 1998;339(14): 947–52.
71. Land C, Rauch F, Munns CF, et al. Vertebral morphometry in children and adolescents with osteogenesis imperfecta: effect of intravenous pamidronate treatment. Bone 2006;39(4):901–6.
72. Lowing K, Astrom E, Oscarsson KA, et al. Effect of intravenous pamidronate therapy on everyday activities in children with osteogenesis imperfecta. Acta Paediatr 2007;96(8):1180–3.
73. Ward LM, Rauch F, Whyte MP, et al. Alendronate for the treatment of pediatric osteogenesis imperfecta: a randomized placebo-controlled study. J Clin Endocrinol Metab 2011;96(2):355–64.
74. Letocha AD, Cintas HL, Troendle JF, et al. Controlled trial of pamidronate in children with types III and IV osteogenesis imperfecta confirms vertebral gains but not short-term functional improvement. J Bone Miner Res 2005;20(6):977–86.
75. Fehlings D, Switzer L, Agarwal P, et al. Informing evidence-based clinical practice guidelines for children with cerebral palsy at risk of osteoporosis: a systematic review. Dev Med Child Neurol 2012;54(2):106–16.
76. Thornton J, Ashcroft DM, Mughal MZ, et al. Systematic review of effectiveness of bisphosphonates in treatment of low bone mineral density and fragility fractures in juvenile idiopathic arthritis. Arch Dis Child 2006;91(9):753–61.

Preventing Diabetic Ketoacidosis

Craig A. Jefferies, MBChB, MD[a,b,][*,1], Meranda Nakhla, MSc, MD, FRCPC[c,1],
José G.B. Derraik, PhD[b], Alistair J. Gunn, MBChB, PhD[a,d],
Denis Daneman, MBBCh, FRCPC, DSc (Med)[e], Wayne S. Cutfield, MBChB, MD[a,b]

KEYWORDS

- Type 1 diabetes mellitus • Diabetic ketoacidosis • Prevention • Education
- Recurrent • Noncompliance • Girls

KEY POINTS

- Diabetic ketoacidosis (DKA) is a complication of severe insulin deficiency leading to hyperglycemia, with its attendant glycosuria, dehydration, and ketogenesis, leading to acidosis.
- DKA is associated with significant morbidity, non-negligible mortality, and excessive health care expenditures.
- DKA is largely an avoidable and preventable complication of type 1 diabetes mellitus (T1DM).
- Risk factors associated with DKA at diagnosis of T1DM include age less than 5 years old, lack of private health insurance, lower socioeconomic status (SES), misdiagnosis, delayed diagnosis, and living in regions with a low background incidence of T1DM.
- Factors associated with increased DKA risk in children with established T1DM include age greater than 13 years, female gender, low SES, lack of private health insurance, poor family functioning, psychiatric disorders, higher reported insulin dose, and poor glycemic control.

Competing Interests: The authors have no financial or nonfinancial conflicts of interest to disclose that may be relevant to this work.
[a] Paediatric Endocrinology Service, Starship Children's Hospital, Auckland District Health Board, 2 Park Road, Auckland, 1023, New Zealand; [b] Liggins Institute, University of Auckland, 85 Park Road, Auckland, 1023, New Zealand; [c] Department of Paediatrics, Montreal Children's Hospital, McGill University, 2300 Tupper Street, H3H 1P3, Montreal, Canada; [d] Department of Physiology, University of Auckland, 85 Park Road, Auckland, 1023, New Zealand; [e] Department of Pediatrics, The Hospital for Sick Children, University of Toronto, 555 University Avenue, M5G 1X8, Toronto, Canada
[1] Coprimary authors.
* Corresponding author. Starship Children's Health, Private Bag 92024, Auckland 1142, New Zealand.
E-mail address: CraigJ@adhb.govt.nz

Pediatr Clin N Am 62 (2015) 857–871
http://dx.doi.org/10.1016/j.pcl.2015.04.002
0031-3955/15/$ – see front matter © 2015 Elsevier Inc. All rights reserved.

INTRODUCTION

T1DM is one of the most common chronic diseases of childhood with significant morbidity and non-negligible mortality.[1,2] The global incidence of T1DM is increasing by 3% per year in children and adolescents and by 5% per year in preschoolers.[3,4] Acute complications, such as DKA, are potentially avoidable causes of hospitalizations and mortality in children and adolescents with T1DM. DKA occurs in the presence of severe insulinopenia and is characterized by hyperglycemia, acidosis, and ketosis.

The early development of T1DM involves progressive insulin deficiency, leading to weeks of symptomatic hyperglycemia with polyuria, polydipsia, and weight loss.[5,6] If left untreated, the combination of insulin deficiency and stress (mediated through increased circulating levels of counter-regulatory hormones, including cortisol, catecholamines, growth hormone, and glucagon) leads to lipolysis. Hepatic metabolism of free fatty acids as an alternative energy source (ie, ketogenesis) results in accumulation of acidic intermediate and end metabolites (ie, ketones and ketoacids). The predominant ketones in the body are β-hydroxybutyrate, acetate, and acetoacetate.[5,6] In DKA, the ratio of β-hydroxybutyrate to acetoacetate increases from equimolar amounts (1:1) up to 1.3:1 to 5.5:1.[7] Accumulation of ketoacids is due to their rate-limiting metabolism. Diagnosis of DKA has been traditionally made with a combination of hyperglycemia (blood glucose >11 mmol/L or 200 mg/dL), venous pH less than 7.3 and bicarbonate levels less than 15 mmol/L.[8]

DKA at initial presentation is common, but rates vary strikingly between countries, ranging from approximately 13% to 80%.[9–11] The highest rates are typically seen in the developing world, not surprisingly given the resource constraints.[11] DKA in children previously diagnosed with T1DM is also unfortunately common, with highly variable rates between centers and countries.[11,12] DKA remains the most common cause of mortality in T1DM. The most devastating consequence of DKA is cerebral edema with an incidence of 0.5% to 0.9%.[13,14] The mortality rate from cerebral edema is 21% to 24%, and morbidity from serious neurologic sequelae occurs in 15% to 35% of cases.[11,12] Furthermore, DKA has a long-term impact on cognitive function, including a fall in IQ and persistent loss of short-term memory. The health care expenditures associated with 1 episode of DKA are substantial, estimated at more than $3500.[15]

EPIDEMIOLOGY AND CAUSES OF DIABETIC KETOACIDOSIS

DKA occurs generally under 2 circumstances and in a limited number of situations:

1. At diagnosis
2. In those with established diabetes
   a. As a result of accidental or deliberate insulin omission or
   b. Inappropriate management of intercurrent illness

Most, if not all, episodes of DKA can be prevented. These episodes generally represent a failure of timely diagnosis and/or management of T1DM. Understanding the epidemiology and factors associated with the onset of DKA is essential in developing measures to prevent these episodes.

DIABETIC KETOACIDOSIS AT DIAGNOSIS

Symptoms of new-onset T1DM typically develop over a few days to weeks before presentation, whereas DKA rapidly evolves once ketones accumulate[16]: 75% of patients with new cases of T1DM in the EURODIAB (the Epidemiology and Prevention of

Diabetes) project had symptoms for more than 2 weeks before diagnosis.[17] Thus, DKA at diagnosis of new T1DM ultimately reflects lack of awareness by parents and primary care physicians of the evolving symptoms of T1DM.[17]

A systematic review in 2011 identified 46 studies, including more than 24,000 children with T1DM from 31 countries[18]: the frequency of DKA at diagnosis varied 6-fold, from 12.8% to 80% (**Table 1**).[16] Rates were lowest in Sweden, and Canada and highest in the United Arab Emirates, Saudi Arabia, and Romania. There was an inverse correlation between DKA frequency at diagnosis and the regional background incidence of T1DM, findings that are consistent with previous studies from Europe. This may be explained by an overall increased awareness of T1DM and its presenting symptoms, leading to earlier recognition and diagnosis. DKA frequencies were also found to be lower in countries further from the equator and with a higher gross domestic product (GDP).[12] There are several explanations for this association. Latitude may represent a group of characteristics, including economy, health care provision, and disease burden.[12] Usher-Smith and colleagues[12] found a colinearity between latitude and a country's GDP, suggesting that the variation in latitude may be explained more by a country's economy and health care provision than distance from the equator. In addition, in a recent report analyzing data from countries identified as "wealthy" by the Organisation for Economic Co-operation and Development, a close correlation was found between DKA risk at disease onset and income inequality, defined as the difference in average incomes between a nation's highest and lowest income earners.[19] Among the countries included in the analysis, the frequency of DKA at diagnosis ranged from 16% to 54%, with countries with the lowest income inequality having lower DKA frequencies.

Table 1
Frequency of diabetic ketoacidosis at disease onset of type 1 diabetes mellitus

Country	Diabetic Ketoacidosis (%)
United Arab Emirates	80
Romania	67
Saudi Arabia	40–77
France	54
Kuwait	38–49
Poland	33–54
China	42
Oman	42
Lithuania	35
Austria	37
Italy	32–41
Bulgaria	35
Germany	26–53
United States	27–44
Turkey	29
United Kingdom	25–38
Ireland	25
Finland	19–22
Canada	18.6
Sweden	13–14

The key individual factors associated with greater risk of DKA were being less than 2 years old at presentation, being incorrectly diagnosed or having treatment delayed, belonging to an ethnic minority, lower SES, lack of health insurance in the United States, lower parental education, lower body mass index, and preceding infection.[20] Conversely, having a first-degree relative with T1DM was protective (odds ratio [OR] 0.33).

A small qualitative study (16 children) within the East of England found that the families were aware of symptoms for several weeks before a trigger, such as weight loss, led them to seek medical advice.[21] At the time of presentation, many families suspected the diagnosis. A strong protective effect of a family history of T1DM has been noted in several studies.[21–23] This relationship is unlikely to be genetic, because although high-risk genotypes are associated with DKA risk, having even 1 first-degree family member with T1DM is associated with dramatically reduced risk of DKA.[24] Furthermore, participating in a long-term follow-up study, The Environmental Determinants of Diabetes in the Young, was associated with reduced risk of DKA.[25] Thus, this protective relationship is almost certainly due to greater family awareness of the symptoms of diabetes.

Supporting this proposal, studies have found an overall fall in the risk of DKA over a 20-year interval in northern Finland,[26] consistent with the overall increase in incidence of T1DM over this period. There are some contradictory findings, however. In some countries, the rate of new-onset DKA has not fallen over time despite a temporal increase in incidence, even where there are highly organized and easily accessible health care systems. In Austria for example, the risk of DKA on a prospectively recorded country-wide register remained similar between 2005 to 2009 and 2010 to 2011.[27] A single-center study from Australia found no change in the risk of DKA in 1073 children and adolescents ages up to 18 years with newly diagnosed T1DM from 1998 to 2010.[28] Similarly, in Auckland, the largest city in New Zealand, the incidence and severity of new-onset DKA remained stable at approximately 27% over the past 15 years[29] and are similar to the previous review in 1995 to 1996.[10] These findings suggest that health care providers and families are failing to recognize the early symptoms of T1DM.

Age

Several studies have consistently demonstrated that younger age at diagnosis of T1DM is a significant risk factor in the development of DKA. Usher-Smith and colleagues[18] conducted a meta-analysis consisting of 32 studies and found that children ages less than 2 years old had 3 times the risk of presenting with DKA as children ages greater than 2 years old (OR 3.41; 95% CI, 2.54–4.59). This increased risk continued up to age 5 years (OR 1.59; 95% CI, 1.38–1.84). In general, studies have demonstrated that the frequency of DKA at diagnosis decreases significantly with age from 37% to 40% (95% CI, 32.9%–41.8%) in children ages 0 to 4 years old to 14.7% to 23.6% (95% CI, 11.7%–17.7%) in children ages 15 to 19 years old.[23,30] The higher rates of DKA in the younger age groups may be related to several factors, including (1) the classic symptoms of T1DM may not be obvious and easily distinguishable from other common acute illnesses, resulting in a delay in diagnosis; (2) clinicians may have a lower index of suspicion for T1DM among younger children, particularly in the under 2-year age group;[3,25] (3) younger children have a less developed mechanism of metabolic compensation resulting in faster development of acidosis and dehydration;[23,31] and (4) β-cell destruction[4] may be more aggressive in younger children because serum levels of C-peptide are lowest in the under 2-year age group at diagnosis of T1DM compared with older age groups.[32]

Ethnic Minority

Studies in both the United States and United Kingdom have demonstrated an increased risk of DKA among ethnic minorities. A recent multicenter US study found that nonwhite youth were more at risk of presenting with DKA at diagnosis compared with non-Hispanic white youth, independent of SES and age (OR 1.21; 95% CI, 1.03–1.43).[20] A study in the United Kingdom reported a higher frequency of DKA at diagnosis among ethnic minorities (41.3%) compared with non-Hispanic white patients (21.4%) (P = .03).[33] In addition, a study in New Zealand showed that non-Europeans were more likely to present in DKA than those of European ethnicity (OR 1.52; P = .048).[29] These disparities may be due to cultural or language barriers, lack of access to health care services, or lack of awareness of T1DM in ethnic minorities.

Lower Socioeconomic Status

Lower SES as measured by family income or neighborhood income is associated with an increased risk of DKA at diagnosis.[34] One US study found that the frequency of DKA was 70% to 80% higher in patients with a family income below $50,000 compared with those with a family income greater than $50,000 (higher income).[20] In Canada, where patients enjoy universal access to health care, patients with low SES, as measured by neighborhood income quintiles, were more likely to present with DKA at diagnosis compared with the highest income quintiles (OR 1.39; 95% CI, 1.17-1.63).[34]

Lack of Private Health Insurance

In countries without universal health coverage, lack of private health insurance has been consistently found to be a significant risk factor for DKA at diagnosis.[35,36] For instance, study in the United States found that patients with private health insurance were least likely to present with DKA.[35] Patients with no health insurance were 60% more likely to present with DKA compared with those with health insurance coverage. Furthermore, when uninsured patients presented with DKA, they were more likely to present with severe DKA.[37] The odds of uninsured patients presenting with severe DKA (ie, venous pH <7.10; serum bicarbonate <5 mmol/L) were 6 times (OR 6.09; 95% CI, 3.21–11.56) the odds for insured patients.[36] These findings suggest that patients without health insurance may delay seeking timely medical care and thus present with severe DKA.

Delayed Diagnosis

A delay of more than 24 hours between the initial presentation to a primary or secondary care provider and referral to a multidisciplinary diabetes team in the United Kingdom has been reported associated with an increased risk of presenting with DKA (52.3% vs 20.5%, P<.05).[33] The most common reason cited for the delayed diagnosis was arrangement for a fasting blood sugar prior to referral to a multidisciplinary team.

Diagnostic Error

Several retrospective cohort studies have reported an increased risk of DKA in children not diagnosed with T1DM at first presentation to the health care system due to either a misdiagnosis or lack of recognition of the symptoms of T1DM.[33,34] In Ontario, Canada, the authors previously reported that children with DKA at diabetes diagnosis were more likely to have seen a health care professional on 1 or more occasions in the weeks prior, at which time the diagnosis of T1DM was missed.[34] Diagnostic error at first presentation to the health care system has been associated with a 3-fold increased risk of presenting with DKA (OR 3.35; 95% CI, 2.35-5.79), independent of the presence of a preceding infectious illness.[1] Misdiagnosis was more likely to occur among younger children. In 1 study, patients with DKA in whom the diagnosis of diabetes was missed at initial presentation tended to be younger (mean age 5.4 ± 4.4 years old) compared with those in whom the diagnosis was not missed (mean age 8.8 ± 4.0 years old) (P<.001). Younger children tended to be misdiagnosed with urinary tract infection, upper respiratory tract infection, gastroenteritis, or otitis media.[34]

Preceding Infectious Illness

The presence of a concomitant infection may mask the early symptoms of diabetes or delaying the diagnosis resulting in an increased risk of DKA.[20] Furthermore, an infectious or febrile illness generally increases the counter-regulatory response, resulting in insulin resistance and metabolic decompensation.

Protective Factors

The protective factors associated with a decreased risk of DKA at disease onset include first-degree relative with T1DM and higher parental education. Having a higher awareness and better recognition of the signs and symptoms of hyperglycemia likely explain the decreased risk of DKA among families with a first-degree relative with diabetes.[1,30,32] Children from families in which parents had greater than a postsecondary education or had at least 1 parent with an academic degree are at a decreased risk of DKA at diagnosis.[18,30,32]

Can Diabetic Ketoacidosis Be Prevented at Diagnosis?

In light of the existing evidence, it is highly plausible that improving community and medical awareness of the presenting features of T1DM in children may help prevent DKA. There have been few studies, however, on community education with indirect and unmonitored methods used, which have led to inconclusive results.

A small study from Parma, Italy,[38] involved providing a poster to primary and secondary public schools and providing local pediatricians with equipment for measuring urine and blood glucose and patient cards. Over the subsequent 8 years, the rate of DKA in children ages 6 to 14 years was 12.5% (3/24) in Parma compared with 83% (25/30) in nearby areas, where children did not receive the information. Furthermore, the duration of symptoms was much shorter in the Parma area (mean 5 vs 28 days), and the length of hospitalization was also shortened. Despite its encouraging results, this study was limited by its small size and the high baseline rate of DKA compared with typical European rates.

Another small prospective study also suggested significant benefit from an educational campaign in Australia. In this study, a 2-year control period was followed by a 2-year intervention[37] in 1 region (Gosford) but not in 2 others (Newcastle and Sydney). Posters were provided to childcare centers, schools, and doctors' offices, with doctors also given glucose and ketone testing equipment. The proportion of children with DKA decreased in the intervention region from 38% (15/40) to 14% (4/29), whereas there was no change in DKA rates in the control regions (37% [46/123] and 39% [49/127]). Unexpectedly, the incidence of T1DM in Gosford also fell by 28%, raising the possibility that the reduction in new-onset DKA might have partly reflected redirection of patients to other larger, children's hospitals in the region.

In contrast, a national study in Wales found no benefit.[39] Posters were sent to every pharmacy, school, and general practitioner surgery across Wales, and the campaign publicized with radio interviews. Before the campaign, the risk of DKA was approximately 25% from 1991 to 2009, with no temporal change. After the campaign, from 2008 to 2009, 26% of children diagnosed with T1DM had DKA. Questionnaires suggested that few families were aware of the campaign. Thus, it seems that the format of the campaign without more direct engagement with the community may not be effective.

Furthermore, another nationwide prospective study in Austria involving 4038 children with new-onset T1DM also found no effect of community education.[27] This study attempted greater penetration than other studies, and posters were given to all kindergartens, schools, pharmacies, pediatricians, and general practitioners in 2009. In addition, medical officers in schools received education twice a year, and there was national media publicity. Before the campaign (2005–2009), 26% of children had mild DKA and 12% had severe DKA compared with 27% mild and 9.5% severe cases afterward (2010–2011). Although DKA was more common in younger children, there was no effect of stratification by age. This study suggests that a primarily poster-based education campaign is insufficient, possibly because of greater competition for parent's attention. Regional differences cannot be excluded, however, and it is also possible that simply displaying posters was the wrong media tool for the modern generation.

Thus, there is at best limited evidence that community-based mass campaigns improve the risk of DKA in new-onset T1DM. Critical to any mass educational program is a clear simple message. It is worth reflecting that in the Parma study, approximately 90% of children had bed wetting at diagnosis.[38] Similarly, in Auckland, a local audit from 2000 to 2009 suggests that more than 95% of children newly diagnosed with T1DM had bed wetting or increased night-time urination (Starship Children's Hospital, unpublished data). The authors speculate that a focus on such a simplified message may be more effective for community education and should be tested.

DIABETIC KETOACIDOSIS IN ESTABLISHED TYPE 1 DIABETES MELLITUS

Diabetes mellitus management in children is complex and requires intense resources as well as regular access to timely and effective health care services to prevent complications. T1DM is an ambulatory-care sensitive condition, defined as a group of medical conditions typically managed in an ambulatory setting, whereby an admission to hospital indicates a potentially avoidable complication and is an indirect indicator of access and overall quality of outpatient care.[40,41] DKA is generally avoidable and its occurrence in children and adolescence with established T1DM may indicate poor outpatient diabetes mellitus care and could be prevented with comprehensive multidisciplinary outpatient care and improved adherence to diabetes management. **Table 2** outlines the risk factors for DKA among youth with established T1DM.

Epidemiology

Globally, reported rates of DKA in children with established T1DM range between 1 per 100 patient-years in a Swedish cohort[35] to 12 episodes per 100 patient-years in US cohort.[36,42] A retrospective cohort study conducted in the United States by Rewers and colleagues[36] determined that the incidence of DKA was 8 per 100 patient-years in 1243 children from 1996 to 2000. This incidence increased in age among girls (4 per 100 patient-years in <7 year olds; 8 in 7–12 year olds; and 12 in ≥13 year olds) but not boys. In addition, approximately 60% of the DKA episodes occurred in 5% of children with recurrent events (>2 episodes). In a more recent retrospective cohort study from Europe (1995–2008), the incidence of DKA among 28,770 patients with T1DM was 6.3 per 100 patient-years and remained relatively unchanged over the study period, with recurrent episodes seen in 1% of patients.[43] The overall incidence of DKA was slightly higher in girls (7% vs 5.8%) and in immigrants, but there

Table 2
Risk factors associated with new-onset diabetic ketoacidosis versus recurrent diabetic ketoacidosis

New-onset Diabetic Ketoacidosis	Recurrent Diabetic Ketoacidosis
Young age (especially <2 y)	Older age (especially adolescents)
Lack of access to medical care	Lack of access to medical care
Lack of awareness of diabetes	Psychiatric disorders
Lack of family history of T1DM	Low SES
Delayed medical diagnosis of T1DM	Low family cohesion
Low parental education	Higher HbA$_{1c}$
Recent infection	Low income
Minority ethnic groups	Minority ethnic groups
—	High insulin doses and noncompliance with insulin therapy

was no effect of treatment type or duration of diabetes. Recurrent DKA was associated with older age (in particular the early teenage years), higher hemoglobin A$_{1c}$ (HbA$_{1c}$) levels, and higher insulin doses.

In the United States, in the T1D Exchange Clinic Registry of 13,487 children and young adults (<26 years of age) with T1DM for at least 2 years,[35] DKA was most frequent in adolescents and associated with higher HbA$_{1c}$, nonwhite race, lack of private health insurance, and lower household income. A small Swedish study identified 142 episodes of DKA in 1990 to 2000; subjects were aged 14.6 years on average with a mean T1DM duration of 6.6 years.[44] The reported triggers of DKA included missed insulin doses (48.6%), gastroenteritis (14.1%), technical pump problems (12.7%), infections (13.4%), and social problems (1.4%). Pump users had approximately double the rate of DKA compared with patients using intermittent injections. This finding is not universal, however, and may reflect an improved understanding of insulin pumping and early testing for blood ketones.[44] Although the risk of DKA increases with duration of diabetes, there is an appreciable rate in the first year after diagnosis. In a population-based study in Germany, 373 subjects with newly diagnosed T1DM aged less than 15 years who were followed for a mean of 1 year had 4.7 times higher risk of hospitalization.[45]

Risk Factors in Children with Established Type 1 Diabetes Mellitus

In a prospective cohort study of 1243 children and youth with T1DM, the risk of DKA increased with higher HbA$_{1c}$ and higher reported insulin doses among children ages less than 13 years old (see **Table 2**).[45,46] Among older children (>13 years old), the risk of DKA increased with higher HbA$_{1c}$ (relative risk [RR] 1.43 per 1% increase; 95% CI, 1.3–1.6), higher reported insulin dose, underinsurance, and the presence of psychiatric disorders, including major depression, bipolar or anxiety disorder, and/or use of psychotropic medications. These factors were also found to confer an increased risk of recurrent DKA. Other studies have also found similar risk factors for DKA.[35,42,45]

The higher risk of DKA among adolescent girls may be related to body image issues, whereby 10% of adolescent girls with T1DM meet *Diagnostic and Statistical Manual of Mental Disorders*[47] criteria for eating disorders compared with 4% of their age-matched controls without diabetes.[48] One aspect of T1DM that contributes to the development of an eating disorder is that adolescent girls may deliberately omit insulin as a unique and readily available way to control weight through induced hyperglycemia and glycosuria, increasing the risk of DKA.[49–51]

Higher reported insulin dose may represent either lower endogenous insulin secretion with longer duration of T1DM or insulin resistance related to puberty or obesity.[45] Alternatively, in patients who omit insulin, a higher prescribed insulin dose may not be the actual dose taken.

Psychiatric conditions are a significant risk factor for DKA, particularly among adolescent girls (RR 3.22; 95% CI, 2.25–4.61).[8,52] This association may be due to nonadherence to diabetes self-management and to insulin omission.[53]

Lower SES as measured by lack of private health insurance, head-of-household unemployment, or low household income has consistently been found associated with an increased risk of DKA.[36] This association maybe driven by factors, such as compliance with medical care, including decreased blood glucose monitoring, access to transportation, and irregular physician visits.

Additional risk factors include longer diabetes duration,[54] family functioning, the transition to adult care,[55] and insulin pump therapy.[46] Several studies suggest that family functioning is associated with DKA risk. In 1 study, children who had an episode of DKA were more likely to perceive their parents as less warm and caring toward their diabetes management (measure of diabetes-specific family support) and had caregivers who rated themselves as less supportive of their child's diabetes care (measure of parental negativity) compared with children who did not have a DKA episode.[55]

The transition to adult care occurs during a critical and vulnerable period for those with T1DM. The authors' data from the province of Ontario, Canada, identified a small but significant increase in DKA rates as youth with T1DM transitioned from a pediatric to adult health care team. Furthermore, the authors found that girls and lower SES, as measured by neighborhood level income, decreased local medical resources, and previous hospitalizations for DKA, were significant predictors of post-transition DKA episodes.[55]

In summary, DKA in children and adolescents with established T1DM is an avoidable complication that can be prevented through appropriate education and psychosocial support, consistent self-monitoring of blood glucose and ketones, and improved adherence to diabetes self-management.

Poor glycemic control

Poor glycemic control is a major risk factor for recurrent DKA in teenagers.[49] In turn, poor glycemic control is directly related to poor adherence with insulin treatment. For example, in Scotland, in a cohort of 89 patients at a mean age 16 years, there was a significant inverse association between HbA$_{1c}$ and adherence ($r^2 = 0.39$).[40] Not surprisingly, poor adherence was associated with more admissions for DKA and the secular trend for deterioration in glycemic control from 10 to 20 years.

Small studies in which children were studied in more detail have highlighted a clear role for underlying behavioral and psychological stresses in association with recurrent DKA. In a sample of 92 school-age children followed for an average of 9 years from diagnosis, 28% had 3 or more admissions for DKA. Recurrent DKA was associated with higher HbA$_{1c}$ levels, more behavioral problems, younger age at diagnosis, and lower SES.[54] Similarly, in a cohort of 61 children and adolescents followed for 8 years after diagnosis, 28% had 1 or more episode of DKA.[56,57] DKA was more common in girls and was associated with more behavior problems and lower social competence, higher levels of reported family conflict, and lower levels of family cohesion, expressiveness, and organization in year 1.

These studies indicated that a mixture of poor background glycemic control, disadvantaged groups, and (particularly in the United States) lack of medical insurance as key risk factors for recurrent DKA. Nonetheless, even countries with comprehensive medical systems have found little change in the rate of DKA over time. For example, in Ontario, Canada, there were 5008 hospital admissions for DKA in children younger than 19 years from 1991 to 1999, with no change in the admission rate or the case fatality rate of 0.18% over this time.[57]

Prevention of recurrent diabetic ketoacidosis

The existing evidence suggests that there are 2 broad targets for preventing recurrent DKA: improving access to medical care and improving management of individual patient approach to diabetes. The impact of social and access issues in deprived populations is substantial. For example, among adult urban African Americans who developed DKA, more than two-thirds of cases occurred due to cessation of insulin therapy because of lack of money for insulin or transportation to the hospital as well as limited self-care skills.[38] A recent study in the same setting again highlighted the strong link between DKA and lack of adherence to insulin treatment in adult inner-city minority patients in the United States.[58] Once more, two-thirds of cases of DKA were due to cessation of insulin therapy and were linked to depression, alcohol and drug abuse, and homelessness (but not psychiatric illnesses). Such high-risk populations would benefit from practical, targeted assistance.

The more common background for recurrent DKA, however, is teenage patients from nondisadvantaged populations. A systematic review in 2000 identified 24 randomized controlled trials of behavioral interventions for adolescents with T1DM.[53] The effect on DKA rates was rarely examined in the individual studies; therefore, DKA was not a focus of the review. The effect on glycemic control was small and notably heterogeneous, equivalent to a reduction in HbA$_{1c}$ of 0.3%. Furthermore, the studies were small, there were few common outcomes to allow direct comparison of interventions, and there was no long-term follow-up. Moreover, the most effective interventions seem to involve such high institutional and patient commitments that it is questionable whether they could be translated to routine care.

Subsequently, there have been several small studies with similar limitations. For example, a small study in which 17 children received ten 90-minute sessions of in-home behavioral family systems therapy had no effect on glycemic control.[59,60] A modified version of this program in 104 families (involving either educational support for multiple families or 12 sessions over 6 months) was associated with improved glycemic control up to 18 months from the start of the program, but its cost-effectiveness and effect on DKA risk are still unclear. Scheduled bimonthly telephone calls over 17 months from a pediatric diabetes educator did not improve glycemic control or reduce rates of hospital admission in 123 patients at a mean age of 12 years.[61] A more ambitious program consisted of a 6-month home-based intervention for 37 adolescents with poorly controlled T1DM (HbA$_{1c}$ >9.0%), involving monthly home visits and weekly phone contact.[62] In comparison to 32 adolescents in routine care only, there was a modest improvement in HbA$_{1c}$, from 11.1% to 9.7% at 6 months, that was not maintained at 12 and 18 months. It is unknown whether continuing treatment would have been more effective.

In contrast, recent larger studies of behavioral interventions have yielded encouraging results. In a randomized controlled trial in 127 adolescents with poorly controlled T1DM, intensive home-based psychotherapy over 2 years was associated with sustained reduction in hospital admissions compared with baseline or to controls over the full period.[41] This intensive intervention was expensive ($6934 per patient), but this cost was offset by reduced admissions for DKA. A subsequent trial in 146 adolescents with T1DM or type 2 diabetes mellitus showed that this approach was superior to telephone support in improving glycemic control over 12 months.[63] Another study involved more general training in adolescents before 20 years of age, based on 6 small group sessions and monthly follow-up, including social problem solving, cognitive behavior modification, and conflict resolution.[64] There was an associated improvement in glycemic control, and the impact of diabetes on their quality of life was lessened compared with intensive diabetes management alone. This intervention, however, did not reduce the rate of DKA.

On the other hand, in patients with recurrent DKA, Golden and colleagues[65] demonstrated a significant decrease in DKA episodes among patients who were given their insulin injections by a responsible adult. Similarly, Nguyen and colleagues[66] demonstrated a significant improvement in HbA$_{1c}$ levels when teens with persistently poor metabolic control received a dose of long-acting insulin analog at lunchtime by a school nurse.

SUMMARY

The factors associated with DKA at presentation and recurrent DKA after diagnosis are different. Broadly, DKA at presentation seems to be a problem of lack of awareness of the symptoms of T1DM, whereas recurrent DKA in patient with established diabetes seems primarily related to omission of insulin, augmented by social issues. In cases of DKA at presentation, despite promising results from 2 community education projects, nationwide educational campaigns have been ineffective. The authors speculate that simplified messages and better ways of increasing awareness are needed.

In contrast, recurrent DKA is a problem of a minority, in particular girls in early adolescence with related family and behavioral issues, often from disadvantaged backgrounds. The key to reducing recurrent DKA is likely to be achieved by providing targeted intervention for high-risk patients. There is increasing evidence that several forms of support can modestly reduce DKA, but the most promising interventions involve a substantial and expensive commitment and have not been validated in large trials. The challenge for future research is to find programs that are not only efficacious but also readily applicable in routine clinical practice.

REFERENCES

1. Edge JA, Ford-Adams ME, Dunger DB. Causes of death in children with insulin dependent diabetes 1990-96. Arch Dis Child 1999;81(4):318–23.
2. Dahlquist G, Kallen B. Mortality in childhood-onset type 1 diabetes: a population-based study. Diabetes Care 2005;28(10):2384–7.
3. Patterson CC, Dahlquist GG, Gyurus E, et al. Incidence trends for childhood type 1 diabetes in Europe during 1989-2003 and predicted new cases 2005-20: a multicentre prospective registration study. Lancet 2009;373(9680):2027–33.
4. The Diamond Project Group. Incidence and trends of childhood Type 1 diabetes worldwide 1990-1999. Diabet Med 2006;23(8):857–66.
5. Lawrence SE, Cummings EA, Gaboury I, et al. Population-based study of incidence and risk factors for cerebral edema in pediatric diabetic ketoacidosis. J Pediatr 2005;146(5):688–92.
6. Edge JA, Hawkins MM, Winter DL, et al. The risk and outcome of cerebral oedema developing during diabetic ketoacidosis. Arch Dis Child 2001;85(1): 16–22.

7. Wolfsdorf JI. The International Society of Pediatric and Adolescent Diabetes guidelines for management of diabetic ketoacidosis: Do the guidelines need to be modified? Pediatr Diabetes 2014;15(4):277–86.

8. Wolfsdorf JI, Allgrove J, Craig ME, et al. Diabetic ketoacidosis and hyperglycemic hyperosmolar state. Pediatr Diabetes 2014;15(Suppl 20):154–79.

9. Dunger DB, Sperling MA, Acerini CL, et al. ESPE/LWPES consensus statement on diabetic ketoacidosis in children and adolescents. Arch Dis Child 2004;89:188–94.

10. Jackson W, Hofman PL, Robinson EM, et al. The changing presentation of children with newly diagnosed type 1 diabetes mellitus. Pediatr Diabetes 2001;2: 154–9.

11. Onyiriuka AN, Ifebi E. Ketoacidosis at diagnosis of type 1 diabetes in children and adolescents: frequency and clinical characteristics. J Diabetes Metab Disord 2013;12:47.

12. Usher-Smith JA, Thompson M, Ercole A, et al. Variation between countries in the frequency of diabetic ketoacidosis at first presentation of type 1 diabetes in children: a systematic review. Diabetologia 2012;55(11):2878–94.

13. Cameron FJ, Scratch SE, Nadebaum C, et al. Neurological consequences of diabetic ketoacidosis at initial presentation of type 1 diabetes in a prospective cohort study of children. Diabetes Care 2014;37(6):1554–62.

14. Glaser N, Barnett P, McCaslin I, et al. Risk factors for cerebral edema in children with diabetic ketoacidosis. N Engl J Med 2001;344(4):264–9.

15. Tieder JS, McLeod L, Keren R, et al. Variation in resource use and readmission for diabetic ketoacidosis in children's hospitals. Pediatrics 2013;132:229–36.

16. Wolfsdorf J, Craig ME, Daneman D, et al. Diabetic ketoacidosis. Pediatr Diabetes 2007;8:28–43.

17. Levy-Marchal C, Patterson CC, Green A. Geographical variation of presentation at diagnosis of type I diabetes in children: the EURODIAB study. Diabetologia 2001;44(Suppl 3):B75–80.

18. Usher-Smith JA, Thompson MJ, Sharp SJ, et al. Factors associated with the presence of diabetic ketoacidosis at diagnosis of diabetes in children and young adults: a systematic review. BMJ 2011;343:d4092.

19. Limenis E, Shulman R, Daneman D. Is the frequency of ketoacidosis at onset of type 1 diabetes a child health indicator that is related to income inequality? Diabetes Care 2012;35(2):e5.

20. Dabelea D, Rewers A, Stafford JM, et al. Trends in the prevalence of ketoacidosis at diabetes diagnosis: the SEARCH for diabetes in youth study. Pediatrics 2014; 133(4):e938–945.

21. Usher-Smith JA, Thompson MJ, Walter FM. 'Looking for the needle in the haystack': a qualitative study of the pathway to diagnosis of type 1 diabetes in children. BMJ Open 2013;3:e004068.

22. Choleau C, Maitre J, Filipovic Pierucci A, et al. Ketoacidosis at diagnosis of type 1 diabetes in French children and adolescents. Diabetes Metab 2014;40: 137–42.

23. de Vries L, Oren L, Lazar L, et al. Factors associated with diabetic ketoacidosis at onset of Type 1 diabetes in children and adolescents. Diabet Med 2013;30:1360–6.

24. Marigliano M, Morandi A, Maschio M, et al. Diabetic ketoacidosis at diagnosis: role of family history and class II HLA genotypes. Eur J Endocrinol 2013;168: 107–11.

25. Elding Larsson H, Vehik K, Bell R, et al. Reduced prevalence of diabetic ketoacidosis at diagnosis of type 1 diabetes in young children participating in longitudinal follow-up. Diabetes Care 2011;34:2347–52.

26. Hekkala A, Knip M, Veijola R. Ketoacidosis at diagnosis of type 1 diabetes in children in northern Finland: temporal changes over 20 years. Diabetes Care 2007; 30:861–6.
27. Fritsch M, Schober E, Rami-Merhar B, et al. Diabetic ketoacidosis at diagnosis in Austrian children: a population-based analysis, 1989-2011. J Pediatr 2013;163: 1484–8.e1.
28. Claessen FM, Donaghue K, Craig M. Consistently high incidence of diabetic ketoacidosis in children with newly diagnosed type 1 diabetes. Med J Aust 2012;197:216.
29. Jefferies CA, Cutfield SW, Derraik JGB, et al. 15-year incidence of diabetic ketoacidosis at onset of type 1 diabetes in children from a regional setting (Auckland, New Zealand). Sci Rep 2015;5:10358.
30. Rewers A, Klingensmith G, Davis C, et al. Presence of diabetic ketoacidosis at diagnosis of diabetes mellitus in youth: the Search for Diabetes in Youth Study. Pediatrics 2008;121(5):e1258–66.
31. Abdul-Rasoul M, Al-Mahdi M, Al-Qattan H, et al. Ketoacidosis at presentation of type 1 diabetes in children in Kuwait: frequency and clinical characteristics. Pediatr Diabetes 2010;11(5):351–6.
32. Komulainen J, Kulmala P, Savola K, et al. Clinical, autoimmune, and genetic characteristics of very young children with type 1 diabetes. Childhood Diabetes in Finland (DiMe) Study Group. Diabetes Care 1999;22(12):1950–5.
33. Sundaram PC, Day E, Kirk JM. Delayed diagnosis in type 1 diabetes mellitus. Arch Dis Child 2009;94(2):151–2.
34. Bui H, To T, Stein R, et al. Is diabetic ketoacidosis at disease onset a result of missed diagnosis? J Pediatr 2010;156(3):472–7.
35. Cengiz E, Xing D, Wong JC, et al. Severe hypoglycemia and diabetic ketoacidosis among youth with type 1 diabetes in the T1DM Exchange clinic registry. Pediatr Diabetes 2013;14(6):447–54.
36. Rewers A, Chase HP, Mackenzie T, et al. Predictors of acute complications in children with type 1 diabetes. JAMA 2002;287(19):2511–8.
37. King BR, Howard NJ, Verge CF, et al. A diabetes awareness campaign prevents diabetic ketoacidosis in children at their initial presentation with type 1 diabetes. Pediatr Diabetes 2012;13:647–51.
38. Vanelli M, Chiari G, Ghizzoni L, et al. Effectiveness of a prevention program for diabetic ketoacidosis in children. An 8-year study in schools and private practices. Diabetes Care 1999;22:7–9.
39. Lansdown AJ, Barton J, Warner J, et al. Prevalence of ketoacidosis at diagnosis of childhood onset Type 1 diabetes in Wales from 1991 to 2009 and effect of a publicity campaign. Diabet Med 2012;29:1506–9.
40. Morris AD, Boyle DI, McMahon AD, et al. Adherence to insulin treatment, glycaemic control, and ketoacidosis in insulin-dependent diabetes mellitus. The DARTS/MEMO Collaboration. Diabetes Audit and Research in Tayside Scotland. Medicines Monitoring Unit. Lancet 1997;350:1505–10.
41. Ellis D, Naar-King S, Templin T, et al. Multisystemic therapy for adolescents with poorly controlled type 1 diabetes: reduced diabetic ketoacidosis admissions and related costs over 24 months. Diabetes Care 2008;31:1746–7.
42. Estrada CL, Danielson KK, Drum ML, et al. Hospitalization subsequent to diagnosis in young patients with diabetes in Chicago, Illinois. Pediatrics 2009;124(3):926–34.
43. Fritsch M, Rosenbauer J, Schober E, et al. Predictors of diabetic ketoacidosis in children and adolescents with type 1 diabetes. Experience from a large multicentre database. Pediatr Diabetes 2011;12:307–12.

44. Hanas R, Lindgren F, Lindblad B. A 2-yr national population study of pediatric ketoacidosis in Sweden: predisposing conditions and insulin pump use. Pediatr Diabetes 2009;10(1):33–7.

45. Icks A, Rosenbauer J, Haastert B, et al. Hospitalization among diabetic children and adolescents and non-diabetic control subjects: a prospective population-based study. Diabetologia 2001;44(Suppl 3):B87–92.

46. Liberatore R Jr, Perlman K, Buccino J, et al. Continuous subcutaneous insulin infusion pump treatment in children with type 1 diabetes mellitus. J Pediatr Endocrinol Metab 2004;17(2):223–6.

47. American Psychiatric Association. Diagnostic and Statistical Manual of Mental Disorders. 4th edition. Washington, DC; 2000.

48. Jones JM, Lawson ML, Daneman D, et al. Eating disorders in adolescent females with and without type 1 diabetes: cross sectional study. BMJ 2000;320(7249): 1563–6.

49. Daneman D, Olmsted M, Rydall A, et al. Eating disorders in young women with type 1 diabetes. Prevalence, problems and prevention. Horm Res 1998; 50(Suppl 1):79–86.

50. Garrison MM, Katon WJ, Richardson LP. The impact of psychiatric comorbidities on readmissions for diabetes in youth. Diabetes Care 2005;28(9):2150–4.

51. Stewart SM, Rao U, Emslie GJ, et al. Depressive symptoms predict hospitalization for adolescents with type 1 diabetes mellitus. Pediatrics 2005;115(5): 1315–9.

52. Geffken GR, Heather L, Walker KN, et al. Family functioning processes and diabetic ketoacidosis in youths with type I diabetes. Rehabil Psychol 2008;53(2): 231–7.

53. Hampson SE, Skinner TC, Hart J, et al. Behavioral interventions for adolescents with type 1 diabetes: how effective are they? Diabetes Care 2000;23: 1416–22.

54. Kovacs M, Charron-Prochownik D, Obrosky DS. A longitudinal study of biomedical and psychosocial predictors of multiple hospitalizations among young people with insulin-dependent diabetes mellitus. Diabet Med 1995;12:142–8.

55. Nakhla M, Daneman D, To T, et al. Transition to adult care for youths with diabetes mellitus: findings from a Universal Health Care System. Pediatrics 2009;124(6): e1134–41.

56. Dumont RH, Jacobson AM, Cole C, et al. Psychosocial predictors of acute complications of diabetes in youth. Diabet Med 1995;12:612–8.

57. Curtis JR, To T, Muirhead S, et al. Recent trends in hospitalization for diabetic ketoacidosis in Ontario children. Diabetes Care 2002;25:1591–6.

58. Randall L, Begovic J, Hudson M, et al. Recurrent diabetic ketoacidosis in inner-city minority patients: behavioral, socioeconomic, and psychosocial factors. Diabetes Care 2011;34:1891–6.

59. Harris MA, Harris BS, Mertlich D. Brief report: in-home family therapy for adolescents with poorly controlled diabetes: failure to maintain benefits at 6-month follow-up. J Pediatr Psychol 2005;30:683–8.

60. Wysocki T, Harris MA, Buckloh LM, et al. Randomized trial of behavioral family systems therapy for diabetes: maintenance of effects on diabetes outcomes in adolescents. Diabetes Care 2007;30:555–60.

61. Nunn E, King B, Smart C, et al. A randomized controlled trial of telephone calls to young patients with poorly controlled type 1 diabetes. Pediatr Diabetes 2006;7: 254–9.

62. Couper JJ, Taylor J, Fotheringham MJ, et al. Failure to maintain the benefits of home-based intervention in adolescents with poorly controlled type 1 diabetes. Diabetes Care 1999;22:1933–7.
63. Ellis DA, Naar-King S, Chen X, et al. Multisystemic therapy compared to telephone support for youth with poorly controlled diabetes: findings from a randomized controlled trial. Ann Behav Med 2012;44:207–15.
64. Grey M, Boland EA, Davidson M, et al. Coping skills training for youth with diabetes mellitus has long-lasting effects on metabolic control and quality of life. J Pediatr 2000;137:107–13.
65. Golden MP, Herrold AJ, Orr DP. An approach to prevention of recurrent diabetic ketoacidosis in the pediatric population. J Pediatr 1985;107(2):195–200.
66. Nguyen TM, Mason KJ, Sanders CG, et al. Targeting blood glucose management in school improves glycemic control in children with poorly controlled type 1 diabetes mellitus. J Pediatr 2008;153(4):575–8.

The Impact of Technology on Current Diabetes Management

Katharine Garvey, MD, MPH[a,b,*], Joseph I. Wolfsdorf, MB, BCh[a,b]

KEYWORDS

- Technology • Type 1 diabetes mellitus • Children • Adolescents • Insulin analogues
- Insulin pump • Continuous glucose monitoring • Artificial pancreas

KEY POINTS

- Rapid-acting insulin analogues are more convenient to use than regular insulin. Long-acting analogues decrease nocturnal hypoglycemia. Insulin analogues are more expensive than regular and neutral protamine Hagedorn insulin.
- Compared with multiple daily injections, insulin pump therapy is associated with a modest improvement in glycemic control and may be associated with decreased frequency of severe hypoglycemia; available evidence suggests that quality of life is improved and the rate of pump discontinuation is low.
- Continuous glucose monitoring can improve glycemic control in children without increased hypoglycemia. The sensor-augmented insulin pump with low glucose suspension reduces rates of severe hypoglycemia and nocturnal hypoglycemia. Although technological innovations can improve diabetes outcomes and quality of life, maintenance of optimal glycemic control continues to be largely dependent on patient and family motivation, competence, and adherence to daily diabetes care requirements.
- The effective translation of technological advances into clinical practice is costly and requires a substantial investment in education of both practitioners and patients/families.
- Closed-loop "artificial pancreas" systems are currently in development and show great promise to automate insulin delivery with minimal patient intervention.

INTRODUCTION

In the past 2 decades, technological innovations have revolutionized the treatment of type 1 diabetes (T1D). Most recently, new insulin analogues and continuous glucose

The authors declare no conflicts of interest.
[a] Division of Endocrinology, Department of Medicine, Boston Children's Hospital, 300 Longwood Avenue, Boston, MA 02115, USA; [b] Department of Pediatrics, Harvard Medical School, 25 Shattuck St, Boston, MA 02115, USA
* Corresponding author. Division of Endocrinology, Boston Children's Hospital, Harvard Medical School, 300 Longwood Avenue, Boston, MA 02115.
E-mail address: katharine.garvey@childrens.harvard.edu

Pediatr Clin N Am 62 (2015) 873–888
http://dx.doi.org/10.1016/j.pcl.2015.04.005
0031-3955/15/$ – see front matter © 2015 Elsevier Inc. All rights reserved.

pediatric.theclinics.com

monitors (CGM) have become available to complement improvements in glucose meters, insulin pumps, and pen delivery systems. In clinical trials, these technological advances have been shown to improve clinical outcomes; however, their effective translation into clinical practice is both costly and requires substantial investment in education of both practitioners and patients/families, and has had only a modest impact on clinical outcomes. For example, only 25% of youth with T1D enrolled in the Type 1 Diabetes Exchange Clinic registry in the United States meet the International Society of Pediatric and Adolescent Diabetes hemoglobin A1c (HbA1c) target of less than 7.5%.[1]

The aphorism "A tool is only as good as the person using it" is true for management of T1D in children and adolescents. Advances in technology offer potential opportunities to improve diabetes outcomes; however, successful intensive diabetes management continues to be driven by the competence of the patient/family and their motivation to devote the considerable time and effort required to maintain blood glucose (BG) levels in the near-normal range. Excellent glycemic control is largely contingent on specific self-management behaviors, including, but not limited to, frequent self-monitoring of BG (SMBG) levels, administering insulin before meals, and not missing insulin boluses.[2]

This article focuses on recent technological innovations; however, it is important to appreciate that technology has the potential to improve diabetes outcomes only when the fundamental requirements of effective self-care are firmly in place. Motivated and empowered patients require extensive diabetes self-management education and support to achieve the glycemic goals of intensive diabetes treatment.

NEW INSULINS

After the introduction of insulin in 1922, management of T1D consisted of injections of regular insulin before main meals and an additional injection in the middle of the night; however, after intermediate-acting and long-acting insulins were developed, most patients were treated with only 1 or 2 injections daily. In 1993, the Diabetes Control and Complications Trial (DCCT) showed that maintenance of near-normal glycemia with intensive diabetes therapy reduces the risk of microvascular complications[3] and was the major impetus to develop better insulins, insulin-delivery systems, and insulin-replacement strategies that enable patients to more closely mimic physiologic insulin secretion.

Basal-bolus regimens with multiple daily insulin injections (MDI) or continuous subcutaneous (SC) insulin infusion (CSII, insulin pump), referred to as intensive insulin therapy, aim to mimic normal insulin production, which has 2 principal components: (1) basal insulin secretion suppresses lipolysis and balances hepatic glucose production with glucose utilization, and (2) prandial insulin secretion inhibits hepatic glucose production and stimulates glucose disposal after eating. The ability to simulate endogenous insulin production via SC insulin administration is limited by 2 factors: (1) inability to precisely reproduce the 2 distinct phases of prandial insulin release (a rapid first-phase followed by a more prolonged second-phase), and (2) insulin delivery into the systemic and not into the portal circulation.[4]

In the 1980s, human regular (soluble) insulin produced by recombinant DNA technology was introduced into clinical practice and rapidly replaced animal source insulins. Regular insulin is a short-acting prandial insulin, but its rate of entry into the circulation is too slow to match the absorption of glucose, and it remains in the circulation between meals, imparting a substantial basal component (**Table 1**). This mismatch leads to postprandial hyperglycemia unless injected at least 30 to

Table 1
Pharmacodynamic profiles and retail prices of commonly used insulins

Insulin	Onset of Action	Peak Action	Effective Duration	Retail Price per 10 mL Vial US$[a]
Regular (soluble)	30–60 min	2–3 h	5–8 h	121–125
Lispro[b]	5–15 min	30–90 min	4–6 h	221
Aspart[b]	10–20 min	60–180 min	3–5 h	232
Glulisine	5–15 min	30–90 min	4–6 h	191
NPH or isophane	2–4 h	4–10 h	12–16 h	121–124
Glargine	2–4 h	No peak	20–24 h	278
Detemir	2–3 h	No peak	16–24 h	279

Abbreviation: NPH, neutral protamine Hagedorn.

[a] Source: http://www.goodrx.com/ (accessed July 13, 2014); estimated retail cash price of commonly used insulins at a major national pharmacy chain operating in the vicinity of the authors' institution. Also available as 3-mL (300-unit) cartridges for use in nondisposable insulin pens and as 3-mL (300-unit) prefilled disposable pens. Cost per unit of rapid-acting analogue in prefilled disposable pens is approximately 25% more than vials, whereas the cost per unit of long-acting analogues in prefilled disposable pens is approximately 5%–8% less than vials.

[b] According to manufacturers' data; equivalent pharmacodynamic effects.[20] Serum insulin profiles are usually based on an SC injection of 0.1 to 0.2 unit per kilogram of body weight; large variations may be observed within and between individuals, and smaller doses typically have a shorter duration of effect.

60 minutes before a meal and increases the risk of hypoglycemia between meals unless snacks are consumed.

Neutral protamine Hagedorn (NPH) or isophane insulin is a suspension that had been widely used to provide the basal component of insulin regimens. Its inconsistent absorption and action profile results in highly variable intraindividual and interindividual pharmacodynamic effects (see **Table 1**)[5] requiring patients to eat snacks between meals to prevent hypoglycemia. When given before dinner or at bedtime, NPH has an unphysiological and undesirable peak action overnight that is associated with a considerable risk of nocturnal hypoglycemia.[6] Because of these characteristics of regular and NPH insulins, the timing and content of meals and snacks must be consistent from day-to-day, and it is challenging to meticulously balance insulin replacement with diet and exercise and achieve optimal glycemic targets without postprandial hyperglycemia, interprandial hypoglycemia, and excessive weight gain in patients with severe insulin deficiency. Insulin analogues were developed in an attempt to overcome these limitations of human regular and NPH insulins and afford patients greater lifestyle flexibility.[7]

The first rapid-acting analogue (RAA), insulin lispro, was introduced in the mid-1990s, and subsequently 2 additional RAAs (insulin aspart and insulin glulisine) and 3 long-acting analogues (LAAs), insulin glargine, insulin detemir, and insulin degludec, have entered the clinical arena as alternatives to regular and NPH insulin, respectively (see **Table 1**).[4] Insulin degludec is still in clinical trials in pediatrics and is not discussed further.

Despite their considerably greater cost (see **Table 1**), worldwide use of insulin analogues has increased enormously,[8] and analogues are the first and virtually the only choice for treatment of T1D in children and adolescents in many pediatric diabetes centers. Data from the T1D Exchange Clinic registry indicate that 98.6% of the 9919 participants younger than 18 years are exclusively using insulin analogues (T. Riddelsworth, PhD, written communication, 2014). A frequently asked question is: "Do their putative benefits justify their higher cost?"

RAPID-ACTING ANALOGUES

Compared with regular insulin, RAAs exist as monomers that are rapidly absorbed from SC tissue, resulting in a faster onset and shorter duration of action and, unlike regular insulin, their time to peak action is independent of dose.[4,9–11] Intraindividual and interindividual absorption of RAAs are also less variable than regular insulin.[12] For these reasons, they have been recommended as first-line prandial or bolus insulins. RAAs should be administered approximately 15 to 20 minutes before meals to match glucose absorption and limit postprandial glucose excursions.[13,14] This is a major practical advantage compared with regular insulin, which should be injected at least 30 minutes before a meal.[15,16]

In special circumstances (eg, very young children, sick day management, gastroparesis), RAAs may be administered after eating to safely manage unpredictable food intake and absorption.[13,17,18] It is important to note, however, that a bolus of RAA injected either with a syringe or an insulin pump approximately 15 to 20 minutes before starting a meal results in considerably better postprandial glucose control than when the insulin bolus is given immediately before or 20 minutes after meal initiation.[19]

Although the RAAs are modified human insulins with different chemical properties, their pharmacodynamic profiles (see **Table 1**) are not significantly different.[20–22] In children and adolescents with T1D using a basal-bolus regimen (with glargine or NPH), insulin glulisine is comparable to insulin aspart both in terms of efficacy and safety[23]; and an industry-sponsored study comparing insulin aspart with insulin lispro (both delivered with a pump) showed comparable glycemic efficacy and frequency of hypoglycemia.[24]

Although short-term studies show that they reduce postprandial glucose excursions, several meta-analyses show no significant difference in glycemic control as measured by HbA1c when RAAs are compared with regular insulin in children and adolescents (**Table 2**).[25–28] Furthermore, in an analysis of observational data representing "real life" collected over 12 years from 275 German and Austrian centers (37,206 children and adolescents 0–20 years) registered in the Diabetes Patienten Verlaufsdokumentation (DPV) database (corrected for age, center, and diabetes duration), HbA1c was statistically significantly lower in patients using regular insulin as compared with RAAs, 8.18% versus 8.32%, respectively.[8]

Compared with regular insulin, RAAs in combination with either NPH or ultralente as the basal insulin are associated with a significant reduction (3.1% vs 4.4%) in the occurrence of severe hypoglycemia in adults,[29] including patients with a history of recurrent severe hypoglycemia.[30] However, no such difference in the frequency of severe hypoglycemia has been shown in children or adolescents.[25–27] Insulin lispro in combination with NPH has been associated with a decreased frequency of symptomatic or biochemical hypoglycemia and nocturnal hypoglycemia in adolescents,[31] but not in prepubertal children. Furthermore, in a 26-week study of preschool children, comparing basal-bolus MDI therapy with mealtime insulin aspart or human regular insulin (both with basal NPH insulin), or CSII with insulin aspart, metabolic control parameters remained unchanged and equivalent (see **Table 2**).[32]

In open-label studies in adults, RAAs have been associated with modest improvements in quality of life (QOL) attributable to the convenience of more flexible regimens and the shorter interval between insulin administration and food consumption[25,33]; however, a randomized controlled trial (RCT) in adults with T1D did not show a significant improvement in QOL with RAAs.[34] There are no comparable QOL data for children and adolescents. Nonetheless, treatment flexibility related to convenience with respect to the timing of administration is an important consideration that should not be underestimated.

Table 2
Meta-analyses of randomized controlled trials examining the effect of insulin analogues on HbA1c and hypoglycemia in children and adolescents with type 1 diabetes mellitus

	Study	HbA1c	Frequency of hypoglycemia		Quality of life
			Severe	Nocturnal	
Rapid-acting analogues	Plank et al[25]	No difference	a	—	No data
	Siebenhofer et al[26]	No difference	No difference	No difference to decreased[b,c]	
	Singh et al[27]	No difference	No difference	No difference[c], decreased[b,d]	
	WHO[28]	No difference	No difference	Decreased[b,d]	
Long-acting analogues	Singh et al[27]	No difference	No difference	No difference[e], decreased[f]	No data
	WHO[28]	No difference	No difference	No difference[e], decreased[f]	

Comparisons are between rapid-acting insulin analogues (insulin lispro and insulin aspart) and regular human insulin and between long-acting analogues (insulin glargine and insulin detemir) and neutral protamine Hagedorn.

Statistically significant advantages associated with analogues are generally less than clinically important minimal differences, and advantages with respect to hypoglycemia are not consistent across comparisons.

[a] The overall rate of hypoglycemic episodes per patient per month did not differ significantly in prepubertal children. In adolescents, the event rate of overall hypoglycemia per patient per month was significantly reduced with insulin analogue.[25]

[b] Insulin lispro.

[c] Insulin aspart.

[d] Adolescents but not children.

[e] Insulin glargine.

[f] Insulin detemir.

LONG-ACTING INSULINS

In contrast to NPH, the LAAs are relatively peakless and have more reproducible pharmacodynamic profiles.[35,36] Although dose-dependent, their duration of action is longer than that of NPH, and in some patients once-daily administration can achieve satisfactory 24-hour basal coverage. The duration of action of insulin detemir is shorter than that of glargine (see **Table 1**),[37] and many patients with severe insulin deficiency require 2 injections of detemir daily to provide stable 24-hour basal coverage. One industry-sponsored study has shown that insulin detemir has a more reproducible pharmacokinetic profile (less variable absorption) than glargine in children and adolescents with T1D.[38]

Some observational studies have reported HbA1c improvements of 0.5% to 1.0% with LAAs compared with NPH,[39–41] whereas others have shown no significant difference.[42–46] Meta-analyses show that LAAs are associated with modest (~0.1%) or no reduction in HbA1c when compared with NPH insulin (see **Table 2**).[27,28] In the large observational DPV database, HbA1c was significantly lower, 8.09% versus 8.4%, in patients treated with NPH compared with LAAs, respectively.[8]

LAAs do not reduce the risk of severe hypoglycemia in children and adolescents, but insulin detemir, in particular, is associated with decreased occurrence of nocturnal hypoglycemia (and less weight gain).[27,28,47] A recent multinational RCT again showed that HbA1c levels were similar in preschool-age children and in older children and adolescents when insulin detemir, as compared with NPH (both in combination with mealtime insulin aspart), was used for basal-bolus treatment. However, there was less weight gain and a lower risk of hypoglycemia with insulin detemir, attributed to its peakless and more consistent pharmacologic profile.[48,49]

Insulin glargine may cause a sensation of stinging or pain at the injection site. Careful analyses have concluded that glargine is safe, and concerns about its mitogenic and carcinogenic potential are unfounded.[50]

Cost-effectiveness analyses performed in adults show widely varying incremental cost-effectiveness ratios; however, no such analyses have been specifically performed in pediatric T1D.[28]

CONTINUOUS SUBCUTANEOUS INSULIN INFUSION

CSII, or insulin pump therapy, was introduced to treat T1D in the late 1970s and became widely used in pediatric practice only after publication of the DCCT results in 1993.[51] In 1996, fewer than 5% of patients who started CSII were younger than 20 years. Over the intervening years, there has been a dramatic increase in the number of children and adolescents using pump therapy[52]; in the Type 1 Diabetes Exchange, representing 67 clinics in the United States, 55% of 13,316 participants younger than 20 years with T1D for more than 1 year were using an insulin pump.[1] Successful use of CSII requires patients and families to receive intensive self-management education and ongoing support from an experienced diabetes team.

CSII mimics the normal pattern of insulin secretion, providing a continuous basal insulin infusion with superimposed boluses for food or correction of hyperglycemia. A major advantage of CSII is the ability to program changes in basal rates (eg, increase the basal rate from 4 AM to 9 AM to combat the dawn phenomenon or, conversely, decrease the infusion rate or temporarily suspend insulin infusion for physical exercise). In addition, pumps precisely calculate bolus doses and provide the option to extend bolus delivery over a variable time period to account for delayed digestion and nutrient absorption (eg, a meal such as pizza rich in protein and fat). **Table 3** details the technological features of insulin pumps.

Table 3
Technological features of insulin pumps

Insulin delivery	• Low basal rates (0.025–0.05 units/h) • Multiple different basal rates • Temporary basal rates and basal suspension • Small bolus increments (0.025–0.10 units) • Extended boluses for delayed digestion • Bolus calculator (based on BG level and carbohydrate quantity) • Multiple insulin: carbohydrate ratios, sensitivity factors, BG targets • Missed meal bolus reminder
Safety features	• Alarms for occlusion and low insulin reservoir • Active insulin calculation (prevents insulin stacking) • Keypad lock (useful for toddlers) • Waterproof or watertight
Interface with BG monitoring	• Electronic logbook software • Reminder alarms for BG checks, bolus doses • Wireless communication with remote BG meter • Integration with continuous glucose monitoring technology

Abbreviation: BG, blood glucose.

Adapted from Mehta SN, Wolfsdorf JI. Contemporary management of patients with type 1 diabetes. Endocrinol Metab Clin North Am 2010;39(3):584; with permission.

Insulin pump systems include the pump itself, a disposable reservoir for insulin, and an infusion set (consisting of a tube that connects the reservoir with a cannula inserted into the SC tissue). A disposable, tubeless patch pump also has been approved for use in children. Infusion sets and patch pumps are changed every 2 to 3 days. The average list price of an insulin pump is approximately $6500 for individuals without insurance and a typical warranty lasts approximately 4 years. The actual price varies depending on the brand and unique features of the pump. Related pump supplies typically cost approximately $1500 to $2000 per year. The patch pump has a lower initial cost, but a comparable total cost over the course of the warranty period.

Impact of Continuous Subcutaneous Insulin Infusion on Glycemic Control

Multiple pediatric studies have reported decreases in HbA1c with CSII; however, many of these studies are limited by small sample sizes, observational or retrospective design, short duration, or lack of control groups. A meta-analysis of observational and interventional pediatric and adult studies showed a 0.6% improvement in HbA1c with CSII compared with MDI therapy.[53] A systematic review and meta-analysis of 6 short-term RCTs comparing CSII with MDI exclusively in children (165 participants) showed a statistically significant reduction in HbA1c with CSII (–0.24%), and there were no differences in the incidence of diabetic ketoacidosis (DKA) or severe hypoglycemia events.[54] A recent prospective 7-year follow-up study of 345 pediatric patients using CSII in Australia showed that mean HbA1c was 0.6% lower in the pump cohort compared with controls (matched for age, duration of diabetes, and baseline HbA1c) who injected insulin.[55]

Impact of Continuous Subcutaneous Insulin Infusion on the Frequency of Acute Complications

Because RAAs are typically used in CSII, any interruption in basal insulin delivery rapidly leads to metabolic decompensation. To reduce this risk, BG levels must be measured at least 4 to 6 times daily. Early observational studies suggested an increased risk of DKA in pediatric patients using CSII[56]; however, in the recent aforementioned prospective Australian analysis, the rate of hospitalization for DKA was 50% lower (2.3 vs 4.7 per 100 patient-years).[55] The decreased rate of DKA is probably a result of focused patient education and greater patient and family awareness of the consequences of interrupted insulin delivery with CSII.

RCTs in adults have shown decreased rates of severe hypoglycemia with CSII compared with MDI,[57] but pediatric data are inconsistent. Pediatric observational studies have shown a decrease in the rate of severe hypoglycemia in patients using CSII[55,58]; however, the short-term pediatric RCT data in children have not shown significant differences in the occurrence of severe hypoglycemia between CSII and MDI (see Ref.[52] for a detailed review), which may be attributable to the infrequency of severe hypoglycemia events and the lack of statistical power of small studies.

Impact of Continuous Subcutaneous Insulin Infusion on Quality of Life

Studies examining the psychosocial impact of CSII in children and adolescents have shown conflicting results. Several studies have documented improvement in children's QOL or decreased parental anxiety with use of CSII.[59–61] A recent German prospective multicenter study reported significantly increased QOL scores in preschool, school-age, and adolescent patients with T1D after using CSII for 6 months.[62] Other studies, however, have shown no difference in QOL after initiating CSII.[63,64] Inconsistent results and conclusions among these QOL studies may be ascribed to differences in methods and survey instruments in the various studies, as well as age differences in the samples. Methods using qualitative analysis or open-ended questions may yield different results; for instance, describing their experiences in qualitative interviews, parents of young children with T1D reported that switching from MDI to CSII offered more freedom, flexibility around mealtimes, and spontaneity in their lives, as well as decreased worry.[65] It is also noteworthy that the reported rates of discontinuation of pump therapy is low, ranging from 11%[66] and 18%[67] in single-clinic reports to 4% (463 of 11,710) in the large multicenter DPV database in Germany and Austria.[68] These observations have been interpreted as suggesting that pump therapy improves patient satisfaction and quality life.

A systematic review and economic evaluation published in 2010 concluded that based on the totality of evidence, using observational studies to supplement the limited data from RCTs comparing CSII with optimal MDI in T1D, CSII provides some advantages over MDI (**Box 1**). The benefits were estimated to come at an extra cost of approximately £1700 (or approximately US$3000) per annum.[69]

CONTINUOUS MONITORING SYSTEMS AND CLOSED-LOOP THERAPY
Continuous Glucose Monitoring Systems

Real-time CGM devices measure glucose in the interstitial fluid every 5 minutes for up to 7 days via a short, thin subcutaneous probe (glucose sensor). There is a several-minute lag between plasma and interstitial glucose concentrations. SMBG values are still needed to calibrate CGM devices and to confirm glucose levels before an insulin bolus is administered or to confirm hypoglycemia before treatment. At this time, CGM devices cannot substitute for SMBG, but are valuable in providing detailed information on BG trends in the intervals between SMBG values, especially after meals and overnight.[70,71]

A number of recent studies have assessed the impact of CGM on glycemic control in T1D.[72] In the Juvenile Diabetes Research Foundation (JDRF)-sponsored study of CGM, an RCT comparing CGM with conventional SMBG in T1D subjects 8 years or older, adults who used CGM had a greater reduction in HbA1c with no increase in hypoglycemia. Although a clear benefit was not seen in the overall pediatric cohort (likely because of less frequent CGM use), more children (8–14 years) using CGM achieved a statistically significant HbA1c reduction compared with those using SMBG alone.

Box 1
Potential advantages of continuous subcutaneous insulin infusion compared with multiple daily injections

- Better blood glucose control as reflected by hemoglobin A1c
- Reduced glycemic variability
- Ability to combat dawn phenomenon
- Ability to decrease or suspend insulin infusion for physical exercise
- Reduced hypoglycemia
- Improved quality of life
  - Reduced fear of hypoglycemia
  - Greater lifestyle flexibility
- Benefits for parents
- Lower total daily insulin dose

Note that this result was not observed in adolescents older than 14 years.[73] In another RCT (the Sensor-Augmented Pump Therapy for A1C Reduction 3 [STAR3] study), sensor-augmented insulin pump (SAP) therapy showed significant improvement in HbA1c levels in both adults and children (7–18 years) compared with a regimen of MDI and conventional SMBG; again, children were more likely to reach HbA1c targets than adolescents.[74] In both of these trials, despite perceived value on the part of patients and parents, the frequency of CGM use decreased during the study period. Other studies also have shown that near-daily CGM use improves HbA1c levels.[75,76] The data are less clear on the value of CGM alone in reducing the frequency of hypoglycemia in children and adolescents. In the JDRF and STAR3 trials described previously,[73,74] rates of severe hypoglycemia were low and did not differ between CGM and non-CGM pediatric groups; however, these analyses were limited by very small numbers of severe hypoglycemia events.

In the STAR3 study, QOL analyses showed no significant differences in overall health-related QOL between SAP and MDI arms. However, caregivers in the SAP group had significantly improved scores on a survey measuring maladaptive behaviors around hypoglycemia prevention (eg, overtreating hypoglycemia or inappropriately reducing insulin delivery). In addition, key treatment satisfaction measures improved more in the SAP group.[77]

It is noteworthy that despite the potential benefits of CGM, most pediatric patients with T1D are not using this technology. In a recent analysis of 17,317 patients younger than 26 years in the Type 1 Diabetes Exchange, 6% of children younger than 13 years, 4% of adolescents 13 to younger than 18 years, and 6% of young adults 18 to younger than 26 years had used CGM during the previous 30 days.[78] Patients and families report barriers to CGM use, including insertion pain, alarm fatigue, accuracy issues, and skin irritation. Another major drawback is cost; in addition to the cost of the consumables (sensors and transmitters), the cost of a CGM receiver itself is typically $1000 or more. Health insurance plan coverage of CGM systems is variable.

Overcoming the barriers that prevent use of CGM data in daily T1D management is challenging. Irrespective of cost considerations, improvement in CGM devices and strategies for patient and family support are needed to increase the acceptability of CGM devices for long-term use in more youth with T1D.

Sensor-Augmented Pump Therapy with Low Glucose Insulin Suspension

New insulin pump systems offer automatic suspension of insulin delivery for up to 2 hours when a preset CGM glucose threshold is reached. This is an important advance toward automation of insulin delivery in patients with T1D,[79] and studies have demonstrated a reduction in severe hypoglycemia and nocturnal hypoglycemia.[80–83] In a recent 6-month RCT comparing insulin pumps only and automated insulin suspension in 95 children and adults with impaired hypoglycemia awareness, the combined rate of severe and moderate hypoglycemia was significantly reduced in subjects using automated insulin suspension (adjusted incidence rate 9.5 vs 34.2 per 100 patient-months).[81] In an RCT of 45 patients with T1D ages 15 to 45 years studied in their homes, a predictive algorithm was used to suspend insulin delivery before hypoglycemia occurred. Participants had significantly fewer nights (21% vs 33%) with at least 1 sensor value of 60 mg/dL or lower on intervention (predictive algorithm) nights compared with control nights, without an associated risk of morning ketosis.[83]

Closed-Loop Insulin-Delivery Systems

Closed-loop systems, also referred to as an "artificial pancreas," feature continuous glucose sensing and automated insulin delivery with minimal patient intervention. Early studies of closed-loop systems have shown great promise. In an RCT in adults, over-night closed-loop insulin delivery improved glucose control and reduced hypoglyce-mia, even after a large carbohydrate meal with alcohol.[84] In a multinational trial comparing a closed-loop system with SAP therapy in children ages 10 to 18 years at a diabetes camp, subjects using closed-loop had better overnight glycemic control with less nocturnal hypoglycemia.[85] Likewise, even in children younger than 7 years, closed-loop insulin delivery in a hospital study decreased the severity of overnight hyperglycemia without increasing hypoglycemia.[86] Finally, recent trials show near-normal glucose levels in adults with T1D using a bihormonal (insulin and glucagon) closed-loop system.[87,88] This system was recently also evaluated in adolescents (12–21 years) in a summer camp crossover study. In the adolescent population, comparing a 5-day closed-loop period to a control period, the mean plasma glucose was lower, 138 versus 157 mg/dL, but the percentage of time with a low plasma glucose reading was similar during the 2 periods.[89] In sum, closed-loop systems improve the safety and efficacy of insulin therapy. Additional studies are in progress to refine closed-loop algorithms and further evaluate their performance in pediatric patients in the home setting.

SUMMARY

Several prospective observational studies show that over the past 2 decades, HbA1c levels have significantly improved and, equally important, rates of severe hypoglyce-mia have simultaneously decreased in pediatric T1D.[90–94] Moreover, rates of micro-vascular complications have improved over this period.[95,96] It is noteworthy, however, that in a study of more than 30,000 children and adolescents with T1D, pub-lished in 2012, the average HbA1c level was not different between treatment regi-mens, suggesting that the improvement in HbA1c cannot be completely explained by changes in the mode of insulin treatment per se (ie, increased use of MDI and CSII).[91] It seems likely that improved health outcomes are largely attributable to widespread adoption and implementation of the principles of intensive diabetes man-agement, including multidisciplinary team care, intensive patient education and self-management training, establishment of treatment goals, and more frequent SMBG to guide optimal insulin-dose selection.[97] A critical review of the empiric data suggests that use of more physiologic insulin-replacement regimens with MDI and pumps, increased use of insulin analogues, and, most recently, use of CGM have contributed only modesty to lower HbA1c levels.

It is appropriate to ask why diabetes care providers so enthusiastically embrace new and expensive technologies when the "real-life" advantage of each is relatively small. The answer to this question is complex. One possible explanation includes the impact of marketing on health care providers and directly to patients and the influ-ence of thought leaders (investigators) who conduct clinical trials under ideal condi-tions on selected, motivated patients. In addition, although QOL analyses in pediatric patients with T1D using pumps and CGM have yielded inconsistent results, providers may receive positive feedback from patients and families regarding "lifestyle" benefits of these technologies that serves to reinforce their prescribing pat-terns. However, many pediatric diabetes clinics do not have sufficient personnel resources required to optimally educate and train patients and families in intensive diabetes management using pumps and CGM, which requires a considerable and ongoing investment of time in patient education and support.

Looking ahead, the pace of current research suggests that within the next several years, "artificial pancreas" systems may become available that will reduce the burden of care and enable children with T1D to maintain near-normal glycemia, especially overnight, with minimal risk of severe hypoglycemia. Meanwhile, as Skinner and Cameron have eloquently stated, it is important not to allow pharmacologic and technological considerations to subvert the critically important elements of comprehensive pediatric diabetes care, which include setting appropriate individualized treatment goals, a cohesive multidisciplinary diabetes team that shares a common philosophy of care, and psychosocial support.[98]

REFERENCES

1. Wood JR, Miller KM, Maahs DM, et al. Most youth with type 1 diabetes in the T1D Exchange Clinic Registry do not meet American Diabetes Association or International Society for Pediatric and Adolescent Diabetes clinical guidelines. Diabetes Care 2013;36(7):2035–7.
2. Campbell MS, Schatz DA, Chen V, et al. A contrast between children and adolescents with excellent and poor control: the T1D Exchange clinic registry experience. Pediatr Diabetes 2014;15(2):110–7.
3. The effect of intensive treatment of diabetes on the development and progression of long-term complications in insulin-dependent diabetes mellitus. The Diabetes Control and Complications Trial Research Group. N Engl J Med 1993;329(14):977–86.
4. Hirsch IB. Insulin analogues. N Engl J Med 2005;352(2):174–83.
5. Binder C, Lauritzen T, Faber O, et al. Insulin pharmacokinetics. Diabetes Care 1984;7(2):188–99.
6. Fanelli CG, Pampanelli S, Porcellati F, et al. Administration of neutral protamine Hagedorn insulin at bedtime versus with dinner in type 1 diabetes mellitus to avoid nocturnal hypoglycemia and improve control. A randomized, controlled trial. Ann Intern Med 2002;136(7):504–14.
7. Holt RI. Insulin analogues: a step forward in the care in diabetes. Diabetes Obes Metab 2009;11(1):1–4.
8. Kapellen TM, Wolf J, Rosenbauer J, et al. Changes in the use of analogue insulins in 37 206 children and adolescents with type 1 diabetes in 275 German and Austrian centers during the last twelve years. Exp Clin Endocrinol Diabetes 2009;117(7):329–35.
9. Holleman F, Hoekstra J. Insulin lispro. N Engl J Med 1997;337:176–83.
10. Holmes G, Galitz L, Hu P, et al. Pharmacokinetics of insulin aspart in obesity, renal impairment, or hepatic impairment. Br J Clin Pharmacol 2005;60(5):469–76.
11. Becker RH, Frick AD. Clinical pharmacokinetics and pharmacodynamics of insulin glulisine. Clin Pharmacokinet 2008;47(1):7–20.
12. Howey DC, Bowsher RR, Brunelle RL, et al. [Lys(B28), Pro(B29)]-human insulin. A rapidly absorbed analogue of human insulin. Diabetes 1994;43(3):396–402.
13. Danne T, Aman J, Schober E, et al. A comparison of postprandial and preprandial administration of insulin aspart in children and adolescents with type 1 diabetes. Diabetes Care 2003;26(8):2359–64.
14. Swan KL, Weinzimer SA, Dziura JD, et al. Effect of puberty on the pharmacodynamic and pharmacokinetic properties of insulin pump therapy in youth with type 1 diabetes. Diabetes Care 2008;31(1):44–6.
15. Dimitriadis GD, Gerich JE. Importance of timing of preprandial subcutaneous insulin administration in the management of diabetes mellitus. Diabetes Care 1983;6(4):374–7.
16. Lean ME, Ng LL, Tennison BR. Interval between insulin injection and eating in relation to blood glucose control in adult diabetics. Br Med J (Clin Res Ed) 1985;290(6462):105–8.

17. Deeb LC, Holcombe JH, Brunelle R, et al. Insulin lispro lowers postprandial glucose in prepubertal children with diabetes. Pediatrics 2001;108(5):1175–9.
18. Rutledge KS, Chase HP, Klingensmith GJ, et al. Effectiveness of postprandial Humalog in toddlers with diabetes. Pediatrics 1997;100(6):968–72.
19. Cobry E, McFann K, Messer L, et al. Timing of meal insulin boluses to achieve optimal postprandial glycemic control in patients with type 1 diabetes. Diabetes Technol Ther 2010;12(3):173–7.
20. Plank J, Wutte A, Brunner G, et al. A direct comparison of insulin aspart and insulin lispro in patients with type 1 diabetes. Diabetes Care 2002;25(11):2053–7.
21. Cemeroglu AP, Kleis L, Wood A, et al. Comparison of the effect of insulin glulisine to insulin aspart on breakfast postprandial blood glucose levels in children with type 1 diabetes mellitus on multiple daily injections. Endocr Pract 2013;19(4): 614–9.
22. Heise T, Nosek L, Spitzer H, et al. Insulin glulisine: a faster onset of action compared with insulin lispro. Diabetes Obes Metab 2007;9(5):746–53.
23. Philotheou A, Arslanian S, Blatniczky L, et al. Comparable efficacy and safety of insulin glulisine and insulin lispro when given as part of a basal-bolus insulin regimen in a 26-week trial in pediatric patients with type 1 diabetes. Diabetes Technol Ther 2011;13(3):327–34.
24. Weinzimer SA, Ternand C, Howard C, et al. A randomized trial comparing continuous subcutaneous insulin infusion of insulin aspart versus insulin lispro in children and adolescents with type 1 diabetes. Diabetes Care 2008;31(2):210–5.
25. Plank J, Siebenhofer A, Berghold A, et al. Systematic review and meta-analysis of short-acting insulin analogues in patients with diabetes mellitus. Arch Intern Med 2005;165(12):1337–44.
26. Siebenhofer A, Plank J, Berghold A, et al. Short acting insulin analogues versus regular human insulin in patients with diabetes mellitus. Cochrane Database Syst Rev 2006;(2):CD003287.
27. Singh SR, Ahmad F, Lal A, et al. Efficacy and safety of insulin analogues for the management of diabetes mellitus: a meta-analysis. CMAJ 2009;180(4):385–97.
28. World Health Organization. Review of the evidence comparing insulin (human or animal) with analogue insulins. 2011. Available at: http://www.who.int/selection_medicines/committees/expert/18/applications/Insulin_review.pdf?ua=1. Accessed June 27, 2014.
29. Brunelle BL, Llewelyn J, Anderson JH Jr, et al. Meta-analysis of the effect of insulin lispro on severe hypoglycemia in patients with type 1 diabetes. Diabetes Care 1998;21(10):1726–31.
30. Pedersen-Bjergaard U, Kristensen PL, Beck-Nielsen H, et al. Effect of insulin analogues on risk of severe hypoglycaemia in patients with type 1 diabetes prone to recurrent severe hypoglycaemia (HypoAna trial): a prospective, randomised, open-label, blinded-endpoint crossover trial. Lancet Diabetes Endocrinol 2014; 2(7):553–61.
31. Holcombe JH, Zalani S, Arora VK, et al. Comparison of insulin lispro with regular human insulin for the treatment of type 1 diabetes in adolescents. Clin Ther 2002; 24(4):629–38.
32. Pankowska E, Nazim J, Szalecki M, et al. Equal metabolic control but superior caregiver treatment satisfaction with insulin aspart in preschool children. Diabetes Technol Ther 2010;12(5):413–8.
33. Rachmiel M, Perlman K, Daneman D. Insulin analogues in children and teens with type 1 diabetes: advantages and caveats. Pediatr Clin North Am 2005;52(6): 1651–75.

34. Gale EA. A randomized, controlled trial comparing insulin lispro with human soluble insulin in patients with Type 1 diabetes on intensified insulin therapy. The UK Trial Group. Diabet Med 2000;17(3):209–14.
35. Heise T, Nosek L, Ronn BB, et al. Lower within-subject variability of insulin detemir in comparison to NPH insulin and insulin glargine in people with type 1 diabetes. Diabetes 2004;53(6):1614–20.
36. Lepore M, Pampanelli S, Fanelli C, et al. Pharmacokinetics and pharmacodynamics of subcutaneous injection of long-acting human insulin analog glargine, NPH insulin, and ultralente human insulin and continuous subcutaneous infusion of insulin lispro. Diabetes 2000;49(12):2142–8.
37. Porcellati F, Rossetti P, Busciantella NR, et al. Comparison of pharmacokinetics and dynamics of the long-acting insulin analogs glargine and detemir at steady state in type 1 diabetes: a double-blind, randomized, crossover study. Diabetes Care 2007;30(10):2447–52.
38. Danne T, Datz N, Endahl L, et al. Insulin detemir is characterized by a more reproducible pharmacokinetic profile than insulin glargine in children and adolescents with type 1 diabetes: results from a randomized, double-blind, controlled trial. Pediatr Diabetes 2008;9(6):554–60.
39. Hathout EH, Fujishige L, Geach J, et al. Effect of therapy with insulin glargine (lantus) on glycemic control in toddlers, children, and adolescents with diabetes. Diabetes Technol Ther 2003;5(5):801–6.
40. Colino E, Lopez-Capape M, Golmayo L, et al. Therapy with insulin glargine (Lantus) in toddlers, children and adolescents with type 1 diabetes. Diabetes Res Clin Pract 2005;70(1):1–7.
41. Jackson A, Ternand C, Brunzell C, et al. Insulin glargine improves hemoglobin A1c in children and adolescents with poorly controlled type 1 diabetes. Pediatr Diabetes 2003;4(2):64–9.
42. Schober E, Schoenle E, Van Dyk J, et al. Comparative trial between insulin glargine and NPH insulin in children and adolescents with type 1 diabetes. Diabetes Care 2001;24(11):2005–6.
43. Chase HP, Dixon B, Pearson J, et al. Reduced hypoglycemic episodes and improved glycemic control in children with type 1 diabetes using insulin glargine and neutral protamine Hagedorn insulin. J Pediatr 2003;143(6):737–40.
44. Tan CY, Wilson DM, Buckingham B. Initiation of insulin glargine in children and adolescents with type 1 diabetes. Pediatr Diabetes 2004;5(2):80–6.
45. Dixon B, Peter Chase H, Burdick J, et al. Use of insulin glargine in children under age 6 with type 1 diabetes. Pediatr Diabetes 2005;6(3):150–4.
46. Paivarinta M, Tapanainen P, Veijola R. Basal insulin switch from NPH to glargine in children and adolescents with type 1 diabetes. Pediatr Diabetes 2008;9(3 Pt 2): 83–90.
47. Robertson KJ, Schoenle E, Gucev Z, et al. Insulin detemir compared with NPH insulin in children and adolescents with Type 1 diabetes. Diabet Med 2007;24(1):27–34.
48. Thalange N, Bereket A, Larsen J, et al. Treatment with insulin detemir or NPH insulin in children aged 2-5 yr with type 1 diabetes mellitus. Pediatr Diabetes 2011; 12(7):632–41.
49. Thalange N, Bereket A, Larsen J, et al. Insulin analogues in children with Type 1 diabetes: a 52-week randomized clinical trial. Diabet Med 2013;30(2):216–25.
50. Garg SK, Hirsch IB, Skyler JS. Insulin glargine and cancer–an unsubstantiated allegation. Diabetes Technol Ther 2009;11(8):473–6.
51. Skyler JS. Continuous subcutaneous insulin infusion–an historical perspective. Diabetes Technol Ther 2010;12(Suppl 1):S5–9.

52. Phillip M, Battelino T, Rodriguez H, et al. Use of insulin pump therapy in the pediatric age-group: consensus statement from the European Society for Paediatric Endocrinology, the Lawson Wilkins Pediatric Endocrine Society, and the International Society for Pediatric and Adolescent Diabetes, endorsed by the American Diabetes Association and the European Association for the Study of Diabetes. Diabetes Care 2007;30(6):1653–62.

53. Pickup JC, Sutton AJ. Severe hypoglycaemia and glycaemic control in Type 1 diabetes: meta-analysis of multiple daily insulin injections compared with continuous subcutaneous insulin infusion. Diabet Med 2008;25(7):765–74.

54. Pankowska E, Blazik M, Dziechciarz P, et al. Continuous subcutaneous insulin infusion vs. multiple daily injections in children with type 1 diabetes: a systematic review and meta-analysis of randomized control trials. Pediatr Diabetes 2009;10(1):52–8.

55. Johnson SR, Cooper MN, Jones TW, et al. Long-term outcome of insulin pump therapy in children with type 1 diabetes assessed in a large population-based case-control study. Diabetologia 2013;56(11):2392–400.

56. Hanas R, Ludvigsson J. Hypoglycemia and ketoacidosis with insulin pump therapy in children and adolescents. Pediatr Diabetes 2006;7(Suppl 4):32–8.

57. Hoogma RP, Hammond PJ, Gomis R, et al. Comparison of the effects of continuous subcutaneous insulin infusion (CSII) and NPH-based multiple daily insulin injections (MDI) on glycaemic control and quality of life: results of the 5-nations trial. Diabet Med 2006;23(2):141–7.

58. Nimri R, Weintrob N, Benzaquen H, et al. Insulin pump therapy in youth with type 1 diabetes: a retrospective paired study. Pediatrics 2006;117(6):2126–31.

59. Streisand R, Swift E, Wickmark T, et al. Pediatric parenting stress among parents of children with type 1 diabetes: the role of self-efficacy, responsibility, and fear. J Pediatr Psychol 2005;30(6):513–21.

60. McMahon SK, Airey FL, Marangou DA, et al. Insulin pump therapy in children and adolescents: improvements in key parameters of diabetes management including quality of life. Diabet Med 2005;22(1):92–6.

61. Weinzimer SA, Ahern JH, Doyle EA, et al. Persistence of benefits of continuous subcutaneous insulin infusion in very young children with type 1 diabetes: a follow-up report. Pediatrics 2004;114(6):1601–5.

62. Muller-Godeffroy E, Treichel S, Wagner VM. German Working Group for Paediatric Pump Therapy Investigation of quality of life and family burden issues during insulin pump therapy in children with Type 1 diabetes mellitus–a large-scale multicentre pilot study. Diabet Med 2009;26(5):493–501.

63. Valenzuela JM, Patino AM, McCullough J, et al. Insulin pump therapy and health-related quality of life in children and adolescents with type 1 diabetes. J Pediatr Psychol 2006;31(6):650–60.

64. Weissberg-Benchell J, Antisdel-Lomaglio J, Seshadri R. Insulin Pump Therapy: a meta-analysis. Diabetes Care 2003;26(4):1079–87.

65. Sullivan-Bolyai S, Deatrick J, Gruppuso P, et al. Mothers' experiences raising young children with type 1 diabetes. J Spec Pediatr Nurs 2002;7(3):93–103.

66. de Vries L, Grushka Y, Lebenthal Y, et al. Factors associated with increased risk of insulin pump discontinuation in pediatric patients with type 1 diabetes. Pediatr Diabetes 2011;12(5):506–12.

67. Wood JR, Moreland EC, Volkening LK, et al. Durability of insulin pump use in pediatric patients with type 1 diabetes. Diabetes Care 2006;29(11):2355–60.

68. Hofer SE, Heidtmann B, Raile K, et al. Discontinuation of insulin pump treatment in children, adolescents, and young adults. A multicenter analysis based on the DPV database in Germany and Austria. Pediatr Diabetes 2010;11(2):116–21.

69. Cummins E, Royle P, Snaith A, et al. Clinical effectiveness and cost-effectiveness of continuous subcutaneous insulin infusion for diabetes: systematic review and economic evaluation. Health Technol Assess 2010;14(11):iii–iv, xi–xvi, 1–181.
70. Blevins TC, Bode BW, Garg SK, et al. Statement by the American Association of Clinical Endocrinologists Consensus Panel on continuous glucose monitoring. Endocr Pract 2010;16(5):730–45.
71. Phillip M, Danne T, Shalitin S, et al. Use of continuous glucose monitoring in children and adolescents. Pediatr Diabetes 2012;13(3):215–28.
72. Pickup JC, Freeman SC, Sutton AJ. Glycaemic control in type 1 diabetes during real time continuous glucose monitoring compared with self monitoring of blood glucose: meta-analysis of randomised controlled trials using individual patient data. BMJ 2011;343:d3805.
73. Tamborlane WV, Beck RW, Bode BW, et al. Continuous glucose monitoring and intensive treatment of type 1 diabetes. N Engl J Med 2008;359(14):1464–76.
74. Bergenstal RM, Tamborlane WV, Ahmann A, et al. Effectiveness of sensor-augmented insulin-pump therapy in type 1 diabetes. N Engl J Med 2010;363(4):311–20.
75. Kordonouri O, Pankowska E, Rami B, et al. Sensor-augmented pump therapy from the diagnosis of childhood type 1 diabetes: results of the Paediatric Onset Study (ONSET) after 12 months of treatment. Diabetologia 2010;53(12):2487–95.
76. Beck RW, Buckingham B, Miller K, et al. Factors predictive of use and of benefit from continuous glucose monitoring in type 1 diabetes. Diabetes Care 2009;32(11):1947–53.
77. Rubin RR, Peyrot M, Group SS. Health-related quality of life and treatment satisfaction in the Sensor-Augmented Pump Therapy for A1C Reduction 3 (STAR 3) trial. Diabetes Technol Ther 2012;14(2):143–51.
78. Wong JC, Foster NC, Maahs DM, et al. Real-Time continuous glucose monitoring among participants in the T1D Exchange Clinic Registry. Diabetes Care 2014;37(10):2702–9.
79. Ly TT, Breton MD, Keith-Hynes P, et al. Overnight glucose control with an automated, unified safety system in children and adolescents with type 1 diabetes at diabetes camp. Diabetes Care 2014;37(8):2310–6.
80. Buckingham B, Chase HP, Dassau E, et al. Prevention of nocturnal hypoglycemia using predictive alarm algorithms and insulin pump suspension. Diabetes Care 2010;33(5):1013–7.
81. Bergenstal RM, Klonoff DC, Garg SK, et al. Threshold-based insulin-pump interruption for reduction of hypoglycemia. N Engl J Med 2013;369(3):224–32.
82. Ly TT, Nicholas JA, Retterath A, et al. Effect of sensor-augmented insulin pump therapy and automated insulin suspension vs standard insulin pump therapy on hypoglycemia in patients with type 1 diabetes: a randomized clinical trial. JAMA 2013;310(12):1240–7.
83. Maahs DM, Calhoun P, Buckingham BA, et al. A randomized trial of a home system to reduce nocturnal hypoglycemia in type 1 diabetes. Diabetes Care 2014;37(7):1885–91.
84. Hovorka R, Kumareswaran K, Harris J, et al. Overnight closed loop insulin delivery (artificial pancreas) in adults with type 1 diabetes: crossover randomised controlled studies. BMJ 2011;342:d1855.
85. Phillip M, Battelino T, Atlas E, et al. Nocturnal glucose control with an artificial pancreas at a diabetes camp. N Engl J Med 2013;368(9):824–33.
86. Dauber A, Corcia L, Safer J, et al. Closed-loop insulin therapy improves glycemic control in children aged <7 years: a randomized controlled trial. Diabetes Care 2013;36(2):222–7.

87. Russell SJ, El-Khatib FH, Nathan DM, et al. Blood glucose control in type 1 diabetes with a bihormonal bionic endocrine pancreas. Diabetes Care 2012;35(11): 2148–55.
88. Haidar A, Legault L, Dallaire M, et al. Glucose-responsive insulin and glucagon delivery (dual-hormone artificial pancreas) in adults with type 1 diabetes: a randomized crossover controlled trial. CMAJ 2013;185(4):297–305.
89. Russell SJ, El-Khatib FH, Sinha M, et al. Outpatient glycemic control with a bionic pancreas in type 1 diabetes. N Engl J Med 2014;371(4):313–25.
90. Dovc K, Telic SS, Lusa L, et al. Improved metabolic control in pediatric patients with type 1 diabetes: a nationwide prospective 12-year time trends analysis. Diabetes Technol Ther 2014;16(1):33–40.
91. Rosenbauer J, Dost A, Karges B, et al. Improved metabolic control in children and adolescents with type 1 diabetes: a trend analysis using prospective multicenter data from Germany and Austria. Diabetes Care 2012;35(1):80–6.
92. Margeirsdottir HD, Larsen JR, Kummernes SJ, et al. The establishment of a new national network leads to quality improvement in childhood diabetes: implementation of the ISPAD Guidelines. Pediatr Diabetes 2010;11(2):88–95.
93. Svensson J, Johannesen J, Mortensen HB, et al. Improved metabolic outcome in a Danish diabetic paediatric population aged 0-18 yr: results from a nationwide continuous registration. Pediatr Diabetes 2009;10(7):461–7.
94. O'Connell SM, Cooper MN, Bulsara MK, et al. Reducing rates of severe hypoglycemia in a population-based cohort of children and adolescents with type 1 diabetes over the decade 2000-2009. Diabetes Care 2011;34(11):2379–80.
95. Nordwall M, Bojestig M, Arnqvist HJ, et al. Declining incidence of severe retinopathy and persisting decrease of nephropathy in an unselected population of Type 1 diabetes—the Linkoping Diabetes Complications Study. Diabetologia 2004; 47(7):1266–72.
96. Downie E, Craig ME, Hing S, et al. Continued reduction in the prevalence of retinopathy in adolescents with type 1 diabetes: role of insulin therapy and glycemic control. Diabetes Care 2011;34(11):2368–73.
97. Wolfsdorf JI, editor. Intensive diabetes management. 5th edition. Alexandria (VA): American Diabetes Association; 2012.
98. Skinner TC, Cameron FJ. Improving glycaemic control in children and adolescents: which aspects of therapy really matter? Diabet Med 2010;27(4):369–75.

Long-term Outcomes in Youths with Diabetes Mellitus

Neil H. White, MD, CDE

KEYWORDS

- Diabetes mellitus • Retinopathy • Microalbuminuria • Diabetic neuropathy
- CVD risk factors • Neurocognition • Neuroimaging

KEY POINTS

- Clinically significant diabetes-related complications are uncommon in children and adolescents, but patients with youth-onset diabetes do develop life-altering complications during their young adult years.
- Retinopathy, nephropathy (microalbuminuria), and neuropathy are associated with glycemic control; current levels of glycemic control seem inadequate to completely prevent these complications.
- Cardiovascular disease (CVD) associated with diabetes starts during adolescence, and vigorous attention to CVD risk factors (dyslipidemia and hypertension) is an important component of caring for children and adolescents with diabetes.
- Type 2 diabetes with its onset in youth is likely associated with more and earlier diabetes-related microvascular and macrovascular complications than type 1 diabetes.
- Recent and emerging data show that hyperglycemia as well as hypoglycemia may have lasting effects on brain function and structure, especially in young children.
- Taken together, these considerations support the need for continuing research into new approaches and technology to improve the long-term overall glycemic control of those with diabetes of all ages, including young children.

The Diabetes Control and Complications Trial (DCCT) and its ongoing longitudinal observational follow-up study, the Epidemiology of Diabetes Interventions and Complications (EDIC) study, represent a major turning point in our understanding of the long-term outcomes of type 1 diabetes (T1D). The DCCT clearly demonstrated that intensive therapy for diabetes that lowered hemoglobin A1c (HbA1c) levels by about 2% (9.0%–7.1%) reduced the incidence of onset and progression of diabetic retinopathy (DR), diabetic nephropathy, and diabetic neuropathy by 47% to 54%, 39%, and

Department of Pediatrics, Washington University School of Medicine, 660 South Euclid Avenue, Box 8116, St Louis, MO 63110, USA
E-mail address: white_n@kids.wustl.edu

Pediatr Clin N Am 62 (2015) 889–909
http://dx.doi.org/10.1016/j.pcl.2015.04.004
0031-3955/15/$ – see front matter © 2015 Elsevier Inc. All rights reserved.

60%, respectively, in both young adults (18–39 years old)[1] and adolescents (13–18 years old)[2] with a diabetes duration of 1 to 15 years at the time of enrollment. During the EDIC follow-up study, the benefits on cardiovascular disease (CVD) outcomes also became apparent with a 42% reduction in CVD events after 17 years.[3] The ongoing EDIC study subsequently showed that these benefits not only persisted but indeed widened at 4[4,5] and 10[6,7] years after the end of the DCCT during a time of equivalent glycemic control between the original conventional and intensive groups in the DCCT; this has been called *metabolic memory*. The between-group differences in complication rates in DCCT and EDIC and the metabolic memory phenomenon were almost entirely a result of the differences in HbA1c between the groups during the DCCT.[4–7] Other factors contributed little if any to these differences.

Intensive therapy, as implemented in the DCCT and along with many subsequent pharmacologic and technologic advances, has now become the standard of care for T1D. With this changing standard of care for T1D during the last 2 decades since the release of the DCCT results, the morbidity and mortality associated with the microvascular and macrovascular complication of T1D has been reduced or delayed but not eliminated.[8] Comparing complication rates from about 20 years earlier to those in the DCCT/EDIC cohort after 20 years of follow-up, the cumulative incidence of proliferative DR (PDR) and nephropathy decreased from 50% and 35%, respectively, to 30% and 12%, respectively; the rates of end-stage renal disease (ESRD) requiring dialysis or transplantation have also declined (**Fig. 1**). The rates of other clinically severe complications also decreased dramatically. There remains no cure or prevention of T1D, and indeed the incidence of T1D and the overall impact of its complications seem to be increasing.

Simultaneous with the changing climate surrounding T1D, and along with the increasing prevalence of childhood obesity not only in the United States but also around much of the developed world, the incidence of type 2 diabetes (T2D) is

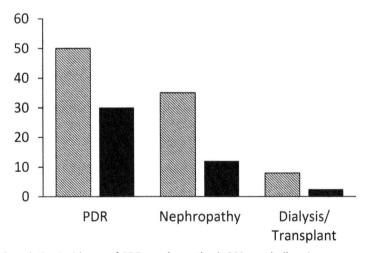

Fig. 1. Cumulative incidence of PDR, nephropathy (≥300 mg/d albumin, serum creatinine ≥2.0 mg/dL, or dialysis/transplantation), and ESRD requiring dialysis or renal transplantation during the pre-DCCT era (*hatched bars*) and the post-DCCT era (*solid bars*). (*Adapted from* Diabetes Control and Complications Trial/Epidemiology of Diabetes Interventions and Complications [DCCT/EDIC] Research Group. Modern-day clinical course of type 1 diabetes mellitus after 30 years' duration. Arch Intern Med 2009;169(14):1306–16.)

increasing. T2D now accounts for a substantial portion of new-onset diabetes in youth. Emerging evidence suggests that T2D starting during childhood or adolescence may have worse long-term outcomes than either T1D in youth or T2D presenting during the adult years (see later discussion).

Here, the author reviews the outcomes of diabetes starting during childhood and adolescence with particular focus on the long-term complications of diabetes (retinopathy, nephropathy, neuropathy, macrovascular disease) and their precursors in T1D starting in youth as well as the emerging, though still inadequate, data related to complications in youths with T2D. Also, the author reviews the recent understanding related to the effects of diabetes on the brain and cognition. This subject warrants important consideration in developing the best targets for managing diabetes in children and adolescents.

OVERVIEW OF DIABETES-RELATED COMPLICATIONS

The outcomes of diabetes in youth include short-term and long-term complications (**Box 1**). Although the long-term complications rarely have clinically important manifestations during the years that youths are under the care of their pediatrician or pediatric endocrinologist, youths with T1D are at risk for the short-term complications every day.

SHORT-TERM COMPLICATIONS OF TYPE 1 DIABETES

Diabetic ketoacidosis is dealt by Jefferies et al. elsewhere in this volume and will not be addressed here.

Some hypoglycemia is unavoidable in most individuals who are insulin treated. Hypoglycemia is best considered an adverse effect of insulin therapy (and potentially

---

Box 1
Overview of diabetes-related complications

Short-term Complications

Diabetic ketoacidosis

Hypoglycemia

Visual

Psychosocial

Long-term Complications

Microvascular

   Retinopathy

   Nephropathy

   Neuropathy

     Peripheral

     Autonomic

Macrovascular

   Coronary artery disease

   Cerebrovascular disease

   Peripheral vascular disease

sulfonylurea therapy as well) instead of a complication of diabetes. Hypoglycemia can cause a myriad of symptoms and signs that are generally divided into neurogenic/autonomic and neuroglycopenic. Neurogenic symptoms are the result of low blood glucose triggering an autonomic response with adrenergic and cholinergic symptoms, including shakiness or tremor, diaphoresis, tachycardia or palpitations, hunger, or irritability. Neuroglycopenic symptoms are the result of reduced availability of glucose to the brain and include sleepiness or lethargy, confusion, loss of consciousness, seizure, coma, and even death. Mild hypoglycemia is generally defined as hypoglycemia that patients recognize because of neurogenic/autonomic symptoms and self-treat with recovery before neuroglycopenic signs or symptoms. Mild hypoglycemia is largely unavoidable in well-managed insulin-treated patients with T1D using currently available treatment modalities. However, see the discussion on "Brain and Cognitive Effects of Diabetes" later.

Severe hypoglycemia, generally defined using the DCCT criteria as hypoglycemia resulting in neuroglycopenic symptoms or signs that render patients unable to treat themselves, represents a more significant concern. Severe hypoglycemia can result in injury (to self or others), seizure, coma, or death. In addition, severe hypoglycemia, especially in young children, may contribute to subsequent neurocognitive deficits and altered regional brain anatomy. Severe hypoglycemia is a complication of diabetes management that should be avoided, and goals of treatment and education should include prevention of severe hypoglycemia.[9,10]

Short-term visual effects of T1D are not uncommon. Blurred vision may be an acute symptom of hypoglycemia in some patients. More commonly, those with high or rapidly fluctuating blood glucose report blurred vision. This effect is usually transient and resolves once the blood glucoses are stable for a while. It is thought that this is caused by changes in the osmotic characteristics of the lens. Refractive error may change acutely with wide fluctuation of blood glucose, and many ophthalmologists and optometrists recommend postponing refraction for the purpose of prescribing glasses or contact lenses until the blood glucose has been stable. In rare cases, cataracts can develop at or soon after the diagnosis of T1D, even in children and teenagers.[11–14] If the visual disturbances do not clear within a couple of months after the onset of diabetes treatment, examination by an eye doctor should be strongly considered.

Psychosocial and behavioral issues are common among children with diabetes and their families. Discussion of these complications and outcomes is beyond the scope of this article; but it should be noted that regardless of whether the disorder or problem predated the onset or presented only after the onset of the diabetes, psychological, behavioral, or emotional problems both interfere with successful management and contribute to worse outcomes associated with poor glycemic control.[15,16]

LONG-TERM COMPLICATIONS OF TYPE 1 DIABETES
Overview

The long-term complications of diabetes are generally divided into microvascular and macrovascular. The microvascular complications include DR, diabetic nephropathy, and diabetic neuropathy. The initial detectable lesions of DR are termed *background DR* (BDR) and include microaneurysms, exudates, and hemorrhages. BDR is generally benign and does not impact on vision. However, it does represent the first readily detectable ocular finding of diabetes in most patients. More sensitive and invasive tests, such as 7-field stereo fundus photography, fluorescein angiography, or vitreous fluorophotometry, are generally not considered the standard of care until retinal lesions are identified and treatment is being considered but are often used as part of interventional or epidemiologic research studies. Swelling of the macula (clinically significant macular edema [CSME]) represents an advanced form of retinopathy that will impact vision if not treated.

Proliferative DR (PDR) represents more advanced disease with neovascularization, vitreous or preretinal hemorrhages, retinal detachment, and other vision-impacting lesions. PDR and CSME warrant evaluation and close follow-up by an experienced ophthalmologist. Laser photocoagulation or other specialized forms of therapy may be necessary to preserve vision. DR is a leading cause of new-onset blindness in adults. However, clinically significant or vision-threatening retinopathy is rarely detected during the years of pediatric follow-up.[17]

The earliest manifestation of renal involvement of T1D in children and adolescents, as well as adults, is hyperfiltration and an elevated renal plasma flow (RPF). Laborde and colleagues[18] found in 45 diabetic children (aged 12.5 ± 4.0 years; duration 4.9 ± 3.5 years) that both the glomerular filtration rate (GFR) (171 ± 31 mL/min/1.73 m^2 and 124 ± 18 mL/min/1.73 m^2, respectively) and RPF (778 ± 172 mL/min/1.73 m^2 and 631 $\pm$ 128 mL/min/1.73 m^2 respectively) were higher in those with T1D than in control nondiabetic children. Studies report that hyperfiltration was associated with an increased risk of developing microalbuminuria (MA).[19,20] Both nephromegaly[21] and higher ambulatory blood pressure[22] precede MA in diabetic children. Nephropathy typically progresses from MA (urinary albumin $\geq$30 mg/d or $\geq$30 mg per gram of creatinine) to macroalbuminuria (urinary albumin $\geq$300 mg/d or $\geq$300 mg per gram of creatinine) to decreasing GFR and ESRD. Without intervention, diabetic nephropathy may progress to ESRD requiring dialysis or renal transplantation. Diabetic nephropathy is a leading cause of ESRD in adults. However, although MA during adolescence is not uncommon, and it may be transient and/or intermittent, it is a predictor of possible future diabetic nephropathy. Macroalbuminuria, hematuria, or renal insufficiency secondary to diabetes are rare during the pediatric years[23]; if present, strong consideration should be given to referral to a renal specialist.

Diabetic neuropathy can be manifest as peripheral neuropathy or autonomic neuropathy. Peripheral neuropathy most frequently presents with symptoms and findings in the feet but can occur in any area of the body. Peripheral diabetic neuropathy is most often manifest with symptoms of numbness, tingling, or burning and signs of reduced or absent reflexes and vibratory or temperature perception. Although the definitive diagnosis of diabetic neuropathy usually requires evaluation by a neurologist and/or a nerve conduction velocity study, screening using the Michigan Neuropathy Screening Instrument[24] has good sensitivity and specificity for the diagnosis of diabetic neuropathy; the use of the 10-g monofilament has good sensitivity for predicting the development of morbidity, such as foot ulcer, infection, or amputation. Peripheral neuropathy, along with poor circulation and wound healing, is a leading cause of nontraumatic amputation in adults.

Diabetic autonomic neuropathy has multiple manifestations, including orthostatic hypotension, gastroparesis, pupillary dysfunction, bowel and bladder dysfunction, cardiac autonomic neuropathy with resting tachycardia and abnormal heart response to breathing and Valsalva, and erectile dysfunction.

Complications affecting the larger blood vessels, macrovascular complications, include coronary artery disease resulting in myocardial infarction, cerebrovascular disease resulting in stroke, and peripheral vascular disease causing poor limb circulation resulting in claudication, infection or gangrene, and amputation. Although these disorders are rarely if ever seen during the time of pediatric follow-up, the CVD risk factors (hypertension and dyslipidemia) and subclinical vascular abnormalities (intimal media thickening, stiffening of blood vessels, atherosclerotic plaque formation) certainly start during the adolescent years.

SCREENING FOR DIABETES COMPLICATIONS IN YOUTHS

Both the American Diabetes Association (ADA) and the International Society for Pediatric and Adolescent Diabetes (ISPAD) have guidelines for screening youths with both T1D and T2D for complications (summarized in **Table 1**).[25,26]

COMPARISON OF OUTCOMES IN THE PRE– AND POST–DIABETES CONTROL AND COMPLICATIONS TRIAL ERAS

During the pre-DCCT era (before the publication of the results of the DCCT in 1993), the prevalence of retinopathy was reported to occur in 27% to 89% of patients with T1D mellitus (TIDM) for 19 to 30 years (**Table 2**).[27–31] The prevalence of MA was reported to be 19% to 28% and macroalbuminuria 16% to 20% after about 15 years' duration (**Table 3**); the prevalence of ESRD was 2.2% and 7.8%, respectively, at 20 and 30 years' duration.[56] Diabetic neuropathy, an outcome that is more difficult to document with certainty, was reported to occur in up to 60% of persons with the onset of T1D during childhood and adolescence (**Table 4**).

During the post-DCCT period, the prevalence of diabetes complications has decreased considerably compared with the pre-DCCT years.[8,56,59,60] Hovind and colleagues[60] reported a reduction in the prevalence of diabetic nephropathy at an average age of 20 years with T1D diagnosed either during 1965 to 1969 or 1970 to 1974. Those diagnosed from 1965 to 1975 had a prevalence of about 40%, whereas those diagnosed in later years (1975–1984) had a prevalence of 13.7% to 18.9%, a 56% reduction. PDR occurred in 30.3% to 32.1% at 20 years for those diagnosed in 1965 to 1974, and the prevalence was about 55% after 40 years. Similar to nephropathy, for those diagnosed during later years, the prevalence of PDR had decreased substantially. Likewise, Nordwall and colleagues[61] reported similar reductions in the prevalence of both diabetic nephropathy and PDR at 25 and 30 years' duration in those diagnosed in 1961 to 1965 compared with those diagnosed in 1970 to 1974.

Table 1 Complication screening recommendations for children and adolescents with T1D		
	ADA Recommendations[25]	**ISPAD Recommendations[26]**
Retinopathy	Annual dilated fundoscopic examination by an eye doctor at or after puberty or at 10 y and 3–5 y of diabetes	Annual fundus photography after 11 y of age and 2 y of diabetes or at 9 y of age and 5 y of diabetes
Nephropathy	Annual urine albumin/creatinine ratio after 5 y of diabetes and after 10 y of age or puberty	Annual urine albumin/creatinine ratio or first morning albumin after 5 y of diabetes and after 10 y of age or puberty
Neuropathy	No specific guidelines in children	No specific guidelines in children
Macrovascular/CVD	Blood pressure annually Lipid profile at 2 y of age with a + family history or 10 y of age or puberty without a + family history; if normal, repeat every 5 y	Blood pressure annually Lipid profile every 5 y starting at 12 y of age

Table 2
Prevalence of DR in youth-onset T1D

Reference, Authors, Year	Number of Subjects	Age at Onset (y) Mean (Range)	Duration (y) Mean (Range)	Percent with DR
Malone et al,[32] 1984	74	Youth	4.9 ± 3.3 (1–13)	BDR: 50.0 PDR: 14.0
Verrotti et al,[33] 1994	55	Children & adolescent	6.9 ± 3.1 (4.8–10)	BDR: 16.4
Kernell et al,[34] 1997	557	14.6	8.0	14.5
d'Annunzio et al,[35] 1997	100	8.3 ± 3.5 (1.2–16.4)	10.4 ± 1.9 (7.3–14.3)	28.0
Bognetti et al,[36] 1997	317	—	—	22.7
Holl et al,[37] 1998	441	Children	7.6 ± 6.3	16.3
Olsen et al,[27,28] 1999, 2000	339	Children & adolescent	13.2	60.0
Skrivarhaug et al,[29] 2006	294	<15	24.3 (19.3–29.9)	BDP: 89.1 PDR: 10.9
Nordwall et al,[30] 2006	80	(7–21)	>13.0	27.0
Majaliwa et al,[38] 2007	99	(5–18)	4.76 ± 3.58	22.7
Nordwall et al,[39] 2009	269	8.6 ± 3.8	25.2 ± 7.6	BDR: 49.6 PDR: 26.1
Mayer-Davis et al,[40] 2012, SEARCH	222	<20	6.8 ± 1.0	17.0
Salardi et al,[31] 2012	105	(16–40)	19.7	56.2
White et al,[7] 2010, DCCT/ EDIC	156	13–18	$\sim$10	Severe BDR: 16.1 PDR: 9.7 CSME: 1.7
			$\sim$16	Severe BDR: 19.5 PDR: 18.2 CSME: 6.9

Fig. 1, using data adapted from reference,[8] compares the cumulative incidence of PDR, nephropathy, and ESRD between the pre-DCCT and the post-DCCT era.

Retinopathy

Reports of the prevalence of DR in patients diagnosed with T1D during childhood and adolescence are summarized is **Table 2**. In these studies, the prevalence of BDR ranges from 14.5% to 50.0% at 5 to 10 years' duration and from 37% to 90% at or beyond 20 years' duration of T1DM. The highest prevalence rates for BDR were from studies published in the 1980s and following patients during the pre-DCCT era. Malone and colleagues[32] reported the prevalence of BDR of 50% at 5 years' duration. However, Verrotti and colleagues[33] and Palmberg and colleagues[62] reported a prevalence of 16.4% and13.0% at 6.2 and 4 to 5 years' duration, respectively; Palmberg and colleagues[62] reported a prevalence of 50% and 95% at 10 to 12 and 26 to 50 years' duration, respectively. The prevalence of PDR was 26% in one study at 26 to

Table 3
Prevalence of MA in youth-onset T1D

Reference, Authors, Year of Report	Number of Subjects	Age of Onset (y) Mean (Range)	Duration (y) Mean (Range)	Percent with MA/MacroA
Joner et al,[41] 1992	371	—	10.5 (6.2–17.3)	12.5
Rudberg et al,[66] 1993	156	<20	6.9 ± 4.5	24.2
Janner et al,[43] 1994	164	Children & Adolescents	—	19.5
Bognetti et al,[36] 1997	317	—	—	11.0
Jones et al,[44] 1998	233	7.7 (median)	8.5	14.5
Schultz et al,[45] 1999	514	<16.0	5.0	12.8
Holl et al,[52] 1999	447	Children	10.0 13.0	5.0 10.0
Olsen et al,[27,28] 1999, 2000	339	Children & adolescent	13.2	Micro: 9.0 Macro: 3.7
Moore et al,[46] 2000	1007	<20.0	7.8 (median) (1.7–15.9)	9.7
Levy-Marchal et al,[47] 2000	702	Children & Adolescents	7.6 ± 3.1	5.1
Dahlquist et al,[67] 2001	60	5.7 ± 3.0	29.0 ± 3.0	Micro: 28.0 Macro: 12.0
Amin et al,[48] 2005	308	9.8 (0.3–15.9)	10.9 (6.0–17.8)	11.4
Nordwall et al,[30] 2006	80	(7–21)	>13.0	5.0
Skrivarhaug et al,[49] 2006	299	<15.0	24.0 (19.3–29.9)	14.9
Gallego et al,[50] 2006	950	<16.0	7.6	13.4
Amin et al,[51] 2009	527	<16.0	10.0	20.9
Raile et al,[42] 2007	27,805	12.9	8.3	Micro: 3.0 Macro: 0.2
Maahs et al,[53] 2007, SEARCH	3259	<20.0	(0–5)	9.2
Chiarelli et al,[54] 2008	340	<18.0	16.0	9.4
Dart et al,[55] 2012	T1D: 1011 T2D: 342	(1–18)	—	13.5 27.1

Abbreviation: MacroA, macroalbuminuria.

Table 4
Prevalence of diabetic neuropathy in youths with T1D

Reference, Authors, Year of Publication	Number of Subjects	Age at Onset (y) Mean (Range)	Duration (y) Mean (Range)	Percent with a Finding Compatible with Diabetic Neuropathy
Bognetti et al,[36] 1997	317	—	—	18.5
Olsen et al,[27,28] 1999, 2000	339	<20	13.2	62.5
Bao et al,[57] 1999	38	<20	7.2	68.4
Nordwall et al,[30] 2006	80	(7–21)	>13	59.0
Jaiswal et al,[58] 2013, SEARCH	329	<20	6.2 ± 0.9	8.2

50 years' duration[62] and varied from 10.9% to 26.1% at and beyond 20 years' duration. It should be noted that Palmberg and colleagues' study[62] reported on those diagnosed before 30 years of age and did not separate out those diagnoses during the pediatric years (defined herein as <20 years); for this reason, Palmberg and colleagues' data are not included in **Table 2**. Although there seems to have been a reduction in the prevalence of BDR from reports during the post-DCCT era, BDR still appears in about 20% by 5 to 10 years and 40% by 20 years.

In all the studies listed in **Table 2** in which it was examined,[28,29,35–40,63,64] poorer glycemic control (higher HbA1c) was consistently associated with a greater risk of retinopathy. Other factors that were reported to be associated include MA,[28,33,63] puberty,[31,35] blood pressure,[63,64] female[29] or male[32] sex, body mass index (BMI),[63] and low-density lipoprotein (LDL) cholesterol[40]; however, these associations were not explored in all studies and not consistently associated when they were explored.

Retinopathy was the primary outcome of the DCCT, and this cohort continues to be followed into EDIC. Of the adolescent participants (enrolled before the age of 18 years), 16.1%, 9.7%, and 1.2% and 19.5%, 19.5%, and 6.9% of the conventional group had developed severe BDR, PDR, and CSME, respectively, at about 10 and about 16 years of T1D, respectively.[7]

DR of any degree is rare in young children. Lueder and colleagues[65] found no cases of retinopathy in 51 children diagnosed before the age of 2 years who were followed and evaluated at a mean duration of 13.7 years. They pointed out that in other studies in the literature at that time, no child less than 10 years old had been identified with DR requiring treatment.

Microalbuminuria

There are many reports of the prevalence of MA or macroalbuminuria in the literature. **Table 3** summarizes those that include patients diagnosed with T1D during childhood and adolescence. Rigorous comparison across studies is difficult because the reported patient characteristics are not standardized and the urine collection techniques and definitions of MA and macroalbuminuria vary somewhat between studies. In addition, many reports use only a single value for microalbumin, whereas other reports use persistent (2 or 3 consecutive elevated values).

The prevalence of MA in these studies of childhood-onset T1D varies from as low as 3% to 5% after a duration of 8 to 13 or more years[30,65,52] to 19% to 29% at 10 to 13 years.[31,42,65] The highest reported prevalence among these studies is 24% to 29% at diabetes durations greater than 15 years.[42,66]

The author examined the prevalence of MA in his entire population of patients seen over a 1-year period (in 2012) in his Pediatric Diabetes Clinic. Of the 836 unique patients with T1D, 572 met the ISPAD criteria[26] for MA screening; of these, 496 (87%) were screened during that year. These patients had a mean (± standard deviation) age of 15.9 ± 8.0 years (range: 3–25) and diabetes duration of 7.9 ± 3.9 years (range: 0–21). The mean age at diabetes onset was 7.9 ± 4.0 years and 52.2% were female. Eighty-eight (17.7%) had a positive urine microalbumin screen (albumin/creatinine ratio ≥30 mg per gram of creatinine); of these, 71 (80.7%) had a second confirmatory determination. Fourteen (19.7%) of these 71 and 2.9% of the entire cohort met the criteria for persistent MA based on 2 consecutive elevated albumin/creatinine ratios. These results are slightly higher though similar to the other reports noted in **Table 3**, though all these patients were diagnosed with diabetes during the post-DCCT era. The presence of MA was associated with higher HbA1c (9.5 ± 1.4% vs 9.1 ± 1.8%; $P = .017$), and persistent MA was associated with even a higher HbA1c (9.8 ± 1.1% at the time of the test and 9.7 ± 1.2% average over the past year). By univariant analysis, longer disease duration, higher systolic (P = .017), but not diastolic (P = .061), blood pressure, and lower height (P = .02) were associated with the presence of a positive MA screen; in this initial analysis, blood pressure and height were not corrected for age or sex, however. When analyzed in a multivariant logistic regression model, only older chronologic age, higher systolic blood pressure, and higher HbA1c were associated with the presence of MA.

In these studies, the most consistent predictor of MA, aside from disease duration, was HbA1c.[34,41,44–46,49,50,52,53,67,68] Systolic, diastolic, and/or mean blood pressure were also associated in some[41,44,47,52,53,67] but not all[68] studies. Female sex is a frequent,[45,65,50,53] but not consistent,[49,52] association. Other factors, such as shorter height, BMI, total or LDL cholesterol, triglycerides, retinopathy, and smoking were not consistently associated with MA in studies in pediatric patients; of course it should be noted that retinopathy is infrequently found and smoking infrequently reported in this age group.

Neuropathy

Reliable and consistent data related to diabetic neuropathy in youths with T1D are limited (see **Table 4**). There are fewer studies than for retinopathy and MA. In addition, many would consider the gold standard for peripheral diabetic neuropathy to include the performance of nerve conduction velocity studies. These studies are expensive, somewhat uncomfortable to painful, and difficult to standardize and, therefore, are infrequently done. The DCCT/EDIC study reported on rates of peripheral and autonomic neuropathy in T1DM; but this cohort is not entirely youth-onset and is, therefore, not discussed directly in this review. Bao and colleagues[57] reported nerve conduction studies in a group of 38 patients with youth-onset T1D and found a high prevalence of abnormalities; but only 2 (5.3%) had symptomatic neuropathy, and there was no control group.

Table 4 summarizes the studies that report the prevalence of findings compatible with peripheral neuropathy in cohorts of youth-onset T1D. The prevalence ranges from 8.2% at a mean duration of about 6 years to about 60.0% by a duration of 13 or more years. Although the DCCT clearly demonstrated that the rate of both peripheral and autonomic neuropathy is reduced by intensive therapy, the cross-sectional studies do not consistently show associations of neuropathy with glycemic control.[58,69,70] Some studies, but not all,[69] report associations with HbA1c,[57] male sex,[28] blood pressure,[28] elevated cholesterol and triglycerides,[57] and the presence of MA.[28,57,58]

Verrotti and colleagues[69] studied cardiovascular autonomic nerve function in 110 children with T1D. Forty-seven (43%) had one or more abnormalities. In this report, there was no association between the abnormal autonomic nervous system findings and glycemic control, sex, diabetes duration, or the presence of retinopathy or MA.

Cardiovascular Disease Risk Factors

CVD risk factors are greater in persons with T1D than in controls, and this is also generally true in youth-onset T1D (**Table 5**). Compared with nondiabetic control children and adolescents, who have been generally well matched for age, sex, and race/ethnicity (but not always for BMI), patients with T1D generally tend to have more CVD risk factors,[72,84,89] higher total cholesterol (TC),[75,78,87] LDL cholesterol,[73,78,87] triglycerides (TG),[75,87] non–high-density lipoprotein (non-HDL) cholesterol,[75,78,87,88] and apolipoprotein B,[78] more small LDL particles,[78] lower HDL cholesterol, and higher adiponectin.[83] However, considerable variability between studies reporting patients

Table 5
CVD risk factors in youths with T1D

Reference, Authors, Year of Publication	CVD Risk Factors Affected
Krantz et al,[71] 2004	↑ cIMT
Rodriguez et al,[72] 2006, SEARCH	25% at age 10–19 had at least 2 CVD risk factors
Kershnar et al,[73] 2006, SEARCH	48% had LDL >100
Schwab et al,[74] 2007	↑ cIMT; ↑ SBP
Petitti et al,[75] 2007, SEARCH	↑ TC, TG, non-HDL
Della Pozza et al,[76] 2007	↑ cIMT
Heilman et al,[77] 2009	↑ cIMT
Guy et al,[78] 2009, SEARCH	↑ TC, ↑ LDL, ↑non-HDL, ↑ apolipoprotein B, ↑ Dense LDL particles
Urbina et al,[79] 2010, SEARCH	↑ Arterial stiffness (PWV)
Babar et al,[80] 2011	↑ cIMT
Della Pozza et al,[81] 2011	↑ cIMT
Wadwa et al,[82] 2012, SEARCH	↓ FMD
Shah et al,[83] 2012, SEARCH	↑ Arterial stiffness (PWV); ↑ adiponectin
Steigleder-Schweiger et al,[84] 2012	76.1% 1+ CVD risk factor 20.8% 2+ CVD risk factors 10.2% 3+ CVD risk factors 4.9% 4+ CVD risk factors
Dabelea et al,[85] 2013, SEARCH	↑ PWV; ↑ SBP
Urbina et al,[86] 2013, SEARCH	↑ cIMT
Maahs et al,[87] 2013, SEARCH	↑ TC,↑ LDL, ↑ TG, ↑non-HDL
Kuryan et al,[88] 2014	↑Non-HDL
Alman et al,[89] 2014	↓ ICH; ↑ PWV

Abbreviations: cIMT, carotid intima-media thickness; FMD, flow-mediated dilation; HDL, high-density lipoprotein cholesterol; ICH, ideal cardiovascular health; non-HDL, non–high-density lipoprotein cholesterol; PWV, pulse wave velocity; SBP, systolic blood pressure; TC, total cholesterol; TG, triglycerides.

during the adolescent years exists. **Table 5** represents a summary of studies reporting CVD risk factors in adolescents with T1D.

In addition to these easily monitored common risk factors for CVD, such as glycemic control, hypertension, and dyslipidemia, direct measures of vascular function have been performed in youths with both T1D and T2D. These measures include ultrasonographically obtained carotid artery intima-media thickness (cIMT), flow-mediated dilation (FMD), and pulse wave velocity (PWV). cIMT was increased,[71,74,81,86] FMD decreased,[80–82] and PWV increased,[77,79,83,85,89] all indicators of vascular dysfunction, in T1D when compared with appropriately matched control subjects. Increased cIMT[90] and PWV[82] were also found in youths with T2D, and these increases persisted after controlling for BMI.

COMPLICATIONS IN YOUTHS WITH TYPE 2 DIABETES MELLITUS

Because T2D among youths has only become prevalent during the last 10 to 20 years, there are less data available about long-term complications in these patients. However, the data available from 3 groups[55,91–94] suggest that the complication risk for these patients may be higher than for patients with T1D diagnosed at a similar age and perhaps occurs earlier in the course of the disease than in adults with T2D. Dart and colleagues[55] from Manitoba Canada (an area where there is a high number of Oji-Cree native Canadians and the incidence of youth-onset T2D is very high) reported a higher burden of renal disease in youth-onset T2D than youth-onset T1D. They compared 1011 subjects with youth-onset T1D with 342 subjects with youth-onset T2D. Not unexpectedly, baseline difference included more girls, higher BMI z-score, and lower socioeconomic status for the T2D group. Persistent MA was present in 26.9% versus 12.7% and persistent macroalbuminuria in 4.7% versus 1.6% (both P<.001) in T2D versus T1D, respectively. The age at onset of MA was similar, but the duration of diabetes was shorter (1.6 ± 1.5 [median 1.2]) in those with T2D than in those with T1D (6.3 ± 3.9 [median 6.0] years). In addition, T2D had an approximate 4-fold increased risk of renal disease (hazard ratio 4.03 [95% confidence interval [CI], 1.64–9.95]) and macroalbuminuria (hazard ratio 3.99 [95% CI, 1.50–10.0]), and a 3- to 5-fold increased risk of developing any renal complications, renal failure, and ESRD for T2D versus T1D at a similar age and diabetes duration. Survival analysis showed 100% renal survival out to 30 years' duration in the T1D group compared with 100% renal survival at 10 years, 91.5% at 15 years, and only 77.5% at 20 years in the T2D group.

Constantino and colleagues[91] from Australia compared the outcomes of 354 patients with T2D with 470 patients with T1D, all diagnosed between 15 and 30 years of age, over a median 21.4-year period (interquartile range 14.0–30.7). Mean age, duration of diabetes, year of diagnosis, HbA1c, and smoking history were similar. As expected, BMI, systolic and diastolic blood pressure, TC, and LDL cholesterol were higher and HDL cholesterol lower in the T2D group. Survival was lower in the T2D group (hazard ratio 2.0 [95% CI 1.2–3.2]; P = .003) with the cumulative mortality rate of 11.0% versus 6.6%; the rate of death caused by CVD was greater (50% vs 30%, P<.035; hazard ratio 3.5 [1.4–8.5], P = .004) in T2D versus T1D. Although retinopathy rates were similar (T2D: 37%; T1D: 41%), albuminuria, albumin/creatinine ratio, and vibratory perception threshold were all higher (all P<.0001) in those with T2D.

In the SEARCH Study,[40] 42% of those with T2D had retinopathy compared with 17% of those with T1D at a similar age and duration. SEARCH also reported a prevalence of peripheral neuropathy of 25.7% in 70 youths with T2D (age 21.6 ± 4.1 years; duration: 7.8 ± 1.8 years) compared with a prevalence of 8.2% in a similar (slightly younger) group of 329 with T1D.[58]

The TODAY (Treatment Options for type 2 Diabetes in Adolescents and Youth) Study can also provide present-day insight into the prevalence of complications in youth-onset T2D. The TODAY Study enrolled 699 subjects with youth-onset T2D mellitus diagnosed at less than 18 years of age and with diabetes duration less than 2 years. At baseline enrollment, the mean age was 14.0 ± 2.0 years and the duration was 7.8 ± 5.9 months. Subjects in the TODAY Study were randomized to 3 treatment groups (metformin alone; metformin + rosiglitazone; metformin + and intensive lifestyle program) and followed for an average of 3.9 years (range: 2–8 years). During the last year of the study, 517 subjects had 7-field stereoscopic fundus photography with centralized reading performed. At an average age of 18.1 ± 2.5 years and an average disease duration of 4.9 ± 1.5 (range: 2.0–8.4) years, 13.7% had mild background retinopathy. None had severe nonproliferative or proliferative retinopathy or macular edema.[92] In the TODAY Study cohort, 11.6% had hypertension at baseline and 33.8% had developed hypertension by the end of the study. Hypertension was more common in boys but did not differ by race/ethnicity, treatment group, glycemic control, or primary treatment outcome. A total of 6.3% had MA (ACR ≥30 mg per gram of creatinine) at baseline; by study end, 16.8% had MA. Fifty-seven (8.2%) developed macroalbuminuria (ACR ≥300 mg per gram of creatinine) and less than 1% had renal insufficiency (GFR <70 mL/min). The incidence of MA was associated with higher HbA1c.[93] At baseline, 4.5% already had an elevated LDL cholesterol; by 36 months of follow-up, this had increased to 10.7%.

In the TODAY Study, LDL and non-HDL cholesterol and apolipoprotein B all increased during the first 12 months of follow-up; this increase was primarily related to HbA1c (P<.0001).[93] Other studies have found similar CVD risk factors and lipid findings in youths with T2D to those seen in TODAY. The SEARCH study[87] found that 92% of youths with T2D, compared with 21% of youths with T1D, had 2 or more CVD risk factors. They also compared the lipid profile from 1680 youths with T1D with 283 youths with T2D who were greater than 10 years old[74] and found that those with T2D had a higher percentage with elevated TC (>200 mg/dL), LDL cholesterol (>130 mg/dL), and TG (>200 mg/dL) and a low HDL cholesterol (<40 mg/dL) than those with T1D. The SEARCH Study[75] also reported that, although the rates of dyslipidemia (elevated levels of TC, LDL, TG, or non-HDL, or lower HDL) were higher in T2D than T1D, the association of dyslipidemia with HbA1c was similar.

The rate of retinopathy in the TODAY cohort is at least as high or higher and the prevalence of MA and cardiovascular risk factors (hypertension and dyslipidemia) seem higher than noted earlier for those with T1D of similar age and duration. Together with the data of Dart and colleagues,[55] Constantino and colleagues,[91] and the SEARCH Study,[40,58] these data strongly suggest that youth-onset T2D is indeed a "more lethal phenotype of diabetes and is associated with a greater mortality, more diabetes complications, and unfavorable CVD risk factors when compared with T1DM"[91] of similar age, duration, and glycemic control.

THE BRAIN AND COGNITIVE EFFECTS OF DIABETES

Since the early reports in the 1980s by Ryan and colleagues[95] and Rovet and colleagues,[96] the effect of diabetes on the brain and cognitive functioning has been an area of vigorous research and controversy. The long history of this subject has been recently extensively reviewed by groups active in this field.[97–101] Reports from the DCCT[102–104] and from Wysocki and colleagues[105] have suggested that there is little if any long-term risk to cognition associated with hypoglycemia occurring in older adolescents and young adults. In the DCCT, there was a slight decline of psychomotor efficiency associated with long-term metabolic control.[104]

There is, however, a robust body of evidence indicating that diabetes with its onset in early childhood is associated with both cognitive deficits and structural changes on MRI. Northam and her colleagues[106] in Australia followed a cohort of children diagnosed with T1D from the time of diagnosis and for another 12 years. The initial mild psychological symptoms observed in children and their parents were largely resolved by 1 year.[106] At 2 years, there were deficits detected in memory and learning.[107] By 6 years, those with T1D had poorer performance on measures of intelligence, attention, processing speed, and executive skills. Attention, processing speed, and executive skills were associated with early onset (<4 years old), whereas intelligence was associated with a history of severe hypoglycemia.[108] At 12 years, these subjects were performing worse than controls on working memory, attention, new learning, and mental efficiency. There was an association of verbal abilities, working memory, and nonverbal processing speed with hypoglycemia and an association of working memory with hyperglycemia.[109] Also, after 12 years, the diabetic subjects had higher rates of mental health referrals and lower school completion.[110] Thus using this cohort followed since the onset of diabetes, Northam and her colleagues[106] have shown the emergence of cognitive deficits in children with T1D over time.

The group at Washington University in St Louis (Hershey, White, and colleagues[111–114]) have also provided a body of data supporting the alteration of cognitive function and brain structure in youths with T1D, most notable those with very early (<5 years old) onset. Hershey and colleagues[110] showed reduced performance on a spatial delayed memory task in early onset children with T1DM and a history of severe hypoglycemia. Perantie and colleagues,[111] in both retrospective and prospective[112] analyses of youths with T1D, showed effects of both hypoglycemia and hyperglycemia on regional brain volumes determined by voxel-based morphometry using MRI. Antenor-Dorsey and colleagues[113] showed alterations in white matter structure using diffusion tensor imaging. As this work has progressed, it has become apparent that both hypoglycemia and hyperglycemia affect brain structure and function, at least in those that develop T1D at a very young age. These data suggest that hypoglycemia and hyperglycemia affect different cognitive domains and different regions of brain, indicating that the mechanisms underlying the effects of hypoglycemia and hyperglycemia may be different.

The DirecNet Study Group has also evaluated brain function and structure in a group of 144 children with T1D onset before 8 years of age and 70 matched nondiabetic controls. Gray matter volumes,[114] white matter structure,[115] and cognitive function[116] were altered in the T1D group (compared with nondiabetic controls). Within the T1D group, these alterations were associated more strongly with hyperglycemia than with hypoglycemia. The mean HbA1c in this group of children was 7.9%, and the associations with hyperglycemia in this group included detailed glycemic assessment using continuous glucose monitors.

Thus, the extant data strongly suggest that even at the current level of glycemic control, there is risk to the brain associated with both hyperglycemia and hypoglycemia, especially in young children. This finding provides further support for the necessity of developing better approaches and technology to achieve blood glucose as close to normal as possible at all ages.

REFERENCES

1. The Diabetes Control and Complications Trial Research Group. The effect of intensive treatment of diabetes on the development and progression of long-term complications in insulin-dependent diabetes mellitus. N Engl J Med 1993;329(14):977–86.
2. The D.C.C.T. Research Group. The effect of intensive treatment on the development and progression of long-term complications in adolescents with insulin-dependent diabetes mellitus: the diabetes control and complications trial. J Pediatr 1994;125:177–88.
3. The Diabetes Control and Complications Trial/Epidemiology of Diabetes Interventions and Complications (DCCT/EDIC) Study Research Group. Intensive diabetes treatment and cardiovascular disease in patients with type 1 diabetes. N Engl J Med 2005;353(25):2643–53.
4. The Diabetes Control and Complications Trial/Epidemiology of Diabetes Interventions and Complications Research Group. Retinopathy and nephropathy in patients with type 1 diabetes four years after a trial of intensive therapy. N Engl J Med 2000;342:381–9.
5. The Diabetes Control and Complications Trial (DCCT)/Epidemiology of Diabetes Interventions and Complications (EDIC) Research Group. Beneficial effects of intensive therapy of diabetes during adolescence: outcomes after the conclusion of the diabetes control and complications trial (DCCT). J Pediatr 2001;139:804–12.

6. Diabetes Control and Complications Trial/Epidemiology of Diabetes Interventions and Complications Research Group. Prolonged effect of intensive therapy on the risk of retinopathy complications in patient with type 1 diabetes mellitus: 10 years after the Diabetes Control and Complications Trial. Arch Ophthalmol 2008;126(12):1707–15.
7. White NH, Sun W, Cleary PA, et al, for the DCCT-EDIC Research Group. Effect of prior intensive therapy in type 1 diabetes on 10-year progression of retinopathy in the DCCT/EDIC: comparison of adults and adolescents. Diabetes 2010;59(5): 1244–53.
8. Diabetes Control and Complications Trial/Epidemiology of Diabetes Interventions and Complications (DCCT/EDIC) Research Group. Modern-day clinical course of type 1 diabetes mellitus after 30 years' duration. Arch Intern Med 2009;169(14):1306–16.
9. Ly TT, Maahs DM, Rewers A, et al. Assessment and management of hypoglycemia. Pediatr Diabetes 2014;15(Suppl 20):180–92.
10. Seaquist ER, Anderson J, Childs B, et al. Hypoglycemia and diabetes: a report of a workgroup of the American Diabetes Association and the Endocrine Society. Diabetes Care 2013;36(5):1384–95.
11. Datta V, Swift PG, Woodruff GH, et al. Metabolic cataracts in newly diagnosed diabetes. Arch Dis Child 1997;76:118–20.
12. Ehlich RM, Kirsch S, Daneman D. Cataracts in children with diabetes mellitus. Diabetes Care 1987;10(6):798–9.
13. Patel CM, Plummer-Smith L, Ugrasbul F. Bilateral metabolic cataracts in 10-yr-old boy with newly diagnosed type 1 diabetes mellitus. Pediatr Diabetes 2009;10(3): 227–9.
14. Kato S, Oshika T, Numaga J, et al. Influence of rapid glycemic control on lens opacity in patients with diabetes mellitus. Ophthalmology 2000;130(3): 354–5.
15. Delamater AM, de Wit M, McDarby V, et al. ISPAD clinical practice consensus guidelines 2014: psychological care of children and adolescents with type 1 diabetes. Pediatr Diabetes 2014;15(Suppl 20):232–44.
16. Anderson BJ, McKay SV. Barriers to glycemic control in youth with type 1 diabetes and type 2 diabetes. Pediatr Diabetes 2011;12(3 Pt 1):197–205.
17. Klein R, Lee KE, Knudtson MD, et al. Changes in visual impairment prevalence by period of diagnosis of diabetes: the Wisconsin Epidemiologic Study of Diabetic Retinopathy. Ophthalmology 2009;116(10):1937–42.
18. Laborde K, Levy-Marchal C, Kindermans C, et al. Glomerular filtration and microalbuminuria in children with insulin-dependent diabetes. Pediatr Nephrol 1990;4(1):39–43.
19. Chiarelli F, Verrotti A, Morgese G. Glomerular hyperfiltration increases the risk of developing microalbuminuria in diabetic children. Pediatr Nephrol 1995;9(2): 154–8.
20. Mauer M, Drummond K, for the International Diabetic Nephropathy Study Group. The early natural history of nephropathy in type 1 diabetes. I. Study design and baseline characteristics of the study participants. Diabetes 2002; 51:1572–9.
21. Lawson ML, Sochett EB, Chait PG, et al. Effect of puberty on markers of glomerular hypertrophy and hypertension in IDDM. Diabetes 1996;45(1):51–5.
22. Garg SK, Chase HP, Icaza G, et al. 24-hour ambulatory blood pressure and renal disease in young subjects with type 1 diabetes. J Diabetes Complications 1997;11(5):263–7.

23. Tuttle KR, Bakris GL, Bilous RW, et al. Diabetic kidney disease: a report from an ADA Consensus Conference. Diabetes Care 2014;37(10):2864–83.
24. Feldman EL, Stevens MJ, Thomas PK, et al. A practical two-step quantitative clinical and electrophysiological assessment for the diagnosis and staging of diabetic neuropathy. Diabetes Care 1994;17(11):1281–9.
25. American Diabetes Association. Standards of medical care in diabetes—2014. Diabetes Care 2014;37(Suppl 1):S14–80.
26. Donaghue KC, Chiarelli F, Trotta D, et al, for ISPAD. Microvascular and macrovascular complications associated with diabetes in children and adolescents. Pediatr Diabetes 2009;10(Suppl 12):195–203.
27. Olsen BS, Johannesen J, Sjolie AK, et al. Metabolic control and prevalence of microvascular complication in young Danish patients with Type 1 diabetes mellitus. Danish Study Group of Diabetes in Childhood. Diabet Med 1999;16(1):79–85.
28. Olsen BS, Sjolie A, Hougard P, et al. A 6-year nationwide cohort study of glycaemic control in young people with type 1 diabetes. Risk markers for the development of retinopathy, nephropathy and neuropathy. Danish Study Group of Diabetes in Childhood. J Diabetes Complications 2000;14(6):295–300.
29. Skrivarhaug T, Fosmark DS, Stene LC, et al. Low cumulative incidence of proliferative retinopathy in childhood-onset type 1 diabetes: a 24-year follow-up study. Diabetologia 2006;49(10):2281–90.
30. Nordwall M, Hyllienmark L, Ludvigsson J. Early diabetic complications in a population of young patients with type 1 diabetes mellitus despite intensive treatment. J Pediatr Endocrinol Metab 2006;19(1):45–54.
31. Salardi S, Porta M, Maltoni G, et al. Diabetes Study Group of the Italian Society of Paediatric Endocrinology and Diabetology. Infant and toddler type 1 diabetes: complications after 20 years' duration. Diabetes Care 2012;35(4):829–33.
32. Malone JI, Grizzard S, Espinoza LR, et al. Risk factors for diabetic retinopathy in youth. Pediatrics 1984;73(6):756–61.
33. Verrotti A, Lobefala L, Chiarelli F, et al. Diabetic retinopathy. Relationship with nephropathy in pediatric age. Panminerva Med 1994;36(4):179–83.
34. Kernell A, Dedorsson I, Joansson B, et al. Prevalence of diabetic retinopathy in children and adolescents with IDDM: a population-based multicentre study. Diabetologia 1997;40(3):307–10.
35. d'Annunzio G, Malvezzi F, Vitali L, et al. A 3-19-year follow-up study on diabetic retinopathy in patients diagnosed in childhood and treated with conventional therapy. Diabet Med 1997;14(11):951–8.
36. Bognetti E, Calori G, Meschi F, et al. Prevalence and correlations of early microvascular complications in young type I diabetic patients: role of puberty. J Pediatr Endocrinol Metab 1997;10(6):587–92.
37. Holl RW, Lang GE, Grabert M, et al. Diabetic retinopathy in pediatric patients with type-1 diabetes: effect of diabetes duration, prepubertal and pubertal onset of diabetes, and metabolic control. J Pediatr 1998;132(5):790–4.
38. Majaliwa ES, Munubhi E, Ramaiya K, et al. Survey on acute and chronic complications in children and adolescents with type 1 diabetes at Muhimbili National Hospital in Dar es Salaam, Tanzania. Diabetes Care 2007;30(9):2187–92.
39. The Microalbumin Cooperative Study Group. Predictors of the development of microalbuminuria in patients with type 1 diabetes mellitus: a seven-year prospective study. Diabet Med 1999;16:918–25.
40. Mayer-Davis EJ, Davis C, Saadine J, et al, SEARCH for Diabetes in Youth Study Group. Diabetic retinopathy in the SEARCH for diabetes in youth cohort: a pilot study. Diabet Med 2012;29(9):1148–52.

41. Joner G, Brinchmann-Hansen O, Torres CG, et al. A nationwide cross-sectional study of retinopathy and microalbuminuria in young Norwegian type 1 (insulin-dependent) diabetic patients. Diabetologia 1992;35(11):1049–54.

42. Raile K, Galler A, Hofer S, et al. Diabetic nephropathy in 27,805 children, adolescents, and adults with type 1 diabetes: effect of diabetes duration, A1C, hypertension, dyslipidemia, diabetes onset, and sex. Diabetes Care 2007;30:2523–8.

43. Janner M, Knill SE, Diem P, et al. Persistent microalbuminuria in adolescents with type I (insulin-dependent) diabetes mellitus is associated to early rather than late puberty. Results of a prospective longitudinal study. Eur J Pediatr 1994;153(6):403–8.

44. Jones CA, Leese GP, Kerr S, et al. Development and progression of microalbuminuria in a clinic sample of patients with insulin dependent diabetes mellitus. Arch Dis Child 1998;78:518–23.

45. Schultz CJ, Konopelska-Bahu T, Dalton RN, et al, for the Oxford Regional Prospecitve Study Group. Microalbuminuria prevalence varies with age, sex, and puberty in children with type 1 diabetes followed from diagnosis in a longitudinal study. Diabetes Care 1999;22(3):495–502.

46. Moore TH, Shield JP, on behalf of the Microalbuminuria in Diabetic Adolescents and Children (MIDAC) research group. Prevalence of abnormal urinary albumin excretion in adolescents and children with insulin dependent diabetes: the MIDAC study. Arch Dis Child 2000;83:239–43.

47. Levy-Marchal C, Sahler C, Cahane M, et al, GECER Study Group. Risk factors for microalbuminuria in children and adolescents with type 1 diabetes. J Pediatr Endocrinol Metab 2000;13(6):613–20.

48. Amin R, Turner C, van Aken S, et al. The relationship between microalbuminuria and glomerular filtration rate in young type 1 diabetic subjects: the Oxford Regional Prospective Study. Kidney Int 2005;68(4):1740–9.

49. Skrivarhaug T, Bangstad HJ, Stene LC, et al. Low risk of overt nephropathy after 24 yr of childhood-onset type 1 diabetes mellitus (T1DM) in Norway. Pediatr Diabetes 2006;7:239–46.

50. Gallego PH, Bulsara MK, Frazer F, et al. Prevalence and risk factors for microalbuminuria in a population-based sample of children and adolescents with T1DM in Western Australia. Pediatr Diabetes 2006;7:165–72.

51. Amin R, Widmer B, Dalton RN, et al. Unchanged incidence of microalbuminuria in children with type 1 diabetes since 1986: a UK based inception cohort. Arch Dis Child 2009;94:258–62.

52. Holl RW, Grabert M, Thon A, et al. Urinary excretion of albumin in adolescents with type 1 diabetes: persistent versus intermittent microalbuminuria and relationship to duration of diabetes, sex and metabolic control. Diabetes Care 1999;22(9):1555–60.

53. Maahs DM, Snively BM, Bell RA, et al. Higher prevalence of elevated albumin excretion in youth with type 2 than type 1 diabetes: the SEARCH for diabetes in youth study. Diabetes Care 2007;30(10):2593–8.

54. Chiarelli F, Giannini C, Verotti A, et al. Increased concentrations of soluble CD40 ligand may help to identify type 1 diabetic adolescents and young adults at risk for developing persistent microalbuminuria. Diabetes Metab Res Rev 2008; 24(7):570–6.

55. Dart AB, Sellers EA, Martens PJ, et al. High burden of kidney disease in youth-onset type 2 diabetes. Diabetes Care 2012;35(6):1265–71.

56. Finne P, Reunanen A, Stenman S, et al. Incidence of end-stage renal disease in patients with type 1 diabetes. JAMA 2005;294:1782–7.

57. Bao XH, Wong V, Wang Q, et al. Prevalence of peripheral neuropathy with insulin-dependent diabetes mellitus. Pediatr Neurol 1999;20(3):204–9.
58. Jaiswal M, Lauer A, Martin CL, et al, SEARCH for Diabetes in Youth Study Group. Peripheral neuropathy in adolescents and young adults with type 1 and type 2 diabetes from the SEARCH for Diabetes in Youth follow-up cohort: a pilot study. Diabetes Care 2013;36(12):3903–8.
59. Pambianco G, Costacou T, Ellis D, et al. The 30-year natural history of type 1 diabetes complications: the Pittsburgh epidemiology of diabetes complications study experience. Diabetes 2006;55:1463–9.
60. Hovind P, Tarnow L, Rossing K, et al. Decreasing incidence of severe diabetic microangiopathy in type 1 diabetes. Diabetes Care 2003;26:1258–64.
61. Nordwall M, Bojestig M, Arnqvist HJ, et al. Declining incidence of severe retinopathy and persisting decrease of nephropathy in an unselected population of type 1 diabetes–the Linkoping Diabetes Complications Study. Diabetologia 2004;47:1266–72.
62. Palmberg P, Smith M, Waltman S, et al. The natural history of retinopathy in insulin-dependent juvenile-onset diabetes. Ophthalmology 1981;88(7): 613–8.
63. Klein R, Knudson MD, Lee KE, et al. The Wisconsin Epidemiologic Study of Diabetic Retinopathy XXII. The twenty-five year progression of retinopathy in persons with type 1 diabetes. Ophthalmology 2008;115:1859–68.
64. Yau J, Rogers S, Kawasaki R, et al. Global prevalence and major risk factors of diabetic retinopathy. Diabetes Care 2012;35(3):556–64.
65. Lueder GT, Pradhan S, White NH. Risk of retinopathy in children with type 1 diabetes mellitus before 2 years of age. Am J Ophthalmol 2005;140(4):930–1.
66. Rudberg S, Ullman E, Dahlquist G. Relationship between early metabolic control and the development of microalbuminuria–a longitudinal study in children with type 1 (insulin-dependent) diabetes mellitus. Diabetologia 1993;36(12): 1309–14.
67. Dahlquist G, Stattin EL, Rudberg S. Urinary albumin excretion rate and glomerular filtration rate in the prediction of diabetic nephropathy; a long-term follow-up study of childhood onset type-1 diabetic patients. Nephrol Dial Tranplant 2001; 16(7):1382–6.
68. Gorman D, Sochett E, Daneman D. The natural history of microalbuminuria in adolescents with type 1 diabetes. J Pediatr 1999;134(3):333–7.
69. Verrotti A, Chiarelli F, Blasetti A, et al. Autonomic neuropathy in diabetic children. J Paediatr Child Health 1995;31(6):545–8.
70. dos Santos LH, Bruck I, Antoniuk SA, et al. Evaluation of sensorimotor polyneuropathy in children and adolescent with type 1 diabetes: associations with microalbuminuria and retinopathy. Pediatr Diabetes 2002;3(2):101–8.
71. Krantz JS, Mack WJ, Hodis HN, et al. Early onset of subclinical atherosclerosis in young persons with type 1 diabetes. J Pediatr 2004;145(4):452–7.
72. Rodriguez BL, Fujimoto WY, Mayer-Davis EJ, et al. Prevalence of cardiovascular disease risk factors in U.S. children and adolescents with diabetes: the SEARCH for Diabetes in Youth Study. Diabetes Care 2006;29(8):1891–6.
73. Kershnar AK, Daniels SR, Imperatore G, et al. Lipid abnormalities are prevalent in youth with type 1 and type 2 diabetes: the SEARCH for Diabetes in Youth Study. J Pediatr 2006;149(30):314–9.
74. Schwab KO, Doefer J, Krebs A, et al. Early atherosclerosis in childhood type 1 diabetes: role of raised blood pressure in the absence of dyslipidemia. Eur J Pediatr 2007;166(6):541–8.

75. Petitti DB, Imperaotore G, Palla SL, et al, SEARCH for Diabetes in YouthStudy Group. Serum lipids and glucose control: the SEARCH for Diabetes in Youth study. Arch Pediatr Adolesc Med 2007;161(2):159–65.
76. Della Pozza R, Bechtold S, Bonfig W, et al. Age of onset of type 1 diabetes in children and carotid intima medial thickness. J Clin Endocrinol Metab 2007; 92(6):2053–7.
77. Heilman K, Zilman M, Zilman K, et al. Arterial stiffness, carotid artery intima-media thickness and plasma myeloperoxidase level in children with type 1 diabetes. Diabetes Res Clin Pract 2009;84(2):168–73.
78. Guy J, Ogden L, Wadwa RP, et al. Lipid and lipoprotein profiles in youth with and without type 1 diabetes: the SEARCH for Diabetes in Youth case-control study. Diabetes Care 2009;32(3):416–20.
79. Urbina EM, Wadwa RP, Davis C, et al. Prevalence of increased arterial stiffness in children with type 1 diabetes mellitus differs by measurement site and sex: the SEARCH for Diabetes in Youth Study. J Pediatr 2010;156(5):731–7.
80. Babar GS, Zidan H, Widlansky ME, et al. Impaired endothelial function in preadolescent children with type 1 diabetes. Diabetes Care 2011;34(3):681–5.
81. Della Pozza R, Beyerlein A, Thilmany C, et al. The effect of cardiovascular risk factors on the longitudinal evolution of the carotid intima medial thickness in children with type 1 diabetes mellitus. Cardiovasc Diabetol 2011;10:53.
82. Wadwa RP, Urbina EM, Anderson AM, et al, SEARCH Study Group. Measures of arterial stiffness in youth with type 1 and type 2 diabetes: the SEARCH for diabetes in youth study. Diabetes Care 2012;33(4):881–6.
83. Shah AS, Dolan LM, Lauer A, et al. Adiponectin and arterial stiffness in youth with type 1 diabetes: the SEARCH for Diabetes in Youth Study. J Pediatr Endocrinol Metab 2012;25(7–8):717–21.
84. Steigleder-Schweiger C, Rami-Merhar B, Waldhor T, et al. Prevalence of cardiovascular risk factors in children and adolescents with type 1 diabetes in Austria. Eur J Pediatr 2012;171(8):1193–202.
85. Dabelea D, Talton JW, D'Agostino R, et al. Cardiovascular risk factors are associated with increased arterial stiffness in youth with type 1 diabetes: the SEARCH CVD study. Diabetes Care 2013;36(12):3838–943.
86. Urbina EM, Dabelea D, D'Agostino RB, et al. Effect of type 1 diabetes on carotid structure and function in adolescents and young adults: the SEARCH CVD study. Diabetes Care 2013;36(9):2597–9.
87. Maahs DM, Dabelea D, D'Agostino RB, et al, SEARCH for Diabetes in Youth Study. Glucose control predicts 2-year change in lipid profile in youth with type 1 diabetes. J Pediatr 2013;162(1):101–7.
88. Kuryan RE, Jacobson MS, Frank GR. Non-HDL-cholesterol in an adolescent diabetes population. J Clin Lipidol 2014;8(2):194–8.
89. Alman AC, Talton JW, Wadwa RP, et al. Cardiovascular health in adolescents with type 1 diabetes: the SEARCH CVD Study. Pediatr Diabetes 2014;15(7):502–10.
90. Shah AS, Dolan LM, Kimball TR, et al. Influence of duration of diabetes, glycemic control, and traditional cardiovascular risk factors on early atherosclerotic vascular changes in adolescents and young adults with type 2 diabetes mellitus. J Clin Endocrinol Metab 2009;94(10):3740–5.
91. Constantino MI, Molyneax L, Limacher-Gisler F, et al. Long-term complications and mortality in young-onset diabetes. Type 2 diabetes is more hazardous and lethal than type 1 diabetes. Diabetes Care 2013;36:3863–9.
92. TODAY Study Group. Retinopathy in youth with type 2 diabetes participating in the TODAY clinical trial. Diabetes Care 2013;36:1772–4.

93. TODAY Study Group. Rapid rise in hypertension and nephropathy in youth with type 2 diabetes: the TODAY clinical trial. Diabetes Care 2013;36:1735–41.

94. TODAY Study Group. Lipid and inflammatory cardiovascular risk worsens over 3 years in youth with type 2 diabetes: the TODAY clinical trial. Diabetes Care 2013;36:1758–64.

95. Ryan C, Vega A, Drash A. Cognitive deficits in adolescents who developed diabetes early in life. Pediatrics 1985;75:921–7.

96. Rovet JF, Ehrlich RM, Hoppe MG. Intellectual deficits associated with the early onset of insulin-dependent diabetes mellitus in children. Diabetes Care 1987;10:510–5.

97. Ryan C. Why is cognitive dysfunction associated with the development of diabetes in early life? The diathesis hypothesis. Pediatr Diabetes 2006;7:289–97.

98. Arbelaez AM, Semenkovich K, Hershey T. Glycemic extremes in youth with T1DM: the structural and functional integrity of the developing brain. Pediatr Diabetes 2013;14:541–53.

99. Ryan C. Does moderately severe hypoglycemia cause cognitive dysfunction in children? Pediatr Diabetes 2004;5:59–62.

100. Biessels GJ, Ryan CM. Cognition and diabetes: a lifespan perspective. Lancet Neurol 2008;7:184–90.

101. McCrimmon RJ, Ryan CM, Frier BM. Diabetes and cognitive dysfunction. Lancet 2012;379:2291–9.

102. Diabetes Control and Complications Trial/Epidemiology of Diabetes Interventions and Complications Study Research Group, Jacobson AM, Musen G, et al. Long-term effect of diabetes and its treatment of cognitive function. N Engl J Med 2009;361(19):1914.

103. Musen G, Jacobson AM, Ryan CM, et al. DCCT/EDIC. Impact of diabetes and its treatment on cognitive function among adolescents who participated in the Diabetes Control and Complications Trial. Diabetes Care 2008;10:1933–8.

104. Jacobson AM, Ryan CM, Cleary PA, et al, Diabetes Control and Complications-Trial/EDIC Research Group. Biomedical risk factors for decreased cognitive functioning in type 1 diabetes: an 18 year follow-up of the Diabetes Control and Complications Trial (DCCT) cohort. Diabetologia 2011;54(2):245–55.

105. Wysocki T, Harris MA, Mauras N, et al. Absence of adverse effects of severe hypoglycemia on cognitive function in school-aged children with diabetes over 18 months. Diabetes Care 2003;6(4):1100–5.

106. Northam E, Anderson P, Adler R, et al. Psychosocial and family functioning in children with insulin-dependent diabetes at diagnosis. J Pediartr Psychol 1996;21(5):699–717.

107. Northam EA, Anderson PJ, Werther GA, et al. Predictors of change in the neuropsychological profiles of children with type 1 diabetes 2 years after disease onset. Diabetes Care 1999;22:1438–44.

108. Northam EA, Anderson PJ, Jacobs R, et al. Neuropsychological profiles of children with type 1 diabetes 6 years after disease onset. Diabetes Care 2001;24:1541–6.

109. Lin A, Northam EA, Rankins D, et al. Neuropsychological profiles of young people with type 1 diabetes 12 yr after disease onset. Pediatr Diabetes 2012;11(4):235–43.

110. Hershey T, Perantie DC, Warren SL, et al. Frequency and timing of severe hypoglycemia affects spatial memory in children with type 1 diabetes mellitus. Diabetes Care 2005;28:2372–7.

111. Perantie DC, Wu J, Koller JM, et al. Regional brain volume differences associated with hyperglycemia and severe hypoglycemia in youth with type 1 diabetes. Diabetes Care 2007;30(9):2331–7.

112. Perantie DC, Koller JM, Weaver PM, et al. Prospectively-determined impact of type 1 diabetes on brain volume during development. Diabetes 2011;60(11): 3006–14.
113. Antenor-Dorsey JA, Meyer E, Rutlin J, et al. White matter microstructural integrity in youth with type 1 diabetes. Diabetes 2013;62(2):581–9.
114. Marzelli MJ, Mazaika PK, Barnea-Goraly N, et al. AL for the Diabetes Research in Children Network (DirecNet). Neuroanatomical correlates of dysglycemia in young children with type 1 diabetes mellitus. Diabetes 2014;63(1):343–53.
115. Barnea-Goraly N, Raman M, Mazaika P, et al, for the Diabetes Research in Children Network (DirecNet). Alterations in white matter structure in young children with type 1 diabetes mellitus. Diabetes Care 2014;37(2):332–40.
116. Cato MA, Mauras N, Ambrosino J, et al, for the Diabetes Research in Children Network (DirecNet). Cognitive functioning in young children with type 1 diabetes. J Int Neuropsychol Soc 2014;20:238–47.

The Impact of Diabetes on Brain Function in Childhood and Adolescence

Fergus J. Cameron, BMedSci, MBBS, DipRACOG, FRACP, MD[a,b],*

KEYWORDS

- Type 1 diabetes • Brain • Cognition • Children • Adolescents

KEY POINTS

- Type 1 diabetes is associated with decrements in cognition during childhood and adolescence.
- The most neurotoxic milieu seems to be young age and/or diabetic ketoacidosis at onset, severe hypoglycemia under the age of 6, followed by chronic hyperglycemia.
- The observed cognitive changes are associated with observable changes in neuroimaging.
- Changes in cognitive performance are 0.3 to 0.8 standard deviations in full-scale IQ, affecting executive functioning, and functional and academic performance.
- There are anatomic and metabolic correlations between adverse cognitive and mental health outcomes.

INTRODUCTION

The primary metabolic fuel for the brain is glucose. In adults, brain energy consumption accounts for 25% of total body glucose utilization.[1] In a developmental context, the pediatric brain dominates whole body metabolism. PET and MRI studies have shown that daily brain use of glucose peaks at 5.2 years at rates of 167 and 146 g/d in males and females, respectively.[2] A constant supply of glucose to the brain

Disclosure Statement: The author has received research support, travel support and honoraria from Novo Nordisk, Lilly, Medtronic, Roche, Abbott, The Juvenile Diabetes Research Foundation and the National Health & Medical Research Council of Australia.
[a] Department of Endocrinology and Diabetes, Royal Children's Hospital, Murdoch Childrens Research Institute, 50 Flemington Road, Parkville, Melbourne 3052, Australia; [b] Department of Paediatrics, University of Melbourne, Melbourne 3010, Australia
* Department of Endocrinology and Diabetes, Royal Children's Hospital, 50 Flemington Road, Parkville, Melbourne 3052, Australia.
E-mail address: fergus.cameron@rch.org.au

is critical for normal cerebral metabolism.[3] Thus, it is not surprising that developing brains in early childhood are more susceptible to metabolic insult, particularly those resulting from perturbations in blood glucose levels. Type 1 diabetes (T1D) is among the most common chronic diseases of childhood[4] and the condition most likely to cause the greatest swings in amplitude in blood glucose on an hour-to-hour basis. Although changes in cognition among children with T1D have been documented for some time, it is only recently that sophisticated neuroimaging techniques have allowed direct measures of the impact of T1D on brain development.

THE EVIDENCE FOR TYPE 1 DIABETES–RELATED BRAIN INJURY
Early Childhood

T1D is not uncommonly diagnosed in early life and in some surveys it is an increased prevalence in the under 5 year old age group that is most commonly seen.[5] This is a particularly vulnerable age in terms of neurodevelopment.[6] A study of preschool-aged children with an average of approximately 2 years' diabetes duration showed them to have similar cognitive function when compared with healthy controls. However, when the group was subanalyzed by metabolic control, those children with higher hemoglobin A1C levels had lower general cognitive abilities, slower fine motor speed, and lower receptive language scores.[7] A similar aged cohort was also found to have no differences overall in full-scale IQ compared with healthy controls; however, there were significant associations with poorer cognitive outcome and severe hypoglycemia[8] or poorer metabolic control.[9] MR studies in this preschool cohort showed lower than predicated white matter volume change with age[8] and lower axial diffusivity values in the temporal and parietal lobes in the T1D group.[9] Children who had a history of severe hypoglycemia had lesser gray and white matter volumes.[8]

Mid Childhood

Group differences in overall cognitive performances between diabetic and nondiabetic cohorts are variably apparent by middle childhood with a history of either diabetic ketoacidosis (DKA) or severe hypoglycemia (especially in early life) being associated with poorer outcome. A cohort of T1D children with a mean age of 10 years performed significantly worse than healthy controls on 11 of 14 cognitive domains. Those children with a history of DKA had the worst outcomes on 8 of these domains.[10] In a larger cohort of T1D children aged 6 to 18 years, children with a history of 3 or more episodes of severe hypoglycemia under the age of 5 years had significantly worse long-delay spatial delayed response performance compared with healthy controls and age- and duration-matched diabetes controls.[11] Another group aged 4 to 10 years with median diabetes duration of 2.5 years did not show differences in IQ, although trends were apparent.[12] MR studies in this age group are again already showing morphologic changes. In a large control study of T1D children with a mean age of 7 years, the T1D group showed gray matter volume change (decreased in the bilateral occipital and cerebellar regions and increased in the left prefrontal, insula, and temporal regions) with association between specific regional volumes and hyperglycemia.[13] This same group also showed white matter change with reductions in white matter diffusivity observed throughout the brain, particularly in the frontal, temporal, parietal, and occipital lobes.[14] White matter diffusivity was associated with hyperglycemia but not severe hypoglycemia. In these studies, the T1D cohort had significantly lesser full-scale IQ scores when compared with the matched healthy controls and this was associated with white matter structural change. Cross-sectional and longitudinal studies of older, peripubertal children with T1D compared with controls again showed changes in specific areas of brain volume, but only after a subanalysis was undertaken for those with a history of severe hypoglycemia and/or chronic hyperglycemia.[15,16]

Adolescence and Early Adulthood

Late adolescence and early adulthood are informative life periods for cognitive study in T1D owing to duration of disease being usually longer and coincident with the time of neuromaturation. The 1 major study reported in this age group was a longitudinal control analysis of diabetic youth from the time of diagnosis to early adulthood. At baseline, both groups were matched for full-scale IQ and socioeconomic status. MR studies 12 years after diagnosis showed that relative to controls the T1D group had spectroscopy profiles consistent with lower neuronal density (reduced N-acety-laspartate) in the frontal lobes and basal ganglia and increase gliosis (increased myoinositol) and demyelination (increased choline) in the frontal, temporal, and parietal lobes.[17] Regional gray and white matter volume changes were noted throughout multiple brain regions.[18] Despite being matched for intelligence at baseline, after 12 years the T1D cohort had lost 0.3 standard deviations (SD) in full-scale IQ points and had twice the rate of school noncompletion.[19,20] Similar spectroscopic changes suggestive of neuronal loss were reported in a case report of an adolescent with recurrent ketoacidosis who showed progressive decline of brain N-acetylaspartate.[21]

Educational and Functional Outcomes

As discussed, measurable neurocognitive deficits have been described frequently in T1D. Metaanalyses of children and adults have shown mild (0.3–0.8 SD) decrements in full-scale IQ.[22–24] Mild and specific deficits have been shown in the areas of attention, executive functions, psychomotor efficiency, and information processing speed. In children, memory and learning deficits were seen only in those with early onset disease and/or a history of severe hypoglycemia. In particular, cognitive outcomes have been found to be worse in those patients diagnosed in early life (<2 years of age).[25] Whether these decrements should be seen as a consequence of disordered brain development or accelerated brain senescence is currently an area of debate.[18,26] Functionally, however, there does seem to be a consequence of even mild decrements in cognition. Both Swedish[27,28] and Finnish[29] population registry–based studies have shown suboptimal academic secondary and primary school outcomes, respectively. A prospective Australian cohort study showed that older adolescents and young adults with T1DM had lower rates of school completion and work/study participation than healthy controls despite having similar IQ at diabetes onset 12 years previously.[20] There is a highly plausible case that, within individuals, suboptimal metabolic control begets ongoing poor metabolic control through deficits in executive skills, such as goal setting, planning, organization, working memory and mental flexibility, reduced treatment adherence,[30] and motivational issues secondary to impaired mental health.

Mental Health

Suboptimal mental health outcomes in children and adolescents with T1D have been well-documented[31,32] with metaanalysis confirming that depression, anxiety, and eating disorders occur more commonly in both children[33] and adults[34,35] with T1D than in healthy controls. These affective disorders are often associated with poor metabolic control. Mental health disorders in T1D have been ascribed hitherto to the existential burden of living with the disease; however, there is an increasing body of evidence that their occurrence may also be linked to pathophysiologic brain changes that affect cognition as described. Corresponding brain regions are involved in cognitive and affective functions, including the hippocampus, prefrontal cortex, and limbic structure. Thus, neuronal injury in these areas is likely to have impacts on both cognition and mental well-being.[36] A recent MR analysis of young adults with T1D and depression showed them to have elevations in prefrontal glutamate–glutamine–γ-aminobutyric acid, which were associated with degree of lifetime hyperglycemia.[37] Finally, there is uncontrolled yet intriguing data showing short- and long-term improvements in behavior, mood, and cognition in children commencing insulin pump therapy.[38,39]

Adulthood

Despite a high frequency of severe hypoglycemia, the Diabetes Control and Complications Trial[40,41] failed to find any evidence of cognitive decline in young adults and adolescents followed prospectively over an 18-year period. Although this was initially reassuring, the baseline line assessment occurred relatively late in the course of neurodevelopment and was not reflective of premorbid cognitive ability. Another study similar to the adolescent cohort of the Diabetes Control and Complications Trial[41] showed that, although there was no evidence of a significant loss in IQ in the overall cohort, episodes of severe hypoglycemia were again prognostic of cognitive outcome. This again was age dependent with severe hypoglycemia under 6 years of age having the most pronounced effect (a loss of 1.3 SD in IQ compared with controls) and episodes between 6 and 10 years of age (a loss of 0.7 SD).[42] A cross-sectional MR study of a slightly older adult cohort showed no differences between T1D patients and controls in white matter; however, the T1D cohort showed reduced gray matter volumes in numerous regions, on this occasion showing association both with exposure to severe hypoglycemia and chronic hyperglycemia.[43,44] In adults, an accelerated aging effect on brain function seems to be also mediated by long-term exposure to hyperglycemia, hypertension, and microvascular disease, including nephropathy, retinopathy, and neuropathy, which are all associated with cognitive deficits.[40,45] There are increasing similarities noted between the brain injury of T1D in adults and Alzheimer's disease, with several shared cerebrospinal fluid biomarkers.[46]

MECHANISMS OF INJURY

Glucose is essential for neuronal metabolism and function. At the cellular level, glucose undergoes glycolysis (a sequence of 10 catalyzed reactions) to generate adenosine triphosphate, and the monocarboxylic acids pyruvate and lactate.[47] Pyruvate and lactate in turn fuel the tricarboxylic acid cycle (generating more adenosine triphosphate). At the neuronal level, adenosine triphosphate is required for transmembrane ion pump activity, which in turn allows for maintenance of transmembrane voltage gradients, action potentials, and subsequent neurotransmission.[1] Pyruvate and lactate are also chemical precursors to the neurotransmitters acetylcholine, glutamate and γ-aminobutyric acid. Pyruvate and lactate, along with ketone bodies (acetoacetate and β-hydroxybutyrate) and free fatty acids (FFAs), are themselves also secondary fuel sources for neurons.[47]

Glucose is taken up by neurons via the glucose transporter proteins (GLUTs 1–12) and the H-myo-inositol transporter.[48] The dominant GLUTs in the central nervous system are GLUT1 and GLUT3, maximally expressed in glial cells and neurons respectively. These 2 transporters are upregulated in response to hypoglycemia and hypoxia in an insulin-independent manner. Both transporters act in a bidirectional fashion that allows for equilibration rather than accumulation of glucose. Secondary fuel sources, pyruvate, lactate, and ketone bodies are transported across neuronal membranes via monocarboxylate transporters.[48] Glucose is presented to the brain from the circulation across the blood–brain barrier, where endothelial junctions are opposed to perivascular astrocytic processes. Brain extracellular fluid levels of glucose are approximately 30% of circulating glucose levels with 20 to 30 minutes' equilibration times during periods of variation in blood glucose.[49] Not all glucose is metabolized immediately, with the main reserve existing in the form of cerebral glycogen. The bulk of this is held within astrocytes at levels several fold greater than cerebral glucose levels under physiologic conditions.[50] In vitro studies have shown that stable glucose levels are essential for neuronal function and activity.[3,51,52] Periods of low or high glucose levels, analogous to hypoglycemia and hyperglycemia, respectively, result in decreased neuronal activity and survival. Periods of rapid glucose fluctuation, analogous to the glycemic variation of diabetic dysglycemia, also result in neuronal injury, perhaps more profoundly so than in a unidimensional glycemic insult.[52]

In periods of sustained insulinopenia or energy restriction, ketone bodies can serve as the primary cerebral energy source, providing up to 60% of metabolic requirements.[53] Ketone bodies can also have direct influences on brain activity by causing increased levels of vascular permeability factor and the vasoconstrictor endothelin-1.[54] In vivo animal studies have shown both benefits and injury to the brain from excessive ketosis, which are again related to context. Although exogenously administered ketones have been shown to reduce infarction and edema in response to hypoxic brain injury,[55] ketones generated in a model of endogenous ketoacidosis resulted in reduced cerebral blood flow and production of high-energy phosphate metabolites.[56]

Alternative cerebral energy resources include triglycerides, FFAs, and amino acids. FFAs are released from the metabolism of triglycerides.[57] Amino acids are both important substrates for gluconeogenesis and neurotransmitters in their own right, and there are several active transport systems for them across the blood–brain barrier.[58] Among the amino acids, glutamate is noteworthy. Glutamate is the most abundant free amino acid in the brain and acts as an excitatory neurotransmitter in the mammalian nervous system.[59] Unlike other amino acids and alternative energy substrates, glutamate does not cross the blood–brain readily and it seems to be present mostly as a consequent rather than precursor metabolite of the tricarboxylic acid cycle.[60] Glutamate, however, is also the precursor metabolite for the dominant inhibitory neurotransmitter γ-aminobutyric acid.[60] Finally, both lactate and pyruvate, the intermediary metabolites between glucose and the tricarboxylic acid pathway, can also act as a reserve energy supply with brain extracellular fluid lactate levels being 3-fold greater than circulating lactate levels under physiologic conditions.[49] FFAs, amino acids, lactate, and pyruvate are efficient secondary metabolic fuel reserves with exogenous administration of each causing cognitive recovery in an insulin clamp model of induced hypoglycemia.[61–64]

Apart from energy metabolites, glucose-regulating hormones also have direct effects on the central nervous system. Both insulin and C-peptide cross the blood–brain barrier. Insulin receptors are widely distributed throughout the brain and, although insulin is not required for glucose uptake by neurons and astrocytes, insulin seems to play an important role in energy homeostasis and cognitive function within the central nervous system.[65] Insulin also increases synapse density and dendritic plasticity in visual pathways as well as glucose utilization of neuronal networks.[66] Decreased brain levels of insulin and C-peptide deficiencies may impact on neural survival through withdrawal of trophic factors (such as insulin-like growth factor-1 and nerve growth factor), leading to gray matter atrophy, and increased oxidative stress leading to neural apoptosis and white matter atrophy.[51] Counterregulatory hormones are also relevant, affecting either directly or indirectly cognitive processes within the brain.[67,68]

Notwithstanding the pleotropic array of potential mechanisms for neuronal injury in T1D, unstable blood glucose levels outside the physiologic range (dysglycemia) are an inevitable consequence of nonphysiologic insulin replacement and the primary insult. Dysglycemia can be characterized as extremes of glycemia—hypoglycemia and hyperglycemia—or rapid variations in glycemia—glycemic variation. Diabetic dysglycemia can be further subcategorized into mild to severe hypoglycemia (with altered conscious state and or seizure), prolonged hyperglycemia with or without ketoacidosis, and intraday or interday glycemic variation.

Hypoglycemia

Hypoglycemia is the form of dysglycemia that is associated most readily with neuronal insult. The cognitive effects of mild hypoglycemia induced by insulin clamp studies have been known for some time. Progressive cognitive dysfunction seems to occur below a blood glucose level of 3.0 to 3.5 mmol/L.[69,70] The cognitive tests affected in these clamp studies included reaction time, trail making, and the Stroop test (**Fig. 1**). These effects seem to be transitory, with rapid recovery occurring upon reestablishment of euglycemia.

Severe hypoglycemia can cause altered conscious state, progressing to seizures or coma and ultimately death.[71] The Diabetes Control and Complications Trial showed that increased rates severe hypoglycemia were an inevitable consequence of lower hemoglobin A1C levels; however, with the advent of greater therapeutic insight, more predictable analog insulins and continuous subcutaneous insulin infusion therapy this paradigm seems to no longer be inevitable.[72] Nonetheless, data from Germany and the United States indicate that severe hypoglycemia still occurs at frequency rates of 2% to 3% per year in pediatric populations under 6 years of age with T1D.[73] An opportunistic study of 4 individuals who had hypoglycemic seizures while wearing continuous glucose monitoring devices has shown that profound hypoglycemia must be continually present for several hours before a seizure occurs (**Fig. 2**).[74] Rat studies have shown that just 1 episode of severe hypoglycemia followed by recovery in nondiabetic Wistar rats results in neuronal apoptosis and gliosis and a marked upregulation in neuronal GLUTs (**Fig. 3**). It is unethical to induce hypoglycemia causing loss of consciousness and/or seizure in humans; thus, the associated acute brain changes have been poorly studied. Severe hypoglycemia seems to cause injury within the cortex, particularly the temporal and hippocampal regions, basal ganglia, and substantia nigra.[75,76] In addition to cortical neuronal injury, there also seems to be subcortical white matter axonal injury involving major white matter tracts, such as the corpus callosum and internal capsule.[77] Very limited studies have shown that these changes may be reversible in part with 1 adult case showing reversal of changes diffusivity.[78] Another series of 3 prepubertal patients who underwent MR brain examination and cognitive assessment within 24 hours of hypoglycemic seizures initially showed altered spectroscopy. Reduced N-acetylaspartate in the frontal lobe was seen in all 3 patients and increased levels of trimethylamines in the temporal lobe were seen in 2 of the 3 patients. These metabolites are markers of neuronal density/activity and membrane turnover, respectively, and they improved over the 6-month follow-up period. Although there was some variation in cognitive function, all 3 patients showed significantly reduced selective attention, which also improved over the follow-up period.[76]

Hyperglycemia and Ketoacidosis

Acute hyperglycemia in and of itself does not result in a severe cognitive phenotype, such as loss of consciousness. Insulin clamp studies, however, have shown acute

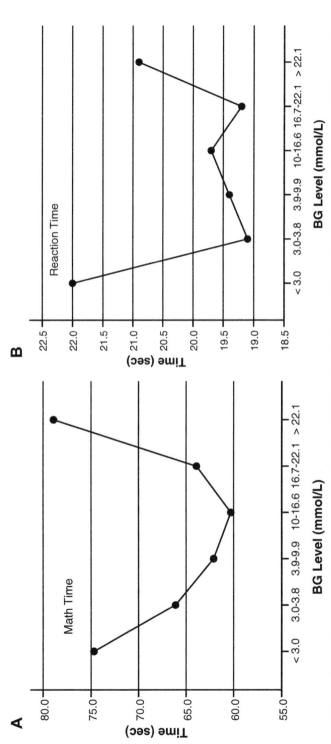

Fig. 1. Glucose thresholds causing alteration in cognitive function. (*A*) Mental math time and (*B*) reaction time across blood glucose (BG) ranges. Sixty-one children with type 1 diabetes (TDM) aged 6 to 11 years took cognitive tests, 70 trials over 4 to 6 weeks with intercurrent BG levels recorded. (*From* Gonder-Frederick LA, Zrebiec JF, Bauchowitz AU, et al. Cognitive function is disrupted by both hypo- and hyperglycemia in school-aged children with type 1 diabetes: a field study. Diabetes Care 2009;32:1003; with permission.)

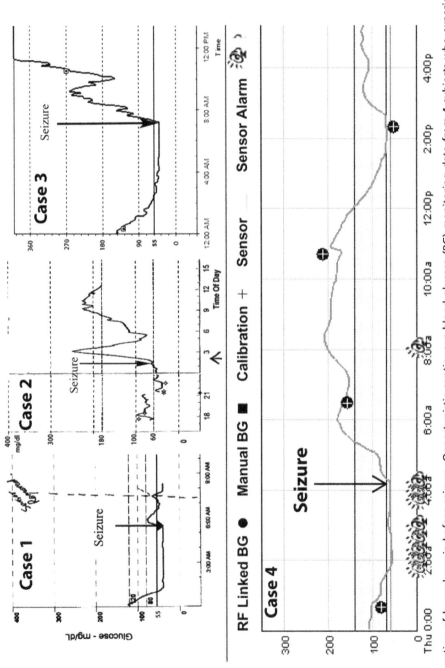

Fig. 2. Duration of hypoglycemia before seizure. Opportunistic continuous blood glucose (BG) monitoring data from 4 subjects who experienced hypoglycemic seizures. Several hours of significant hypoglycemia occurred in all patients before a seizure. (*From* Buckingham B, Wilson DM, Lecher T, et al. Duration of nocturnal hypoglycaemia before seizure. Diabetes Care 2008;31:2111; with permission.)

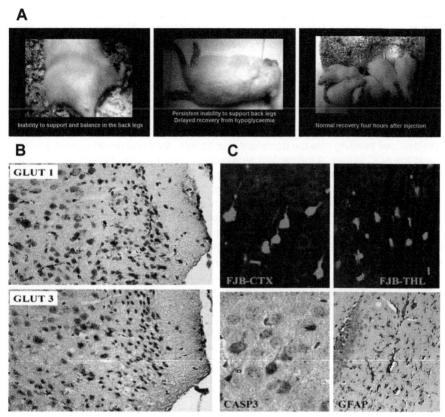

Fig. 3. Effects of a single episode of severe hypoglycemia on a Wistar rat brain. (*A*) Sustained hypoglycemia (<2.8 mmol/L for >1 hour) in 21-day-old Wistar rats (~55 g) using intra-peritoneal insulin injection. (*B*) Activation of glucose transporters. (*C*) Neuronal degenera-tion and apoptosis. CASPASE 3, immunohistochemical marker of apoptosis; CTX, cortex; FJB, histochemical stain marker for neuronal degeneration; GFAP, immunohistochemical marker of gliosis; GLUT, glucose transporter; THL, thalamus.The GLUT-1 stain was with an Anti-GLUT1 (AB1340; Chemicon, Temecula, CA) at 1/500, immunohistochemical staining was performed with Vectastain elite ABC kit (Vector Labs, Burlingame, CA) and slides coun-terstained with Haematoxylin. Magnification was 10× (each of the blue dots, nucleus and the brown stain is about 25 microns in diameter) The neurodegeneration stain (FJB) was performed with with Fluoro-Jade C which stains degenerating/apoptotic neurons. Filter sys-tem was Fluorescein/ FITC, magnification was 40× (each of green neurons are about 25 mi-crons in diameter). Caspase 3 stain was performed with anti-Caspase 3 (SC-7148; Santa Cruz) at 1/500 with immunohistochemical staining performed with Vectastain elite ABC kit (Vector Labs, Burlingame, CA). GFAP stain was with anti GFAP (Chemicon, Temecula, CA) at 1/1000 Immunohistochemical staining performed with Vectastain elite ABC kit (Vector Labs), magnification was 10×. (*Courtesy of* V. Russo, MD.)

subtle cognitive dysfunction[70,79] that mirror the effects of hypoglycemia (see **Fig. 1**). Behavioral changes are also evident. Hyperglycemia measured over 3 days with contin-uous glucose monitoring has been shown to be associated positively with externalizing behavior scores as measured by the Behavior Assessment System for Children.[80]

Hyperglycemia associated with ketoacidosis, on the other hand, can be associated with coma or, in the most clinically feared clinical scenario, cerebral edema. Cerebral edema is a life-threatening, enigmatic complication of DKA that is almost exclusively seen in children and adolescents aged less than 15 years.[81] There has been some debate as to whether the underlying mechanism as vasogenic (leakage of fluid from the vascular space) or cytotoxic (leakage of fluid from hypoxic and ischemic central nervous system cells). Animal models and MR studies have been utilized to investigate these potential mechanisms of injury. MR data from pediatric studies have shown increased apparent diffusion coefficient (ADC) values and increased cerebral blood flow, indicating that the edema developing during DKA treatment may be vasogenic.[82] Increased ADC values are a consequence of increased extravascular water content. If cytotoxic cell swelling was the dominant mechanism, then one would expect a restriction in the ADC values. A further MR study used measures of diffusivity and relaxometry in pediatric patients presenting with severe DKA 6 to 12 hours after initial DKA treatment and stabilization and 96 hours after correction of DKA.[83] Relaxometry measures reflect progression of myelination and normally shorten during childhood development. In this study, relaxometry values were significantly increased during initial DKA resuscitation in both white and gray matter. ADC values were increased, implying a large component of cell membrane water diffusion, and correlated with regional relaxometry changes supporting a mechanism of vasogenic edema. A cytotoxic mechanism of injury, on the other hand, is supported by animal studies that suggest that the characteristics of cerebral perfusion, metabolism, and edema during DKA are similar to those observed during cerebral ischemia and reperfusion. Patients with DKA before resuscitation with intravenous fluids show low cerebral ADC values (suggesting cytotoxic edema) and low cerebral blood flow.[56,84] Brain lactate levels are elevated and levels of high-energy phosphates are decreased.[85] However, after resuscitation has commenced, cerebral blood flow and ADC increase and high-energy phosphates and ratios of N-acetylaspartate to creatinine (an indicator of neuronal health) decline in a similar fashion to that which occurs during the phases of cerebral injury from hypoxia–ischemia.[85] These MR changes do not seem to correlate with speed of rehydration during resuscitation.[86]

DKA can also impact on the brain in the absence of cerebral edema. Numerous biochemical changes occur within the brain at the time of DKA and after resuscitation. Increased levels of ketones and lactate and decreased levels of N-acetylaspartate within the brain at presentation were found to be associated with impaired mental state.[87,88] A recent prospective study of children and adolescents with and without DKA at T1D diagnosis (who did not have cerebral edema) showed that DKA was associated with significant MR brain changes that correlated with cognitive outcome 6 months after diagnosis.[89] In the DKA group, mental state scores were lower at diagnosis. Contemporaneous cerebral white matter volume measured directly and by diffusivity was found to have increased in frontal, temporal, and parietal lobes and in the total brain. By contrast, gray matter volumes were reciprocally decreased so there was no overall impact on total brain volume. Lower levels of N-acetylaspartate were noted in the DKA group at baseline in the frontal gray matter and basal ganglia. These changes correlated positively with younger age and degree of acidosis. Although alterations in brain volumes resolved over the initial postresuscitation period, they were associated with poorer delayed memory recall and poorer sustained and divided attention at 6 months.

Glycemic Variation

There is currently much debate as to the significance of glycemic variation as a determinant of long-term diabetes-related complications.[90] Much of the debate, however, is clouded by a lack of definition of an optimal metric of glycemic variation and a minimal set of standards for a glycemic dataset to be eligible for analysis.[91] Thus, data from clinical enquiries of glycemic variation potentially causing brain injury are lacking. In vitro data, however, are suggestive that significant fluctuations in ambient glucose may be neurotoxic. Neural cell culture models have shown that 6 hourly fluctuations in glucose levels resulted in significantly decreased levels of mitochondrial activity and activation of intrinsic/mitochondrial apoptotic pathways.[52] The degree of neuronal insult induced by fluctuating glucose levels was greater than that seen be either prolonged elevation or depression of glucose levels.[52] Although these changes have been replicated in other in vitro cell systems, such as endothelial cells,[92] the potential role of glycemic variation in brain injury in vivo remains undefined.

IMPLICATIONS FOR MANAGEMENT OF TYPE 1 DIABETES

Arguably the most important developmental imperative is optimal neurodevelopment. Cognitive development, mental health, and personality are fundamental foundations to individual identity and life trajectory. Strategies that reduce the impact of T1D on brain development are thus highly desirable. Such strategies may align with efforts to improve glycemia and may include novel forms of insulin replacement through either mechanical or biological means. As mentioned, there is some preliminary evidence that insulin pump therapy may improve both cognitive and behavioral outcomes, although this remains to be confirmed in controlled trials. Other strategies, however, may be adjunctive and target the brain independently of the glycemic milieu. These remain to be elucidated in humans but in vitro and in vivo animal studies indicate that potential therapies may include alternative energy substrates such as pyruvate, lactate, or FFAs; replacement of neurotrophic hormones such as C-peptide and insulin-like growth factor-1; blockade of neuronal receptors of counterregulatory hormones such as cortisol; and existing neuronal membrane-stabilizing agents. Psychological and cognitive interventions may also play a significant role both in terms of effecting behavioral change to improve overall glycemic control and in assisting recovery after any neurologic injury. To date, much of the adjunctive therapeutic research in T1D has been focused on those organ systems affected by microvascular pathology. The next frontier in T1DM management should now be exploring the utility of therapies that protect neurodevelopment and hinder neurosenescence.

SUMMARY

The evidence of an injurious effect of T1D upon brain development of children and adolescents is now well-established,[24] although the mechanisms, synergies, and hierarchical importance of individual dysglycemic insults remain unclear (**Fig. 4**). Age of T1D onset and subsequent cognitive outcome seems to be the most robust association[93,94] with the magnitude of effects sizes increasing from small to moderate in children with onset before 5 or 6 years compared with age-matched controls.[46] Otherwise, associations between severe hypoglycemia under 5 or 6 years of age and poorer cognition have been documented consistently in the pediatric and adult literature,[8,42,95] particularly compromising verbal intelligence[96] and memory.[11,20,97] Chronic hyperglycemia is now also regarded as a potential contributor with associations appearing between time-weighted hemoglobin A1C levels and cognitive outcomes in childhood and adolescence.[7,8,97] The net contribution of childhood dysglycemia of T1DM on brain development has perhaps been most eloquently described by the "diathesis hypothesis."[98] This model, based on the available evidence, suggests that the most neurotoxic combination is early life severe hypoglycemia followed by chronic hyperglycemia in later life. It is only recently that other clinical

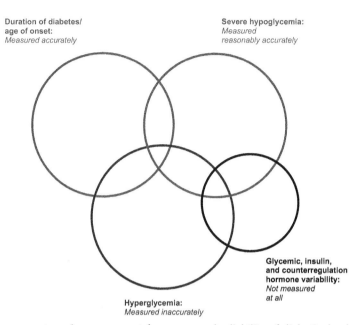

Fig. 4. Components and measurement frequency and reliability of diabetic dysglycemia.

variables, such as ketoacidosis, have also been implicated. The potential impacts of glycemic variation and hormonal variation and their interrelationships have yet to be fully investigated. Although there is an ever increasing armamentarium of imaging tools that can be used to study brain development, the methodologic challenges of truly quantifying dysglycemia remain.[99] However, there is a clear clinical imperative to pursue such research. Optimal brain development must remain the single most important developmental task of childhood and adolescence. In the context of T1D, there is an imperative to define treatments that mitigate aberrant neurochemistry, provide neuroprotection, and decrease cognitive and affective morbidity.

REFERENCES

1. Magistretti PJ, Pellerin L, Martin JL. Brain energy metabolism an integrated cellular perspective. In: Bloom FE, Kupfer DJ, editors. Psychopharmacology: the fourth generation of progress. New York: Raven Press, Ltd; 2000. Available at: http://www.acnp.org/g4/GN401000064/Default.htm.
2. Kuzawa CW, Chugani HT, Grossman LI, et al. Metabolic costs and evolutionary implications of human brain development. Proc Natl Acad Sci U S A 2014;111: 13010–5.
3. Tomlinson DR, Gardiner NJ. Glucose neurotoxicity. Nat Rev Neurosci 2008;9: 36–45.
4. Stanescu DE, Lord K, Lipman TH. The epidemiology of type 1 diabetes in children. Endocrinol Metab Clin North Am 2012;41:679–94.
5. Chong JW, Craig ME, Cameron FJ, et al. Marked increase in type 1 diabetes mellitus in children aged 0-14 yr in Victoria, Australia, from 1999 to 2002. Pediatr Diabetes 2007;8:67–73.
6. Anderson V, Spencer-Smith M, Wood A. Do children really recover better? Neurobehavioural plasticity after early brain insult. Brain 2011;134:2197–221.

7. Patino-Fernandez AM, Delamater AM, Applegate EB, et al. Neurocognitive functioning on preschool-age children with type 1 diabetes. Pediatr Diabetes 2010; 11:424–30.

8. Aye T, Reiss A, Kesler S, et al. The feasibility of detecting neuropsychologic and neuroanatomic effects of type 1 diabetes in young children. Diabetes Care 2011; 34:1458–62.

9. Aye T, Barnea-Goraly N, Ambler C, et al. White matter structural differences in young children with type 1 diabetes: a diffusion tensor imaging study. Diabetes Care 2012;35:2167–73.

10. Shehata G, Eltayeb A. Cognitive function and event-related potentials in children with type 1 diabetes mellitus. J Child Neurol 2010;25:469–74.

11. Hershey T, Perantie DC, Warren SL, et al. Frequency and timing of severe hypoglycaemia affects spatial memory in children with type 1 diabetes. Diabetes Care 2005;28:2372–7.

12. Cato MA, Mauras N, Ambrosino J, et al. Cognitive functioning in young children with type 1 diabetes. J Int Neuropsychol Soc 2014;20:238–47.

13. Marzelli MJ, Mazaika PK, Barnea-Goraly N, et al. Neuroanatomical correlates of dysglycemia in young children with type 1 diabetes. Diabetes 2014;63(1): 343–53.

14. Barnea-Goraly N, Raman M, Mazaika P, et al. Alterations in white matter structure in young children with type 1 diabetes. Diabetes Care 2014;37:332–40.

15. Perantie DC, Wu J, Koller JM, et al. Regional brain volume differences associated with hyperglycemia and severe hypoglycemia in youth with type 1 diabetes. Diabetes Care 2007;30:2331–7.

16. Perantie DC, Koller JM, Weaver PM, et al. Prospectively determined impact of type 1 diabetes on brain volume during development. Diabetes 2011;60:3006–14.

17. Northam EA, Rankins D, Lin A, et al. Central nervous system function in youth with type 1 diabetes 12 years after disease onset. Diabetes Care 2009;32:445–50.

18. Pell GS, Lin A, Wellard RM, et al. Age-related loss of brain volume and T2 relaxation time in youth with type 1 diabetes. Diabetes Care 2012;35:513–9.

19. Lin A, Northam EA, Rankins D, et al. Neuropsychological profiles of young people with type 1 diabetes 12 yr after disease onset. Pediatr Diabetes 2010;11: 235–43.

20. Northam EA, Lin A, Finch S, et al. Psychosocial well-being and functional outcomes in youth with type 1 diabetes 12 years after disease onset. Diabetes Care 2010;33:1430–7.

21. Wootton-Gorges SL, Buonocore MH, Caltagirone RA, et al. Progressive decrease in N-acetylaspartate/Creatine ratio in a teenager with type 1 diabetes and repeated episodes of ketoacidosis without clinically apparent cerebral edema: evidence for permanent brain injury. AJNR Am J Neuroradiol 2010;31:780–1.

22. Gaudieri PA, Greer TF, Chen R, et al. Cognitive function in children with type 1 diabetes: a meta-analysis. Diabetes Care 2008;31:1892–7.

23. Naguib JM, Kulinskaya E, Lomax CL, et al. Neuro-cognitive performance in children with type 1 diabetes – a meta-analysis. J Pediatr Psychol 2009;34: 271–82.

24. Brands AM, Biessels GJ, de Haan EH, et al. The effects of type 1 diabetes on cognitive performance: a meta-analysis. Diabetes Care 2005;28:726–35.

25. McCrimmon RJ, Ryan CM, Frier BM. Diabetes and cognitive dysfunction. Lancet 2012;379:2291–9.

26. Biessels GJ, Staekenborg S, Brunner E, et al. Risk of dementia in diabetes mellitus: a systematic review. Lancet Neurol 2006;5:64–74.

27. Dahlquist G, Källén B. School performance in children with type 1 diabetes-a population-based register study. Diabetologia 2007;50:957–64. Available at: http://www.ncbi.nlm.nih.gov/pubmed?term=Swedish%20Childhood%20Diabetes%20Study%20Group%5BCorporate%20Author%5D.

28. Persson S, Dahlquist G, Gerdtham UG, et al. Impact of childhood-onset type 1 diabetes on schooling: a population-based register study. Diabetologia 2013; 56:1254–62.

29. Hannonen R, Komulainen J, Rikonen R, et al. Academic skills in children with early-onset type 1 diabetes: the effects of diabetes-related risk factors. Dev Med Child Neurol 2012;54:457–63.

30. McNally K, Rohan J, Pendley JS, et al. Executive functioning, treatment adherence, and glycaemic control in children with type 1 diabetes. Diabetes Care 2010;33:1159–62.

31. Cameron FJ, Northam EA, Ambler GR, et al. Routine psychological screening in youth with type 1 diabetes and their parents: a notion whose time has come? Diabetes Care 2007;30:2716–24.

32. Ducat L, Philipson LH, Anderson BJ. The mental health comorbidities of diabetes. JAMA 2014;312:691–2.

33. Reynolds KA, Helgeson V. Children with diabetes compared to peers: depressed? Distressed? Ann Behav Med 2011;42:29–41.

34. Lustman PJ, Anderson RJ, Freedland KE, et al. Depression and poor glycemic control: a meta-analytic review of the literature. Diabetes Care 2000;23:934–42.

35. Anderson RJ, Freedland KE, Clouse RE, et al. The prevalence of comorbid depression in adults with diabetes. Diabetes Care 2001;24:1069–78.

36. McIntyre RS, Kenna HA, Nguyen HT, et al. Brain volume abnormalities and neurocognitive deficits in diabetes mellitus: points of pathophysiological commonality with mood disorders? Adv Ther 2010;27:63–80.

37. Lyoo IK, Yoon SJ, Musen G, et al. Altered prefrontal glutamate-glutamine-gamma-aminobutyric acid levels and relation to low cognitive performance and depressive symptoms in type 1 diabetes mellitus. Arch Gen Psychiatry 2009;66:878–87.

38. Knight S, Northam E, Donath S, et al. Improvements in cognition, mood and behaviour following commencement of continuous subcutaneous insulin infusion therapy in children with type 1 diabetes mellitus: a pilot study. Diabetologia 2009;52:193–8.

39. Knight SJ, Northam EA, Cameron FJ, et al. Behaviour and metabolic control in children with type 1 diabetes mellitus on insulin pump therapy: 2-year follow-up. Diabet Med 2011;28:1109–12.

40. Jacobson AM, Musen G, Ryan CM, et al. Long-term effect of diabetes and its treatment on cognitive function. N Engl J Med 2007;356:1842–52.

41. Musen G, Jacobson AM, Ryan CM, et al. Impact of diabetes and its treatment on cognitive function among adolescents who participated in the diabetes control and complications trial. Diabetes Care 2008;31:1933–8.

42. Asvold B, Sand T, Hestad K, et al. Cognitive function in type 1 diabetic adults with early exposure to severe hypoglycaemia. Diabetes Care 2010;33:1945–7.

43. Musen G, Lyoo IK, Sparks CR, et al. Effects of type 1 diabetes on gray matter density as measured by voxel-based morphometry. Diabetes 2006;55:326–33.

44. Weinger K, Jacobson AM, Musen G, et al. The effects of type 1 diabetes on cerebral white matter. Diabetologia 2008;51:417–25.

45. Ferguson SC, Blane A, Perros P, et al. Cognitive ability and brain structure in type 1 diabetes: relation to microangiopathy and preceding severe hypoglycaemia. Diabetes 2003;52:149–56.

46. Ouwens DM, van Duinkerken E, Schoonenboom SN, et al. Cerebrospinal fluid levels of Alzheimer's disease biomarkers in middle-aged patients with type 1 diabetes. Diabetologia 2014;57:2208–14.
47. Qutub AA, Hunt CA. Glucose transport to the brain: a systems model. Brain Res Brain Res Rev 2005;49:595–617.
48. Simpson IA, Carruthers A, Vannucci SJ. Supply and demand in cerebral energy metabolism: the role of nutrient transporters. J Cereb Blood Flow Metab 2007;27:1766–91.
49. Abi-Saab WM, Maggs DG, Jones T, et al. Striking differences in glucose and lactate levels between brain extracellular fluid and plasma in conscious human subjects: effects of hyperglycemia and hypoglycemia. J Cereb Blood Flow Metab 2002;22:271–9.
50. Oz G, Seaquist ER, Kumar A, et al. Human brain glycogen content and metabolism: implications on its role in brain energy metabolism. Am J Physiol Endocrinol Metab 2007;292:E946–51.
51. Sima AA. Encephalopathies: the emerging diabetic complications. Acta Diabetol 2010;47:279–93.
52. Russo V, Higgins S, Werther GA, et al. Effects of fluctuating glucose levels on neuronal cells in vitro. Neurochem Res 2012;37:1768–82.
53. Owen OE, Morgan AP, Kemp HG, et al. Brain metabolism during fasting. J Clin Invest 1967;46:1589–95.
54. Isales CM, Min L, Hoffman WH. Acetoacetate and beta-hydroxybutyrate differentially regulate endothelin-1 and vascular endothelial growth factor in mouse brain microvascular endothelial cells. J Diabetes Complications 1999;13:91–7.
55. Guzmán M, Blázquez C. Ketone body synthesis in the brain: possible neuroprotective effects. Prostaglandins Leukot Essent Fatty Acids 2004;70:287–92.
56. Glaser N, Ngo C, Anderson S, et al. Effects of hyperglycemia and effects of ketosis on cerebral perfusion, cerebral water distribution, and cerebral metabolism. Diabetes 2012;61:1831–7.
57. Mitchell RW, On NH, Del Bigio MR, et al. Fatty acid transport protein expression in human brain and potential role in fatty acid transport across human brain microvessel endothelial cells. J Neurochem 2011;17:735–46.
58. Gerich JE. Control of glycaemia. Baillieres Clin Endocrinol Metab 1993;7:551–86.
59. Meldrum BS. Glutamate as a neurotransmitter in the brain: review of physiology and pathology. J Nutr 2000;130:1007S–15S.
60. Hawkins RA. The blood-brain barrier and glutamate. Am J Clin Nutr 2009;90:867S–74S.
61. Page KA, Williamson A, Yu N, et al. Medium-chain fatty acids improve cognitive function in intensively treated type 1 diabetic patients and support in vitro synaptic transmission during acute hypoglycemia. Diabetes 2009;58:1237–44.
62. Rossetti P, Porcellati F, Busciantella Ricci N, et al. Effect of oral amino acids on counterregulatory responses and cognitive function during insulin-induced hypoglycemia in nondiabetic and type 1 diabetic people. Diabetes 2008;57:1905–17.
63. Maran A, Cranston I, Lomas J, et al. Protection by lactate of cerebral function during hypoglycaemia. Lancet 1994;343:16–20.
64. Suh SW, Aoyama K, Matsumori Y, et al. Pyruvate administered after severe hypoglycemia reduces neuronal death and cognitive impairment. Diabetes 2005;54:1452–8.
65. Hallschmid M, Schultes B. Central nervous insulin resistance: a promising target in the treatment of metabolic and cognitive disorders? Diabetologia 2009;52:2264–9.

66. Ott V, Benedict C, Schultes B, et al. Intranasal administration of insulin to the brain impacts cognitive function and peripheral metabolism. Diabetes Obes Metab 2012;14:214–21.
67. McGaugh JL, Gold PE, Van Buskirk R, et al. Modulating influences of hormones and catecholamines on memory storage processes. Prog Brain Res 1975;42:151–62.
68. Gomez-Sanchez EP. The mammalian mineralocorticoid receptor: tying down a promiscuous receptor. Exp Physiol 2010;95:13–8.
69. Ryan CM, Atchison J, Puczynski S, et al. Mild hypoglycemia associated with deterioration of mental efficiency in children with insulin-dependent diabetes mellitus. J Pediatr 1990;117:32–8.
70. Gonder-Frederick LA, Zrebiec JF, Bauchowitz AU, et al. Cognitive function is disrupted by both hypo- and hyperglycemia in school-aged children with type 1 diabetes: a field study. Diabetes Care 2009;32:1001–6.
71. Daneman D. Type 1 diabetes. Lancet 2006;367:847–58.
72. Cooper MN, O'Connell SM, Davis EA, et al. A population-based study of risk factors for severe hypoglycaemia in a contemporary cohort of childhood-onset type 1 diabetes. Diabetologia 2013;56:2164–70.
73. Maahs DM, Hermann JM, DuBose SN, et al. Contrasting the clinical care and outcomes of 2,622 children with type 1 diabetes less than 6 years of age in the United States T1D Exchange and German/Austrian DPV registries. Diabetologia 2014;57:1578–85.
74. Buckingham B, Wilson DM, Lecher T, et al. Duration of nocturnal hypoglycaemia before seizure. Diabetes Care 2008;31:2110–2.
75. Jung SL, Kim BS, Lee KS, et al. Magnetic resonance imaging and diffusion-weighted imaging changes after hypoglycemic coma. J Neuroimaging 2005;15:193–6.
76. Rankins D, Wellard RM, Cameron F, et al. The impact of acute hypoglycemia on neuropsychological and neurometabolite profiles in children with type 1 diabetes. Diabetes Care 2005;28:2771–3.
77. Lo L, Tan AC, Umapathi T, et al. Diffusion-weighted MR imaging in early diagnosis and prognosis of hypoglycemia. AJNR Am J Neuroradiol 2006;27:1222–4.
78. Maekawa S, Aibiki M, Kikuchi K, et al. Time related changes in reversible MRI findings after prolonged hypoglycemia. Clin Neurol Neurosurg 2006;108:511–3.
79. Davis EA, Soong SA, Byrne GC, et al. Acute hyperglycaemia impairs cognitive function in children with IDDM. J Pediatr Endocrinol Metab 1996;9:455–61.
80. McDonnell CM, Northam EA, Donath SM, et al. Hyperglycaemia and externalizing behavior in children with type 1 diabetes. Diabetes Care 2007;30:2211–5.
81. Wolfsdorf J, Craig ME, Daneman D. Diabetic ketoacidosis. Pediatr Diabetes 2007;8:28–43.
82. Glaser NS, Wootton-Gorges SL, Marcin JP, et al. Mechanism of cerebral edema in children with diabetic ketoacidosis. J Pediatr 2004;145:164–71.
83. Figueroa RE, Hoffman WH, Momin Z, et al. Study of subclinical cerebral edema in diabetic ketoacidosis by magnetic resonance imaging T2 relaxometry and apparent diffusion coefficient maps. Endocr Res 2005;31:345–55.
84. Yuen N, Anderson SE, Glaser N, et al. Cerebral blood flow and cerebral edema in rats with diabetic ketoacidosis. Diabetes 2008;57:2588–94.
85. Glaser N, Yuen N, Anderson SE, et al. Cerebral metabolic alterations in rats with diabetic ketoacidosis: effects of treatment with insulin and intravenous fluids and effects of bumetanide. Diabetes 2010;59:702–9.

86. Glaser NS, Wootton-Gorges SL, Buonocore MH, et al. Subclinical cerebral edema in children with diabetic ketoacidosis randomized to 2 different rehydration protocols. Pediatrics 2013;131:e73–80.

87. Wootton-Gorges SL, Buonocore MH, Kuppermann N, et al. Detection of cerebral {beta}-hydroxy butyrate, acetoacetate, and lactate on proton MR spectroscopy in children with diabetic ketoacidosis. AJNR Am J Neuroradiol 2005;26:1286–91.

88. Wootton-Gorges SL, Buonocore MH, Kuppermann N, et al. Cerebral proton magnetic resonance spectroscopy in children with diabetic ketoacidosis. AJNR Am J Neuroradiol 2007;28:895–9.

89. Cameron FJ, Scratch S, Nadebaum C, et al. Neurological consequences of diabetic ketoacidosis at initial presentation of type 1 diabetes in childhood. Diabetes Care 2014;37:1554–62.

90. Cameron FJ, Baghurst PA, Rodbard D. Assessing glycaemic variation: why, when and how? Pediatr Endocrinol Rev 2010;7(Suppl 3):432–44.

91. Neylon OM, Baghurst PA, Cameron FJ. The minimum duration of sensor data from which glycaemic variability can be consistently assessed. J Diabetes Sci Technol 2014;8:273–6.

92. Piconi L, Quagliaro L, Assaloni R, et al. Constant and intermittent high glucose enhances endothelial cell apoptosis through mitochondrial superoxide overproduction. Diabetes Metab Res Rev 2006;22:198–203.

93. Ferguson SC, Blane A, Wardlaw J, et al. Influence of an early-onset age of type 1 diabetes on cerebral structure and cognitive function. Diabetes Care 2005;28:1431–7.

94. Kaufmann L, Pixner S, Starke M, et al. Neurocognition and brain structure in pediatric patients with type 1 diabetes. J Pediatr Neuroradiol 2012;1:25–35.

95. Ly T, Anderson M, McNamara K, et al. Neurocognitive outcomes in young adults with early-onset type 1 diabetes. Diabetes Care 2011;34:2192–7.

96. Rovet JF, Ehrlich RM. The effect of hypoglycaemic seizures on cognitive function in children with diabetes: a 7-year prospective study. J Pediatr 1999;134:503–6.

97. Perantie DC, Lim A, Wu J, et al. Effects of prior hypoglycaemia and hyperglycaemia on cognition in children with type 1 diabetes mellitus. Pediatr Diabetes 2008; 9:87–95.

98. Ryan CM. Why is cognitive function associated with the development of diabetes in early life? The diathesis hypothesis. Pediatr Diabetes 2006;7:289–97.

99. Northam EA, Cameron FJ. Understanding the diabetic brain: new technologies but old challenges. Diabetes 2013;62:341–2.

Interpreting Minor Variations in Thyroid Function or Echostructure:
Treating Patients, Not Numbers or Images

Guy Van Vliet, MD[a],*, Johnny Deladoëy, MD, PhD[a,b]

KEYWORDS

• Overt • Thyroid • Children • Hypothyroidism • Hyperthyroidism • Ultrasonography
• Nodule • Incidental

KEY POINTS

• The results of 5% of any laboratory test are outside the reference ranges.
• Without intervention, these results are often within the reference range when repeated.
• Diagnosing Hashimoto thyroiditis does not require ultrasonography imaging.

MINOR VARIATIONS IN THYROID FUNCTION
Introduction

The measurement of serum hormone concentrations on automated analyzers in clinical biochemistry laboratories allows rapid turnaround times, which may have contributed to practitioners requesting these ever more frequently. Because of the high prevalence and nonspecific clinical presentation of thyroid diseases, evaluation of thyroid function figures prominently on the list of blood tests requested. At our institution, a mother-child tertiary care center, serum thyrotropin (TSH) is measured in 55 samples every day, almost 10 times more than serum cortisol (A. Djemli, personal

The authors have no conflicts of interest to disclose.
Disclosure: The authors are supported by a grant from the Canadian Institutes of Health Research (MOP-130390 to J. Deladoëy) and by private donations to the Girafonds/Fondation du Center Hospitalier Universitaire Sainte-Justine (to J. Deladoëy and G.Van Vliet). J. Deladoëy is chercheur-bousier clinicien junior 2 of the Fonds de Recherche du Québec-Santé.
[a] Department of Pediatrics, Endocrinology Service and Research Center, Centre Hospitalier Universitaire Sainte-Justine, 3175 chemin de la Côte-Ste-Catherine, Montréal, Quebec H3T 1C5, Canada; [b] Department of Biochemistry, University of Montreal, 3175 chemin de la Côte-Ste-Catherine, Montréal, Quebec H3T 1C5, Canada.
* Corresponding author. Centre Hospitalier Universitaire Sainte-Justine, Room 1719, 3175 chemin de la Côte-Ste-Catherine, Montréal, Quebec H3T 1C5, Canada.
E-mail address: guy.van.vliet@umontreal.ca

communication, 2013). Ordering clinicians should be aware of intra-assay and interassay variability when interpreting these results. Beyond that, most practitioners are aware that serum cortisol has marked circadian variation, but may not know about the less striking but nevertheless potentially significant circadian rhythm of serum TSH (discussed later). The changes in normal thyroid hormone parameters during growth require better appreciation, but ethical limitations in drawing blood from normal children has hampered the establishment of age-related references ranges.[1,2]

Isolated Hyperthyrotropinemia

Subclinical hypothyroidism is often defined by an increased serum TSH level with a normal serum free thyroxine (fT_4) level. We argue that the descriptive term isolated hyperthyrotropinemia is more appropriate and that subclinical hypothyroidism should only be used for individuals with high TSH and low fT_4 levels but neither sign nor symptom of hypothyroidism. In addition, serum TSH levels in normal individuals decrease progressively with age (**Fig. 1**) and the use of adult reference intervals results in many young children being labeled as having isolated hyperthyrotropinemia.

Aside from age-related changes, there is a nocturnal surge in TSH.[3] This surge may lead to an erroneous interpretation of TSH level being abnormal: a 10-year-old girl was evaluated in our emergency room for an anxiety attack after seeing a horror movie. Because of tachycardia, a sample was drawn at 2:00 AM to rule out hyperthyroidism and serum TSH level was 9.33 mU/L (with a normal fT_4 level of 9.78 pmol/L); there was no goiter on examination, a repeat serum TSH test at 2:00 PM on the same day

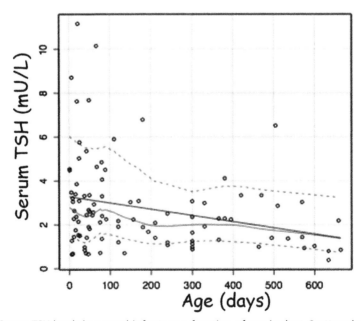

Fig. 1. Serum TSH levels in normal infants as a function of age in days. Scatter plot of individual values (*dots*), regression (*full black line*), lowest fit (*full red line*) and 5th to 95th confidence intervals (*striped red lines*). (*Adapted from* Djemli A, Van Vliet G, Belgoudi J, et al. Reference intervals for free thyroxine, total triiodothyronine, thyrotropin and thyroglobulin for Quebec newborns, children and teenagers. Clin Biochem 2004;37(4):328–30; with permission.)

was normal at 1.79 mU/L and there were no detectable antibodies against thyroperoxidase or thyroglobulin in serum. **Fig. 2** shows the mean ± standard error serum TSH level in normal children over a 24-hour period: to extrapolate to ±2 SD, the normal range of serum TSH at 2:00 AM extends to about 10 mU/L.

Even less well known is the observation of seasonal variation: in the Northern Hemisphere, mean serum TSH is 10% to 15% higher in the winter and, in countries with wide temperature differences, this may lead to overdiagnosing so-called subclinical hypothyroidism.[4]

By far the largest numbers of children referred for isolated hyperthyrotropinemia are those with exogenous obesity. Although excess weight gain caused by hypothyroidism in growing children can easily be distinguished from developing exogenous obesity on clinical grounds alone by assessing height velocity (decreasing in the former, increasing in the latter), many practitioners nevertheless request a serum TSH level, which is occasionally slightly increased. The mechanisms for this association are unclear but serum TSH level decreases if weight loss is achieved and thyroxine treatment in this situation is futile.[5]

Isolated hyperthyrotropinemia in children is often transient, with spontaneous normalization without treatment.[6] In the absence of autoimmunity, a common cause of permanent hyperthyrotropinemia seems to be monoallelic mutations inactivating

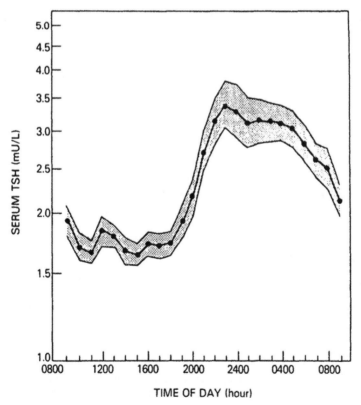

Fig. 2. Mean (± standard error) serum TSH levels in normal children over a 24-hour period. (*From* Rose SR, Nisula BC. Circadian variation of thyrotropin in childhood. J Clin Endocrinol Metab 1989;68(6):1088; with permission.)

the TSH receptor.[7] Because the increase of serum TSH level is an appropriate physiologic response to the relative TSH resistance, which results in normal serum fT_4 concentrations and does not worsen over time, it can be left untreated[8] and serial monitoring of serum TSH is unwarranted, with considerable benefits to the patients and savings to the health care system. A first step in evaluating these children is to obtain a serum TSH level on all first-degree relatives, about 40% of whom also have hyperthyrotropinemia.[7]

Persistent hyperthyrotropinemia of neonatal onset is also observed in some patients with pseudohypoparathyroidism,[9,10] the dysmorphic features becoming more evident as the child ages, or with the brain-lung-thyroid syndrome, in which the respiratory and neurologic phenotypes typically dominate.[11,12] A more complete discussion of the possible causes of isolated, mild neonatal hyperthyrotropinemia and of its likely innocuous nature can be found in our recent review on congenital hypothyroidism.[13]

Isolated Hypothyroxinemia

Isolated hypothyroxinemia is commonly observed in premature neonates. Numerous studies have found the degree of hypothyroxinemia to be correlated with adverse short-term and long-term outcomes. However, correlation does not imply causation, and a landmark double-blind randomized placebo-controlled trial (RCT) showed that thyroxine treatment did not affect outcome.[14] A possible benefit in neonates born before 27 weeks in post-hoc subgroup analyses may be an effect of iodine, not of thyroxine (which contains 66% of iodine by weight). Very premature infants are in negative iodine balance[15] and the results of an RCT comparing the effects of thyroxine and iodine on the neurodevelopmental outcome of such neonates are awaited.[16]

Children with Prader-Willi syndrome often present mild hypothyroxinemia: this is not present on the neonatal screening specimen but develops at older ages, consistent with evolving hypothalamic dysfunction.[17] On stimulation testing with TSH-releasing hormone, the typical hypothalamic profile[18] is only rarely seen. Thus, routine thyroxine administration is not currently recommended for these individuals.[19]

In children receiving growth hormone (GH) replacement for GH deficiency or pharmacologic doses of GH for other conditions, such as Turner syndrome, a slight decrease in fT_4 level is frequently observed. This decrease results from stimulation of deiodination of T_4 to triiodothyronine (T_3) by GH.[20,21] This decrease does not indicate hypothyroidism but these children are nevertheless often given thyroxine. In these cases, previously detectable serum TSH becoming undetectable suggests unjustified or excessive thyroxine treatment, which may be clinically relevant because such treatment advances skeletal maturation more than height itself, therefore potentially decreasing adult height.[22]

Nonthyroidal Illnesses

T_4, a biologically inactive prohormone, can be either activated to T_3 through the actions of deiodinases type 1 and 2 or inactivated to reverse T_3 through deiodinase type 3. Both chronic and acute systemic diseases may result in preferential inactivation of T_4, resulting in the low-T_3 syndrome. When prolonged, severe disease may eventually result in low fT_4 and TSH levels as well, suggesting true central hypothyroidism; this situation is usually seen in patients hospitalized in an intensive care unit (ICU) and is associated with a poor prognosis for survival, but there is no evidence that administering T_4 or T_3 influences outcome.[23] A common cause of suppressed serum TSH in ICUs is the use of dopamine infusions[24]: in 64% of extremely low birth weight neonates, for instance, a dopamine infusion is administered during the first week of life.[25] On recovery from severe nonthyroidal illness, serum TSH levels may be transiently and slightly increased.

Disorders of Thyroid Hormone Metabolism or Transport into the Cells

Over the past decade, the genetic mechanisms underlying 2 seemingly rare syndromes involving disordered thyroid hormone metabolism or transport into the cells have been identified. Deficiency of selenium insertion protein SECISBP2 (also called SBP2), an autosomal recessive condition, may present with a subtle phenotype of an isolated slowing of linear growth and of skeletal maturation.[26] However, consistent with a global effect on selenoproteins, a more severe multisystem disorder can also be observed.[27] Serum selenium level is low and may be the clue to the diagnosis. In contrast, male patients hemizygous for mutations in the gene encoding the monocarboxylate transporter 8 (MCT8, which transports T_3 into certain brain cells) are diagnosed from a dramatic neurologic phenotype known as the Allan-Herndon-Dudley syndrome.[28] The serum levels of thyroid hormones and TSH reflect the different mechanisms of these two conditions: high T_4 and low T_3 in the former, low T_4 and high T_3 in the latter, with normal or slightly increased TSH in both; these abnormalities are often subtle. In boys hemizygous for MCT8 mutations, treatment with diiodothyropropionic acid (a thyroid hormone analogue that does not require MCT8 to enter tissues) normalizes thyroid function and ameliorates metabolism but has no effect on the severe neurologic phenotype.[29] In SBP2 deficiency, T_3 treatment induces transient growth acceleration in children with low serum T_3 levels, whereas selenium replacement increases serum selenium but not selenoproteins synthesis. Antioxidant treatment may be tried in severe cases.[27]

Isolated Serum Thyrotropin Suppression (with Normal or Low Serum Free Thyroxine Level)

In adolescents with anorexia nervosa, a chronically negative caloric balance leads to the low-T_3 syndrome. As in ICU patients, this phenomenon is energy-preserving and should not be treated. In addition, the numerous other endocrine dysfunctions found in anorexia nervosa are thought to have a hypothalamic origin and, consistent with this concept, an isolated decrease in serum TSH level can also be observed. The abnormalities in thyroid function in bulimia nervosa are less well characterized.[30]

Subclinical Hypothyroidism

Worldwide, the commonest cause of subclinical hypothyroidism is iodine deficiency. Although its severe form has been eradicated in many parts of the world where it was previously endemic, its more moderate form is reappearing in some industrialized countries. At the population level, this likely reflects lapses in salt iodization programs[31] but, at the individual level, a dietary history should be obtained to uncover unusual habits.[32]

Among the many challenges pediatricians face in the care of children with Down syndrome is the interpretation of their thyroid function tests. Recent population-based studies[33] do not support earlier claims that overt congenital hypothyroidism is much more common in Down syndrome than in the general population. On the screening specimen, there is a slight shift of the T_4 distribution to the left and of TSH to the right in newborns with Down syndrome compared with normal newborns. These shifts are so mild that they do not result in an increased recall rate after neonatal screening when a TSH cutoff of 15 mU/L is used.[33] They persist throughout growth and are associated with decreased thyroid volume on ultrasonography.[34] This state of relative TSH resistance does not require treatment: another landmark double-blind RCT of thyroxine versus placebo in the Netherlands only found a slight difference favoring thyroxine in one of the motor development subscales at 2 years[35] but this did not translate into higher motor or cognitive scores at age 11 years.[36]

Superimposed on their intrinsic congenital condition and persistent shift in TSH and T_4 distributions, older children of both sexes with Down syndrome (without the female predominance seen in the normal population) have a greater propensity to autoimmune thyroid disease, most commonly Hashimoto thyroiditis.[37] Because some symptoms of hypothyroidism, such as constipation, overlap with characteristics of Down syndrome, regular screening of these children with serum TSH has been advocated. However, this should not distract clinicians from the fact that, as in normal children, slowing of linear growth, which can be observed on Down syndrome–specific growth charts, is the key to making a clinical diagnosis of hypothyroidism in a timely fashion.[38]

Subclinical Hyperthyroidism

Iatrogenic
In a population attending a health fair in Colorado in 1995, 535 of 25,862 adult subjects were found to have subclinical hyperthyroidism. Of subjects taking a thyroid medication, 20.7% had subclinical hyperthyroidism, whereas this was only 0.9% of those who were not taking such medication, suggesting overprescription.[39] This finding was recently confirmed in the general population in the United Kingdom.[40] The overprescription of thyroxine to children has not been specifically studied. However, 38% of children diagnosed as having congenital hypothyroidism (1 in 2300) in the United States have stopped treatment by the age of 4 years,[41] without medical surveillance but without any reports of increased prevalence of recurring hypothyroidism in the ensuing years. By contrast, in the early days of screening, when prevalence was estimated as 1 in 4000 newborns, permanence of hypothyroidism was documented in almost all children.[42] Taken together, this suggests that current screening algorithms have become too sensitive, leading to overdiagnosis and overtreatment.

Neonates born to mothers with Graves disease
Graves disease is often quoted as affecting 1 in 500 pregnant women. However, clinically diagnosed hyperthyroidism in the fetus or in the neonate is exceptional: the computerized database of our service contains 9 such entries over 9 years and our institution provides maternal and neonatal care to a population with about 50,000 births per year, thus validating the often-quoted prevalence of neonatal hyperthyroidism of 1 in 50,000 births. Overt congenital hyperthyroidism is a serious condition in which fetal mortality is still observed, leading to the recommendation that pregnant women with a present or past history of Graves disease should have the titer of TSH receptor antibodies measured in their serum in midpregnancy. However, the justified fear of overt congenital hyperthyroidism should not lead to overdiagnosis and overtreatment. In a recent French series, biochemical hyperthyroidism was present in 7 of 23 neonates born to TSH receptor antibody–positive women but none developed clinical symptoms.[43] Thus, we argue that clinical surveillance (especially of weight gain and heart rate) suffices, being cognizant that, if the mother is treated with antithyroid drugs, hyperthyroidism in her newborn child may be masked during the first few days and become evident later, because of the shorter half-lives of drugs compared with that of TSH receptor–stimulating antibodies.

Hyperfunctioning thyroid nodules
Autonomous thyroid adenomas (or so-called hot nodules) are rare in children and the associated hyperthyroidism is generally mild, with the commonest manifestation being tachycardia. Serum TSH concentrations may be undetectable in spite of normal

fT_4 levels, in which case it is justified to measure serum T_3 (to diagnose T_3 toxicosis).[44,45]

Interference from Cardiovascular, Antiepileptic, and Psychotropic Medications

The most clinically significant interference between nonthyroid medications and thyroid function, TSH suppression by dopamine infusions, was discussed earlier. In addition, several other classes of drugs may interfere with thyroid function testing. Among these, the most widely used are antiepileptic drugs. For instance, serum fT4 level is lower and TSH level higher in epileptic children on valproate than in those on carbamazepine.[46] Newer antipsychotic drugs often induce major weight gain, which may affect serum TSH, as discussed earlier. Less used in children than in adults is the antiarrhythmic drug amiodarone, which has an extremely rich iodine content and may induce both overt hypothyroidism[47] and hyperthyroidism but also more subtle abnormalities in thyroid function tests.[48] Likewise, interferon therapy may induce both overt and subclinical thyroid dysfunction.[49]

MINOR VARIATIONS IN THYROID ECHOSTRUCTURE
Nonpalpable < 1cm Cysts and Nodules

In adults, thyroid abnormalities incidentally discovered on ultrasonography, mostly nonpalpable nodules, have been estimated to occur in a high but variable percentage (13%–67%) of the population. To our knowledge, only 1 clinic-based study has been conducted in children: incidental thyroid findings were observed in 18%. These thyroid findings were mostly cysts and ectopic thymus.[50] Likewise, cysts and ectopic thymus were the commonest findings in a population-based study of Japanese children.[51]

Infracentrimetric cysts within the thyroid are thought to represent degenerated follicles containing serous or colloid fluid, or hemorrhagic debris. Many are hyperechogenic and present the comet-tail artifact (**Fig. 3**), possibly representing microcrystals and indicating a benign lesion. In a limited number of longitudinal observations, these images remained stable or disappeared.[50]

The presence of intrathyroidal thymic tissue is not surprising given the vicinity of the thyroid anlage and of the third branchial pouches during embryogenesis. Consistent

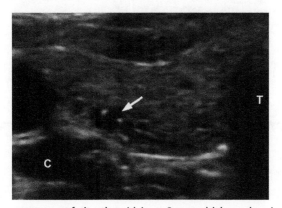

Fig. 3. Transverse sonogram of the thyroid in a 6-year-old boy, showing a cystic lesion (arrow) within the right lobe. In the periphery of the cyst, 2 hyperechoic punctate foci with comet-tail artifact are seen. C, right common carotid artery; T, trachea. (From Avula S, Daneman A, Navarro OM, et al. Incidental thyroid abnormalities identified on neck US for non-thyroid disorders. Pediatr Radiol 2010;40(11):1774–80; with permission.)

with age-related involution of the thymus, ectopic intrathyroidal thymic tissue is more common in young children and decreases in size with age.[52] In contrast with thyroid cysts, which had a female preponderance in the population-based Japanese study,[51] the sex ratio (male/female) for ectopic thyroid thymus was 8:1 in the series from Toronto[50] and 4:5 in the series from Rome.[52] The most important ultrasonography characteristic of this ectopic thymic tissue is that its echostructure is that of normal thymus,[50] just as the echostructure of ectopic thyroid is that of normal thyroid.[13] With age, intrathyroidal ectopic thymic tissue decreases in size and increases in echogenicity (**Fig. 4**).[52] It is therefore reasonable to observe these, with the expectation that they will decrease in size as the child ages, as shown in the longitudinal study of Segni and colleagues[52] (**Table 1**). In a 4-year-old girl with such a lesion, fine-needle aspiration biopsy with flow cytometry analysis allowed clinicians to make the diagnosis without surgery.[53] In a case in Toronto, typical Hassall corpuscles were seen on histopathologic examination.[50] Thyroid scintigraphy is unnecessary in these cases, but if it is performed it reveals, as expected, that the lesion is "cold."[50,53]

Hashimoto Thyroiditis

In contrast with adults with autoimmune hypothyroidism, who present at a more advanced stage of the disease when the thyroid has already atrophied, children and adolescents with Hashimoto thyroiditis most often present with a goiter: 181 of 274 cases (66%) seen over a 5-year period at our institution.[54] Twenty years ago, thyroid scintigraphy was still frequently ordered by referring physicians before consulting a

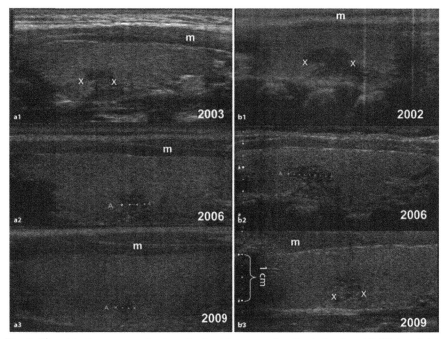

Fig. 4. Thyroid ultrasonography, longitudinal images, of patients 1 (a) and 2 (b) (see table for patient data), show intrathyroidal thymic inclusions that decrease in size and increase in echogenicity over time. m, Muscles. (*From* Segni M, di Nardo R, Pucarelli I, et al. Ectopic intrathyroidal thymus in children: a long-term follow-up study. Horm Res Paediatr 2011;75(4):260; with permission.)

Table 1
Clinical and ultrasonographic characteristics of children with intrathyroidal thymic inclusions (ITI)

Patient No.	Sex	Age at First Observation (y)	Age at Last Observation (y)	Follow-up (mo)	Dimensions of ITI at First Observation (mm)	Dimensions of ITI at Last Observation (mm)
1	M	$11^{7/12}$	$17^{7/12}$	72	R $9.0 \times 7.7 \times 6.4$	$3.9 \times 1.8 \times 2.0$
2	F	6	13	84	R $11 \times 8.0 \times 9.0$	$7 \times 4.5 \times 5.6$
3	F	$1^{1/12}$	$3^{7/12}$	32	R 3.2	$5.6 \times 3.6 \times 3.6$
4	M	$4^{8/12}$	$8^{8/12}$	48	L $10 \times 4.0 \times 2.0$	$6.5 \times 3.4 \times 2.1$
5	M	$4^{2/12}$	$5^{8/12}$	18	L $6.2 \times 3.0 \times 2.1$	$6.0 \times 2.8 \times 2.0$
6	F	6	$9^{2/12}$	38	R $7.0 \times 5.0 \times 6.0$	$6.5 \times 5.0 \times 4.5$
7	F	$4^{2/12}$	$5^{1/12}$	9	L $6.8 \times 9.1 \times 6.0$	$7.0 \times 9.0 \times 6.0$
8	M	$7^{9/12}$	$8^{3/12}$	6	L $4.0 \times 3.7 \times 6.0$	$4.1 \times 3.7 \times 6.0$
9	F	$11^{2/12}$	$11^{9/12}$	6	L $4.6 \times 5.5 \times 2.5$	$3.8 \times 5.4 \times 2.5$

Dimensions are expressed as length × height × depth.
Abbreviations: F, female; L, left lobe; M, male; R, right lobe.
From Segni M, di Nardo R, Pucarelli I, et al. Ectopic intrathyroidal thymus in children: a long-term follow-up study. Horm Res Paediatr 2011;75(4):258–63; with permission.

pediatric endocrinologist, in spite of its uselessness. Over the past 2 decades, this practice has been replaced by the equally useless routine request for thyroid ultrasonography in these patients. The diagnosis of Hashimoto thyroiditis should be based on the clinical finding of a small, generally painless or only mildly sensitive goiter with a firm, pebbly feeling, often accompanied by a delphian node, ranging in size from that of a grain of rice to that of a pea, above the isthmus. The diagnosis can be confirmed by the finding of an increased titer of serum antithyroperoxidase and/or antithyroglobulin antibodies (the former more frequently than the latter). The most commonly associated thyroid dysfunction is hypothyroidism (in our series, 62% of patients, of whom only a third had overt hypothyroidism) but hyperthyroidism (mostly subclinical) can also be observed, albeit rarely (1%).[54]

In spite of the uselessness of ultrasonography examination in the diagnostic work-up for Hashimoto thyroiditis, numerous articles reporting the sonographic characteristics of the thyroid in this condition have been published (reviewed in Ref.[55]). The gland may appear diffusely heterogeneous with a coarse echotexture and multiple discrete hypoechogenic nodules that may reach a diameter of 6 mm, leading to unwarranted concerns about neoplasia.

Another difference between Hashimoto thyroiditis beginning in childhood and adulthood is that the associated hypothyroidism may be more often transient in the former. Complete remission has even been reported with disappearance of the serum thyroid antibodies. Again, thyroid ultrasonography is not required to document remission but sequential images (**Fig. 5**) in one case documented restoration of a normal echostructure.[56]

The Single Thyroid Nodule

A review of the single thyroid nodule measuring more than 1 cm in diameter, which is generally detected clinically and is more often malignant in children than in adults (22% vs 14%),[57] is beyond the scope of this article. However, it is important to

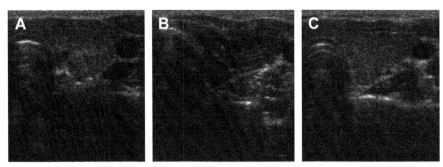

Fig. 5. Representative sequential ultrasonography images of the left lobe of the thyroid in a girl with Hashimoto thyroiditis. (*A*) At age 12 years, when serum antibodies against thyroperoxidase and thyroglobulin were very increased: note thin, patchy texture, slight cystic changes throughout, and pseudonodules. (*B*) Two years later: the gland is slightly bigger and diffusely and markedly hypoechoic. (*C*) One more year later: normal thyroid ultrasonography (and disappearance of the serum antibodies). (*From* Nanan R, Wall JR. Remission of Hashimoto's thyroiditis in a twelve-year-old girl with thyroid changes documented by ultrasonography. Thyroid 2010;20(10):1187–90; with permission.)

remember that, because low-dose external radiation of the neck (including total body irradiation) is a major risk factor for the development of differentiated thyroid carcinoma, children who have been exposed to such radiation should be examined regularly throughout life not only for mild thyroid dysfunction, which is common, but also for the development of thyroid nodules. Careful clinical examination of the neck is therefore mandatory, because ultrasonography screening is not performed routinely.[58] Infracentrimetric nodules are discussed earlier.

Multinodular Goiter

Multinodular goiters are exceeding rare in children[59–61] and are not a minor variation discovered on ultrasonography. As such, they are only mentioned here to underline the novel finding that these may be the sentinel case for identifying pedigrees with the DICER1 cancer predisposition syndrome.[62]

Hemiagenesis

Absence of one of the thyroid lobes, generally the left, is a common congenital anomaly: in 1 population-based study in Belgium, it was present in 1 school-aged child in 500.[63] Most children are euthyroid but hemiagenesis may also be encountered in newborns with a high TSH level at screening.[64,65]

SUMMARY

The increased prescriptions for thyroid function testing and for neck ultrasonography for nonspecific complaints or physical findings predictably generates an increased number of unexpected laboratory results or images. Clinicians should go back to the patient, asking themselves why the test was requested in the first place. Several intellectual concepts and processes are involved in the interpretation of a laboratory result, but common sense remains paramount. In contrast, the discovery of incidental findings on imaging may justify repeating the clinical examination but clinicians should continue to trust their own eyes and fingers more than imaging studies. A continuous dialogue between clinicians, biochemists, and radiologists is also important to evaluate findings of uncertain significance.

REFERENCES

1. Djemli A, Van Vliet G, Belgoudi J, et al. Reference intervals for free thyroxine, total triiodothyronine, thyrotropin and thyroglobulin for Quebec newborns, children and teenagers. Clin Biochem 2004;37(4):328–30.
2. Adeli K. Closing the gaps in pediatric reference intervals: an update on the CALIPER Project. Clin Biochem 2014;47(9):737–9.
3. Rose SR, Nisula BC. Circadian variation of thyrotropin in childhood. J Clin Endocrinol Metab 1989;68(6):1086–90.
4. Kim TH, Kim KW, Ahn HY, et al. Effect of seasonal changes on the transition between subclinical hypothyroid and euthyroid status. J Clin Endocrinol Metab 2013;98(8):3420–9.
5. Reinehr T, de Sousa G, Andler W. Hyperthyrotropinemia in obese children is reversible after weight loss and is not related to lipids. J Clin Endocrinol Metab 2006;91(8):3088–91.
6. Lazar L, Frumkin RB, Battat E, et al. Natural history of thyroid function tests over 5 years in a large pediatric cohort. J Clin Endocrinol Metab 2009;94(5):1678–82.
7. Calebiro D, Gelmini G, Cordella D, et al. Frequent TSH receptor genetic alterations with variable signaling impairment in a large series of children with nonautoimmune isolated hyperthyrotropinemia. J Clin Endocrinol Metab 2012;97(1):E156–60.
8. Lucas-Herald A, Bradley T, Hermanns P, et al. Novel heterozygous thyrotropin receptor mutation presenting with neonatal hyperthyrotropinaemia, mild thyroid hypoplasia and absent uptake on radioisotope scan. J Pediatr Endocrinol Metab 2013;26(5–6):583–6.
9. Yokoro S, Matsuo M, Ohtsuka T, et al. Hyperthyrotropinemia in a neonate with normal thyroid hormone levels: the earliest diagnostic clue for pseudohypoparathyroidism. Biol Neonate 1990;58(2):69–72.
10. Levine MA. An update on the clinical and molecular characteristics of pseudohypoparathyroidism. Curr Opin Endocrinol Diabetes Obes 2012;19(6):443–51.
11. Maquet E, Costagliola S, Parma J, et al. Lethal respiratory failure and mild primary hypothyroidism in a term girl with a de novo heterozygous mutation in the TITF1/NKX2.1 gene. J Clin Endocrinol Metab 2009;94(1):197–203.
12. Carre A, Szinnai G, Castanet M, et al. Five new TTF1/NKX2.1 mutations in brain-lung-thyroid syndrome: rescue by PAX8 synergism in one case. Hum Mol Genet 2009;18(12):2266–76.
13. Deladoey J, Van Vliet G. The changing epidemiology of congenital hypothyroidism: fact or artifact? Expert Rev Endocrinol Metab 2014;9(4):387–95.
14. van Wassenaer AG, Kok JH, de Vijlder JJ, et al. Effects of thyroxine supplementation on neurologic development in infants born at less than 30 weeks' gestation. N Engl J Med 1997;336:21–6.
15. Ares S, Escobar-Morreale HF, Quero J, et al. Neonatal hypothyroxinemia: effects of iodine intake and premature birth. J Clin Endocrinol Metab 1997;82(6):1704–12.
16. La Gamma EF, van Wassenaer AG, Ares S, et al. Phase 1 trial of 4 thyroid hormone regimens for transient hypothyroxinemia in neonates of <28 weeks' gestation. Pediatrics 2009;124(2):e258–68.
17. Fillion M, Deal CL, Van Vliet G. Normal minipuberty of infancy in boys with Prader-Willi syndrome. J Pediatr 2006;149(6):874–6.

18. Costom BH, Grumbach MM, Kaplan SL. Effect of thyrotropin-releasing factor on serum thyroid-stimulating hormone. An approach to distinguishing hypothalamic from pituitary forms of idiopathic hypopituitary dwarfism. J Clin Invest 1971; 50(10):2219–25.
19. Sharkia M, Michaud S, Berthier MT, et al. Thyroid function from birth to adolescence in Prader-Willi syndrome. J Pediatr 2013;163(3):800–5.
20. Jorgensen JO, Pedersen SA, Laurberg P, et al. Effects of growth hormone therapy on thyroid function of growth hormone-deficient adults with and without concomitant thyroxine-substituted central hypothyroidism. J Clin Endocrinol Metab 1989; 69(6):1127–32.
21. Massa G, de Zegher F, Vanderschueren-Lodeweyckx M. Effect of growth hormone therapy on thyroid status of girls with Turner's syndrome. Clin Endocrinol (Oxf) 1991;34(3):205–9.
22. Van den Brande JL, Van Wyk JJ, French FS, et al. Advancement of skeletal age of hypopituitary children treated with thyroid hormone plus cortisone. J Pediatr 1973;82(1):22–7.
23. von Saint Andre-von Arnim A, Farris R, Roberts JS, et al. Common endocrine issues in the pediatric intensive care unit. Crit Care Clin 2013;29(2): 335–58.
24. Williams FL, Ogston SA, van TH, et al. Serum thyroid hormones in preterm infants: associations with postnatal illnesses and drug usage. J Clin Endocrinol Metab 2005;90(11):5954–63.
25. Laughon M, Bose C, Allred E, et al. Factors associated with treatment for hypotension in extremely low gestational age newborns during the first postnatal week. Pediatrics 2007;119(2):273–80.
26. Dumitrescu AM, Liao XH, Abdullah MS, et al. Mutations in SECISBP2 result in abnormal thyroid hormone metabolism. Nat Genet 2005;37(11):1247–52.
27. Schoenmakers E, Agostini M, Mitchell C, et al. Mutations in the selenocysteine insertion sequence-binding protein 2 gene lead to a multisystem selenoprotein deficiency disorder in humans. J Clin Invest 2010;120(12):4220–35.
28. Dumitrescu AM, Liao XH, Best TB, et al. A novel syndrome combining thyroid and neurological abnormalities is associated with mutations in a monocarboxylate transporter gene. Am J Hum Genet 2004;74(1):168–75.
29. Verge CF, Konrad D, Cohen M, et al. Diiodothyropropionic acid (DITPA) in the treatment of MCT8 deficiency. J Clin Endocrinol Metab 2012;97(12):4515–23.
30. Warren MP. Endocrine manifestations of eating disorders. J Clin Endocrinol Metab 2011;96(2):333–43.
31. Pearce EN, Andersson M, Zimmermann MB. Global iodine nutrition: where do we stand in 2013? Thyroid 2013;23(5):523–8.
32. Pacaud D, Van Vliet G, Delvin E, et al. A Third World endocrine disease in a 6-year-old North American boy. J Clin Endocrinol Metab 1995;80(9):2574–6.
33. Deladoey J, Ruel J, Giguere Y, et al. Is the incidence of congenital hypothyroidism really increasing? A 20-year retrospective population-based study in Quebec. J Clin Endocrinol Metab 2011;96(8):2422–9.
34. van Trotsenburg AS, Vulsma T, Van Santen HM, et al. Lower neonatal screening thyroxine concentrations in Down syndrome newborns. J Clin Endocrinol Metab 2003;88(4):1512–5.
35. van Trotsenburg AS, Vulsma T, Rozenburg-Marres SL, et al. The effect of thyroxine treatment started in the neonatal period on development and growth of two-year-old Down syndrome children: a randomized clinical trial. J Clin Endocrinol Metab 2005;90(6):3304–11.

36. Marchal JP, Maurice-Stam H, Ikelaar NA, et al. The effect of early thyroxine treatment on development and growth at the age of 10.7 years: follow-up of a randomized placebo-controlled trial in children with Down syndrome. J Clin Endocrinol Metab 2014;99(12):E2722–9.

37. Popova G, Paterson WF, Brown A, et al. Hashimoto's thyroiditis in Down's syndrome: clinical presentation and evolution. Horm Res 2008;70(5):278–84.

38. Van Vliet G. How often should we screen children with Down's syndrome for hypothyroidism? Arch Dis Child 2005;90(6):557–8.

39. Canaris GJ, Manowitz NR, Mayor G, et al. The Colorado thyroid disease prevalence study. Arch Intern Med 2000;160(4):526–34.

40. Taylor PN, Iqbal A, Minassian C, et al. Falling threshold for treatment of borderline elevated thyrotropin levels-balancing benefits and risks: evidence from a large community-based study. JAMA Intern Med 2014;174(1):32–9.

41. Kemper AR, Ouyang L, Grosse SD. Discontinuation of thyroid hormone treatment among children in the United States with congenital hypothyroidism: findings from health insurance claims data. BMC Pediatr 2010;10:9.

42. Davy T, Daneman D, Walfish PG, et al. Congenital hypothyroidism. The effect of stopping treatment at 3 years of age. Am J Dis Child 1985;139(10):1028–30.

43. Besancon A, Beltrand J, Le Gac I, et al. Management of neonates born to women with Graves' disease: a cohort study. Eur J Endocrinol 2014;170(6):855–62.

44. Mircescu H, Parma J, Huot C, et al. Hyperfunctioning malignant thyroid nodule in an 11-year-old girl: pathologic and molecular studies. J Pediatr 2000;137(4):585–7.

45. Grob F, Deladoey J, Legault L, et al. Autonomous adenomas caused by somatic mutations of the thyroid-stimulating hormone receptor in children. Horm Res Paediatr 2014;29:73–9.

46. Verrotti A, Scardapane A, Manco R, et al. Antiepileptic drugs and thyroid function. J Pediatr Endocrinol Metab 2008;21(5):401–8.

47. Trudel K, Sanatani S, Panagiotopoulos C. Severe amiodarone-induced hypothyroidism in an infant. Pediatr Crit Care Med 2011;12(1):e43–5.

48. Loh KC. Amiodarone-induced thyroid disorders: a clinical review. Postgrad Med J 2000;76(893):133–40.

49. Nair KC, Haamann F, Nienhaus A. Frequency of thyroid dysfunctions during interferon alpha treatment of single and combination therapy in hepatitis C virus-infected patients: a systematic review based analysis. PLoS One 2013;8(2):e55364.

50. Avula S, Daneman A, Navarro OM, et al. Incidental thyroid abnormalities identified on neck US for non-thyroid disorders. Pediatr Radiol 2010;40(11):1774–80.

51. Hayashida N, Imaizumi M, Shimura H, et al. Thyroid ultrasound findings in children from three Japanese prefectures: Aomori, Yamanashi and Nagasaki. PLoS One 2013;8(12):e83220.

52. Segni M, di Nardo R, Pucarelli I, et al. Ectopic intrathyroidal thymus in children: a long-term follow-up study. Horm Res Paediatr 2011;75(4):258–63.

53. Aguayo-Figueroa L, Golightly MG, Hu Y, et al. Cytology and flow cytometry to identify ectopic thymic tissue masquerading as a thyroid nodule in two children. Thyroid 2009;19(4):403–6.

54. Alos N, Huot C, Lambert R, et al. Thyroid scintigraphy in children and adolescents with Hashimoto disease. J Pediatr 1995;127(6):951–3.

55. Chang YW, Hong HS, Choi DL. Sonography of the pediatric thyroid: a pictorial essay. J Clin Ultrasound 2009;37(3):149–57.

56. Nanan R, Wall JR. Remission of Hashimoto's thyroiditis in a twelve-year-old girl with thyroid changes documented by ultrasonography. Thyroid 2010;20(10):1187–90.

57. Gupta A, Ly S, Castroneves LA, et al. A standardized assessment of thyroid nodules in children confirms higher cancer prevalence than in adults. J Clin Endocrinol Metab 2013;98(8):3238–45.

58. Vivanco M, Dalle JH, Alberti C, et al. Malignant and benign thyroid nodules after total body irradiation preceding hematopoietic cell transplantation during childhood. Eur J Endocrinol 2012;167(2):225–33.

59. Leger J, Nihoul-Fekete C, Iris L, et al. Multinodular goiter in children. Arch Fr Pediatr 1987;44(8):579–82 [in French].

60. Al-Fifi S, Rodd C. Multinodular goiter in children. J Pediatr Endocrinol Metab 2001;14(6):749–56.

61. Garcia CJ, Daneman A, Thorner P, et al. Sonography of multinodular thyroid gland in children and adolescents. Am J Dis Child 1992;146(7):811–6.

62. Rath SR, Bartley A, Charles A, et al. Multinodular goiter in children: an important pointer to a germline DICER1 mutation. J Clin Endocrinol Metab 2014;99(6):1947–8.

63. Shabana W, Delange F, Freson M, et al. Prevalence of thyroid hemiagenesis: ultrasound screening in normal children. Eur J Pediatr 2000;159(6):456–8.

64. Devos H, Rodd C, Gagne N, et al. A search for the possible molecular mechanisms of thyroid dysgenesis: sex ratios and associated malformations. J Clin Endocrinol Metab 1999;84(7):2502–6.

65. Castanet M, Leenhardt L, Leger J, et al. Thyroid hemiagenesis is a rare variant of thyroid dysgenesis with a familial component but without Pax8 mutations in a cohort of 22 cases. Pediatr Res 2005;57(6):908–13.

Disorders of Menstruation in Adolescent Girls

Mary Anne Jamieson, MD

KEYWORDS

- Adolescent • Menstrual disturbances • Amenorrhea • Menstruation
- Dysmenorrhea • Abnormal uterine bleeding

KEY POINTS

- Distinguishing whether the teen is ovulatory or not can be helpful in narrowing the differential diagnosis.
- The menstrual cycle can take several months to become regular and ovulatory. Reassurance may be all that is necessary but treat if interfering with activities or depleting the teen (physically and/or emotionally).
- Primary physiologic dysmenorrhea is usually not present at menarche; it accompanies the establishment of ovulatory cycles. Take NSAIDs proactively and be suspicious of endometriosis if properly administered nonsteroidal antiinflammatory drugs (NSAID) in combination with Combined Contraceptives (CCs) fail to control dysmenorrhea. Similarly, be suspicious of outflow obstruction if dysmenorrhea is intractable, if menarche is painful or if puberty is near complete and no menses has occurred.
- CCs offer many benefits but teens and/or parents often have misinformation about safety and side effects that must be addressed.
- Functional amenorrhea is a diagnosis of exclusion and is caused by an imbalance of stress, diet, and/or exercise. These factors can also cause irregular menses.
- It can be difficult to identify polycystic ovarian syndrome (PCOS) patients during adolescence.
- With true menorrhagia, take bleeding history from teen and her family.

INTRODUCTION

Abnormal menstruation in adolescent girls can cause psychological, emotional, and physical strain from excess, unpredictable, painful, or even absent bleeding. This article discusses these common complaints and describes variations of normal, including the maturation of the hypothalamic-pituitary-ovarian (HPO) axis, but goes on to provide indications for reassurance alone versus active intervention. (Figs. 1 and 2) show broad differential diagnoses for common symptoms. It is important for readers to recognize that these key figures and their list of underlying

Department of Obstetrics & Gynecology, Queen's University, 99 University Ave, Kingston, Ontario K7L 3N6, Canada
E-mail address: maj3@queensu.ca

Pediatr Clin N Am 62 (2015) 943–961
http://dx.doi.org/10.1016/j.pcl.2015.04.007
0031-3955/15/$ – see front matter © 2015 Elsevier Inc. All rights reserved.

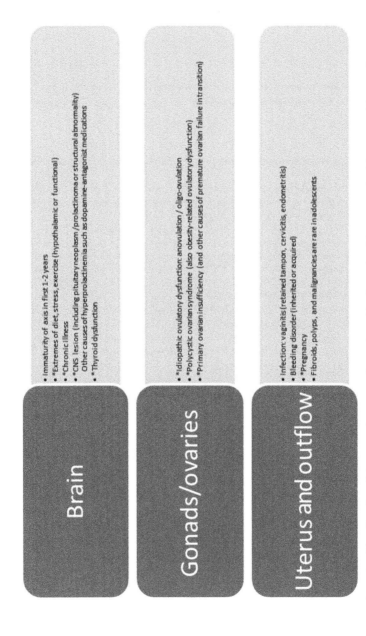

Brain
- Immaturity of axis in first 1-2 years
- *Extremes of diet, stress, exercise (hypothalamic or functional)
- *Chronic illness
- *CNS lesion (including pituitary neoplasm / prolactinoma or structural abnormality)
- Other causes of hyperprolactinemia such as dopamine-antagonist medications
- *Thyroid dysfunction

Gonads/ovaries
- *Idiopathic ovulatory dysfunction: anovulation / oligo-ovulation
- *Polycystic ovarian syndrome (also obesity-related ovulatory dysfunction)
- *Primary ovarian insufficiency (and other causes of premature ovarian failure in transition)

Uterus and outflow
- Infection: vaginitis (retained tampon, cervicitis, endometritis)
- Bleeding disorder (inherited or acquired)
- *Pregnancy
- Fibroids, polyps, and malignancies are rare in adolescents

Fig. 1. Abnormal uterine bleeding in adolescents: heavy, prolonged, and/or irregular (those noted with an asterisk can also present as secondary amenorrhea). CNS, central nervous system.

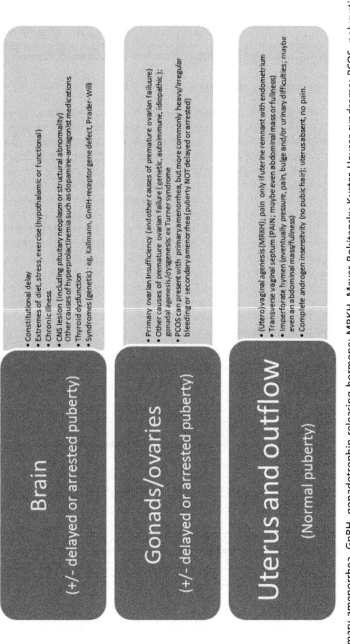

Brain
(+/- delayed or arrested puberty)

- Constitutional delay
- Extremes of diet, stress, exercise (hypothalamic or functional)
- Chronic illness
- CNS lesion (including pituitary neoplasm or structural abnormality)
- Other causes of hyperprolactinemia such as dopamine-antagonist medications
- Thyroid dysfunction
- Syndromes (genetic): eg, Kallmann, GnRH-receptor gene defect, Prader-Willi

Gonads/ovaries
(+/- delayed or arrested puberty)

- Primary ovarian insufficiency (and other causes of premature ovarian failure)
- Other causes of premature ovarian failure (genetic, autoimmune, idiopathic): gonadal agenesis/dysgenesis; ex Turner syndrome
- PCOS can present with primary amenorrhea, but more commonly heavy/irregular bleeding or secondary amenorrhea (puberty NOT delayed or arrested)

Uterus and outflow
(Normal puberty)

- (Utero)vaginal agenesis (MRKH); pain only if uterine remnant with endometrium
- Transverse vaginal septum (PAIN); maybe even abdominal mass or fullness)
- Imperforate hymen (eventually pressure, pain, bulge and/or urinary difficulties; maybe even an abdominal mass/fullness)
- Complete androgen insensitivity (no pubic hair); uterus absent, no pain.

Fig. 2. Primary amenorrhea. GnRH, gonadotrophin-releasing hormone; MRKH, Mayer Rokitansky Kuster Hauser syndrome; PCOS, polycystic ovarian syndrome.

conditions are meant to guide the clinician's history, physical examination, and the choice of investigations. Treatment options are organized according to symptoms and presenting complaints in **Table 1**, which can be referenced regardless of the underlying disorder. The article elaborates on hypothalamic/functional amenorrhea, polycystic ovarian syndrome (PCOS), and primary dysmenorrhea, and applies or adapts the previously described basic principles of history, physical examination, investigations, and treatment to these conditions. To avoid missing the diagnosis, inherited bleeding disorders are discussed.

THE COMMON PRESENTING COMPLAINTS

Care providers for adolescent girls are likely to be confronted with concerns over periods that are perceived as too heavy or prolonged, too painful (dysmenorrhea), irregular (unpredictable, too frequent, or infrequent), and/or nonexistent (primary or secondary amenorrhea). There are many suggested sets of terminology but, to avoid misinterpretation, this article uses lay language descriptors and the term abnormal uterine bleeding (AUB). When it comes to heavy flow, it is often helpful to first elicit evidence of ovulation (classic premenstrual molimina such as breast tenderness, headaches, cyclic mood changes, and cycle regularity). When cycles are regular and ovulatory, but still heavy, the problem is more likely the teen's inability to manage idiopathic heavy flow or a bleeding disorder. In contrast, anovulatory cycles, or cycles triggered by infrequent ovulation, can be heavy and/or prolonged. When ovulation is absent or infrequent, the underlying cause is often endocrinopathy; imbalance or syndrome at the hypothalamus, the pituitary, or at the ovary (see **Fig. 1**). Infections of the lower genital tract (or a retained tampon) tend to cause intermenstrual bleeding, and pregnancy must be considered with almost every change in menstrual cycle or abnormal vaginal bleeding presentation.

Key point/pearl
- Distinguishing whether the teen is ovulatory or not can be helpful in narrowing the differential diagnosis.

Table 1
Medicinal treatment options for problematic menstrual bleeding (symptom based)

Heavy (and/or Prolonged) Flow	Irregular: Infrequent and Unpredictable	Irregular: Frequent (± Prolonged)	Painful/ Crampy
CCs	CCs	CCs	CCs
Antifibrinolytic	Cyclic oral progestins	Antifibrinolytic	—
NSAIDs (proactive)	Maybe do nothing if ≥4 cycles/y	—	NSAIDs ± acetaminophen
LAP	—	LAP	LAP
Course of oral progestin (if isolated prolonged bleed; discussed later)	—	—	—

Options need not be tried in the order listed.
   Antifibrinolytics are tranexamic acid or aminocaproic acid.
   Abbreviations: CCs, combined contraceptives (eg, oral pill, transdermal patch, vaginal ring); LAPs, long-acting progestins (ie, depomedroxyprogesterone acetate or levonorgestrel intrauterine system); NSAIDs, nonsteroidal antiinflammatory drugs.

WHAT IS NORMAL, AND THE MATURATION OF THE HYPOTHALAMIC-PITUITARY-OVARIAN AXIS

Although there may be trends toward earlier puberty, the average age at menarche has been fairly stable between ages of 12 and 13 years in Canada and the United States. More than 90% of adolescent girls have had menarche by 14 years of age. It is generally accepted that most menarchal bleeds are the result of endometrial proliferation from estrogen. Both thelarche and leukorrhea are evidence of estrogen exposure and precede menarche by 1 to 2 years. Menarche is an anovulatory bleed; often the result of erratic sloughing of the proliferative endometrium as opposed to a synchronous slough 2 weeks after ovulation, which explains why, for many young teens, the bleed can be prolonged and heavy but, at the same time, usually fairly painless (discussed later). It is also generally agreed that the HPO axis needs time to mature, averaging 6 months to 3 years before regular ovulatory cycles are established. The earlier menarche occurs, the sooner cycles regulate. During these months immediately after menarche, teens can experience cycles consistent with ovulatory dysfunction: irregular and unpredictable (frequent or infrequent), heavy and prolonged, but intervals between menses are seldom greater than 3 months. It is well recognized that teens and their parents may have misinformation or misguided expectations about what is normal. Education and reassurance are sometimes all that is necessary if the girl is otherwise coping. They may report her to be irregular if the cycle is not exactly every 30 days and they may report her to be experiencing heavy bleeding because she is having menstrual accidents but she is still learning how and when to use pads/tampons. Regular ovulatory cycles typically occur every 21 to 34 days and blood loss is less than 80 mL. Trying to determine which teens are experiencing abnormally heavy flow (and among them, which may have an inherited bleeding disorder [discussed later]) can be challenging. Looking for anemia and clarifying the number of saturated pads/tampons required in a day and the number/size of clots can be helpful but how it affects the girl's life is paramount. However, having to change a pad/tampon every 1 to 2 hours and greater than 7 days' moderate/heavy flow is likely excessive. Whether the teen is merely experiencing HPO axis maturation, or whether she has an underlying disorder, treatment should be indicated if the problem is causing distress or dysfunction. The American College of Obstetricians and Gynecologists' committee on Adolescent Health care has a useful summary of the menstrual cycle as a vital sign, which outlines expectations and causes for concern,[1] and Wilkinson and Kadir[2] reviewed adolescent menstrual disorders in a supplement of the *Journal of Pediatric & Adolescent Gynecology* that is dedicated to this topic and inherited bleeding disorders.

Menstrual Cramps (Dysmenorrhea)

With the establishment of ovulatory cycles, the teen may begin to experience dysmenorrhea. Primary dysmenorrhea refers to prostaglandin-mediated physiologic menstrual cramping typical of ovulatory cycles. Dysmenorrhea is typically absent from the first several menses because they are often anovulatory, and it is concerning when the menarchal bleed is very painful because it can be the result of obstructed outflow (discussed later).

Key point/pearl
- The menstrual cycle takes 6 months to 3 years on average to become regular and ovulatory.
- Reassurance may or may not be all that is necessary even if symptoms are considered a physiologic variant. Treat if interfering with activities or depleting the teen (physically and/or emotionally).

- Underlying disorders (see **Fig. 1**) such as disordered eating, PCOS, pregnancy, and bleeding disorders can be present during the first few years after menarche. Immaturity of the HPO axis is a default diagnosis.
- Primary physiologic dysmenorrhea is usually not present at menarche; it accompanies the establishment of ovulatory cycles.
- Helpful patient/parent information is available:
  - http://www.naspag.org/index.php/patients[3]
  - http://www.sexualityandu.ca/parents/discussing-menstruation[4]
  - http://www.youngwomenshealth.org[5]

Interpreting and Using the Figures

Fig. 1 provides a broad differential for heavy bleeding, prolonged bleeding, and/or irregular bleeding. The conditions noted by an asterisk (*) can also cause secondary amenorrhea. Secondary amenorrhea traditionally was a term reserved for cessation of menses of 6 months or more. Many clinicians now advocate for the criterion to be only 3 months or 90 days. Although there is less chance of disorder, this more lenient criterion affords more opportunity for early recognition of pregnancy, eating disorders, and so forth. **Fig. 2** provides a broad differential for primary amenorrhea, which may or may not be accompanied by delayed or arrested puberty. Although definitions vary, delayed puberty in a girl refers to absence of breast development (thelarche) by age 13 years. Neither figure includes the hypothalamic-pituitary-adrenal axis, but conditions such as congenital adrenal hyperplasia, Cushing, and tumors (adrenal gland and ovary) need to be considered when there is significant androgenization/virilization or other stigmata. Chronic illness can include disorders such as type 1 diabetes, renal failure, and inflammatory bowel disease. Both hyperthyroid and hypothyroid disease can affect the HPO axis functionality and thus both figures mention thyroid endocrinopathy. Both figures list premature ovarian failure (POF), which can be idiopathic or caused by gonadal dysgenesis/agenesis (ex Turner syndrome), fragile X premutation, cancer therapies (chemotherapy, radiation), autoimmune oophoritis, and so forth. Autoimmune POF often coexists with other autoimmune conditions in the patient and/or her family. Primary ovarian insufficiency is an entity in itself but for the purposes of this article it should be considered a mild form of POF or a state of transition. Remember that these figures are meant to guide the history, physical examination, and choice of investigations.

ABNORMAL UTERINE BLEEDING: THE GENERIC ASSESSMENT
History: Key Features

- Explicit description of menstrual complaints, perceived menstrual cycle, and time elapsed since menarche: if heavy, try to establish how heavy by inquiring about the frequency required for changing pads/tampons, number and size of clots, and the duration of flow. Recall that changing pads/tampons every 1 to 2 hours and consistently greater than 7 days' heavy flow is likely excessive. If irregular, try to establish how irregular by inquiring about the longest and shortest intervals between menses. Recall that normal menses occur every 21 to 34 days and although it can take up to 3 years to establish a normal regular cycle, irregularity should prompt inquiry guided by the disorders listed in **Fig. 1**. For both heavy and irregular menses, try to ascertain whether the girl is ovulatory by asking about molimina such as breast tenderness, cyclic mood changes, and cramping. If painful, try to establish whether the pain is consistent with physiologic dysmenorrhea and treatments tried and how they were used (discussed elsewhere in the article). If absent (amenorrhea), establish whether it is primary (never menstruated), or secondary (>90 days warrants assessment). Other

important clues include the mother's age at menarche, any history of pelvic pain, the subjective impression of pubertal progression, and any chance of pregnancy.
- Review of systems using **Fig. 1** or **2** as a guide looking for symptoms of endocrinopathy or syndromes such as dieting, thyroid imbalance, or PCOS.
- Sexual history and need for contraception.
- Traditional past medical history, past surgical history, medications, smoking/risk taking, allergies, and related family history.

Physical Examination

Depending on the presenting complaint, clinicians should use **Fig. 1** or **2** as a guide when looking for physical stigmata of endocrinopathy or syndromes such as short stature (Turner syndrome), underweight (eating disorder), goiter (thyroid condition), and hirsutism/obesity (PCOS).

Physical Examination: Key Features

- Height, weight, body mass index (BMI) (calculate percentage and plot on growth chart), blood pressure (especially if the patient is obese or has PCOS features, and/or if combined contraceptives [CCs] will be prescribed).
- Secondary sexual characteristics/Tanner staging, if applicable.
- Abdominal examination.
- If menses are absent, introital examination must be included and consider single-digit vaginal examination. Is there a vagina, patent hymen, leukorrhea? Leukorrhea is suggestive of current estrogen.
- Speculum examination is not always indicated (recall, Pap smear is no longer indicated in teens, and urine can be sent for some sexually transmitted infection [STI] screening).
- If there is intermenstrual bleeding, and/or the girl is sexually active, consider a speculum examination, but, if the teen is precoital, choose a narrow speculum (if deemed necessary).

Investigations and Diagnostic Tools

It is hoped that, through history and physical examination, the differential diagnosis has been narrowed, but the clinician usually needs to choose from the following list of investigations to confirm or refute plausible conditions.

Investigations and Diagnostic Tools to Consider

- Urine human chorionic gonadotropin (HCG)
- Complete blood count, ferritin
  - Anemia might corroborate abnormally heavy flow and raise the suspicion of a bleeding disorder or add justification for treatment
- Thyroid-stimulating hormone (TSH) (free T4), plus or minus prolactin
- Follicle-stimulating hormone (FSH), luteinizing hormone (LH)
  - High (menopausal) gonadotropin levels confirm gonadal or ovarian insufficiency or failure (discussed elsewhere in the article). If LH and FSH are both less than 1 the clinician can be confident that the problem is hypothalamic or pituitary dysfunction, but often low normal values are difficult to interpret.
- Ultrasonography pelvis.
- Clinicians should individualize the need for cervix and/or vaginal swabs, and pregnancy testing. Although urine can be tested for gonorrhea and *Chlamydia*, *Trichomonas* requires a vaginal swab.
  - Examples of accessory testing to consider:

- If functional or hypothalamic amenorrhea, PCOS, or bleeding disorder is suspected, see the relevant parts of this article outlining other warranted investigations.
- If there are central nervous system (CNS) symptoms or hyperprolactinemia, consider brain imaging.
- If there is gonadal insufficiency or failure, order karyotype and consider referral (pediatric endocrine, pediatric/adolescent gynecology, genetics).
- If there is profound or marked hyperandrogenism/virilization, consider serum androgens plus or minus adrenocorticotropic hormone (ACTH) stimulation and imaging adrenals. This situation is likely to warrant referral (pediatric endocrine or gynecology).
- If there is intractable dysmenorrhea or primary amenorrhea suggestive of müllerian anomaly, consider MRI pelvis and referral (pediatric/adolescent gynecology or gynecology).

Also consider referral (eg, gynecology, pediatric gynecology, pediatric endocrine, genetics hematology, psychiatry, as indicated) for:

1. Delayed or arrested puberty
2. True eating disorder or elite athlete
3. Inherited bleeding disorder
4. Complex or confusing scenarios in which investigations or response to traditional therapies are unsuccessful

For more detailed reviews of delayed puberty, primary ovarian insufficiency, and POF in adolescents see Refs.[6–14]

Treatment (in General)

Table 1 presents a symptom-based chart of several useful medicinal treatment options that can be used and referred to by clinicians almost independent of underlying condition. The following list elaborates further on these treatment modalities and a series of questions is provided to help the clinician choose from the various reasonable medications for any particular menstrual complaint/symptom.

Treatment Options (in General)

- Nonsteroidal antiinflammatory drugs (NSAIDs): ibuprofen, mefenamic acid, naproxen sodium, ketorolac
- CCs: daily pill, weekly patch, monthly vaginal ring
  - Consider extended cycle: gradually increase the number of consecutive weeks between hormone-free intervals (HFIs), when either the HFI or the withdrawal bleed are still problematic.
  - Consider shortening the HFI when either the HFI or the withdrawal bleed are still problematic. For example, 4 days off instead of 7.
- Cyclic oral progestins: 5 to 10 mg of medroxyprogesterone acetate or 200 mg of progesterone X for 10 to 14 days. These progestins can be used to induce a withdrawal bleed in teens whose menstruation is heavy and prolonged but infrequent. A single course can also be useful as a medical dilatation and curettage for isolated anovulatory bleeds that continue for several weeks.
- Depomedroxyprogesterone acetate (DMPA) 150 mg intramuscularly every 10–13 weeks.
  - Informed choice about weight gain, side effects (including irregular bleeding or amenorrhea), bone density

- Levonorgestrel intrauterine system (LIUS)
  - Patient must be properly selected and counseled
  - Adolescent age is not a contraindication to intrauterine device or system
  - Nulligravid patients may experience more cramping and higher expulsion rate
- Antifibrinolytics: tranexamic acid 1 to 1.5 grams p.o. 3 to 4 times/d, aminocaproic acid 2 to 4 grams p.o. 4 to 6 times/d.

Consider referral when there are contraindications to CCs or for LIUS insertion. When using **Table 1**, ask:

1. What are the symptoms of priority? Heavy? Irregular? Painful?
2. What are the patient's preconceived ideas about, and past successes/failures with, methods?
3. Can the patient/family afford it? Is subsidy available?
4. Will the patient adhere to or accept it (eg, would she take a daily pill or accept an injectable method)?
5. Are there any contraindications (eg, CCs and migraines with complex neurologic features, LIUS and current STI cervicitis)?
6. Are there any other noncontraceptive benefits to be exploited (eg, CCs and acne or hirsutism)?
7. Does the patient also need reliable family planning/contraception? Private time with patient alone should be part of the routine to allow for open discussion and to reinforce healthy sexual choices and advise dual protection (advised).
8. Does the patient also need an iron supplement?

Other key points/pearls (for treatment in general)
- NSAIDs work best if they are taken proactively (and combined when necessary with acetaminophen).
- CCs offer cycle regulation, reduced flow, reduced cramps, and reduced acne/hirsutism with a single medication, but teens and/or parents often have misinformation or misperceptions about safety and side effects that must be addressed to facilitate compliance/adherence. For example, confidently reassure that CCs do not cause significant weight gain or cancer.[15,16]
- If planning to use CCs in an extended cycle fashion, slowly increase the number of consecutive weeks between HFIs. Continuous use from the outset often involves persistent breakthrough bleeding that frustrates the teen and leads her to abandon the treatment plan.
- There is still a role for DMPA in properly selected and fully informed adolescents.
- Pelvic examination is not a prerequisite for hormonal methods (except intrauterine).

ABNORMAL UTERINE BLEEDING: CAUSES WORTHY OF PARTICULAR MENTION

Functional hypothalamic amenorrhea, PCOS, dysmenorrhea and inherited bleeding disorders.

Functional Hypothalamic Amenorrhea (and Disordered Menstruation)

Functional (hypothalamic) amenorrhea refers to the absence of menses as a result of an imbalance of stress, dietary intake, and exercise. With respect to dietary intake and exercise, it is generally accepted that there is insufficient nutritional intake to match the energy expenditure, thus resulting in a deficit. Eating disorders or disordered eating are common but not always present, and weight loss may have occurred but is not a necessity. Gonadotrophin-releasing hormone ceases to pulse effectively (if at all) and the HPO axis gets suppressed or becomes ineffective. The patient's presentation depends on when the problem is acquired in relation to puberty and menarche, and how severe the extremes of diet/stress/exercise are. The patient may present with delayed puberty or arrested puberty and primary amenorrhea but secondary amenorrhea is far more common and consistent. Disordered menstruation with irregular or infrequent cycles can occur initially or when the imbalance is less severe. Catherine Gordon[17] has written an outstanding review of hypothalamic functional amenorrhea for the *New England Journal of Medicine*.

When the teen presents with delayed menarche (primary amenorrhea) the health care provider must consider other differential diagnoses such as (but not limited to) Kallmann syndrome (hypothalamic), POF (gonadal), or a müllerian anomaly (outflow tract) (see **Fig. 2**). Obstructing anomalies such as imperforate hymen and transverse vaginal septum should be easy to eliminate with a mini–genital examination, especially if there is no history of pelvic pain despite significant pubertal development. **Fig. 3** shows some of these anomalies, but more detailed reviews of müllerian anomalies (obstructive and nonobstructive) were published as clinical recommendations in the *Journal of Pediatric & Adolescent Gynecology* December 2014.[18,19] Vaginal agenesis [Mayer Rokitansky Kuster Hauser (MRKH) syndrome] can exist with or without a uterus and that uterus may or may not have a nidus of functional endometrium. Thus, whereas/although vaginal agenesis always presents with normal puberty, there may or may not be any pelvic pain complaints. If there is little or no pubertal development, attention should be focused on hypothalamic and ovarian causes (see **Fig. 2**).

Clues on history corroborating functional/hypothalamic disorder

Patients often report that cycles were regular and then disappeared or became very infrequent (sudden or gradual). Inquiry might identify weight loss, eating disorder, psychosocial stress or anxiety, performance pressure, and exercise for health, weight loss, or competitive athletics. A validated eating aptitudes test could be used.[20]

Health care providers who care for teens should make regular inquiries about the presence of menstrual cycles and consider this a fifth vital sign.[1] Similarly, diet, exercise, and body image are important topics for routine inquiry. Teens who are not menstruating may not be acquiring bone density at the intended rate. Although there

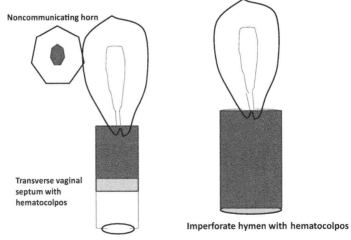

Noncommunicating horn

Transverse vaginal septum with hematocolpos

Imperforate hymen with hematocolpos

Fig. 3. Examples of obstructive anomalies.

can be denial and a lack of insight, pressing for a detailed dietary log and exercise schedule plus exploring psychosocial stressors and anxiety is important in recognizing and confidently diagnosing functional/hypothalamic amenorrhea.

Clues on physical examination corroborating functional/hypothalamic disorder BMI tends to be low. Look for signs of eating disorders and compensatory behaviors, absent or arrested puberty, and absent estrogen at introitus (eg, red hyperemic, tissues less plump, few rugae). None of these features are compulsory in making the diagnosis but be sure to rule out signs of other endocrinopathies or syndromes (see **Figs. 1** and **2**), such as hyperthyroidism or hypothyroidism and PCOS or a true eating disorder. Eating disorder reviews provide extensive lists of stigmata.[21,22]

Clues from investigations that corroborate functional/hypothalamic disorder Clues include low or undetectable FSH level and low or undetectable LH level, although other investigations, such as TSH, prolactin, and pelvic ultrasonography, will be normal. Once the diagnosis is made, other investigations may be indicated, such as bone density or complete blood count.

Management of functional/hypothalamic amenorrhea
Clinicians should also focus on the menstrual complaints and symptoms and use the guide to general treatment options in **Table 1**. For example, if the teen has stress-related or diet-related unpredictable and infrequent menses, she could use CCs or cyclic progestins (if she does not need birth control), but this does not address the causative imbalance.

For functional hypothalamic amenorrhea (or disordered menses), the patient needs to understand her condition and be motivated to make changes. She may need counseling or strategies to deal with stress, or more likely she will need to increase caloric and nutritional intake or reduce the amount of vigorous exercise she is doing. A consultation and follow-up with a dietician (who has some understanding of this condition) may increase the likelihood of resumption of menses, but the patient should know that it can take some time. Multidisciplinary care may be warranted, especially if there is an underlying eating disorder, an anxiety disorder, or elite athleticism. There is still debate about whether a critical weight or body fat percentage needs to be reached, but, if weight loss was involved in the original cessation of menses, the teen may need to regain that weight and a bit more. Bone health is at risk while the amenorrhea persists and CCs have not been shown to be protective in this setting. This author finds it helpful to conceptualize when explaining this condition and recovery to patients and their parents. Explain that the brain is unwilling to allow fertility until it is convinced that it can trust the adolescent to provide it with regular adequate nutrition (no deficit) and that she is coping better with life. This concept seems to make sense in its simplicity but the addendum always worth mentioning to teens who are (or are going to become) sexually active is that it is not a reliable form of pregnancy prevention.

Key points/pearls
- Functional hypothalamic amenorrhea is a diagnosis of exclusion and is caused by an imbalance of stress, diet, and/or exercise.
- Hypothalamic or brain issues can cause ovulatory dysfunction without necessarily being severe enough to completely suppress the HPO axis. These causes can present with irregular bleeding or amenorrhea.
- Be suspicious if the patient is fully pubertal but has not experienced menarche; ask about pelvic pain, which might signify obstructive müllerian anomaly or müllerian agenesis.

- There are 2 specific groups worthy of mention but that are beyond the scope of this article: the female athletic triad and patients with eating disorders (especially anorexia). When exploring history and performing physical examination for amenorrhea and/or disordered menses, health care providers may identify one (or both; they can coexist) of these diagnoses. The female athletic triad refers to absent menses in an athlete with osteopenia and low energy availability (imbalance of nutrition vs energy expenditure but not always with coexistent eating disorder).
- Select articles are provided and recommended for more detailed review of eating disorders.[21–23] Dr Catherine Gordon's[17] review of functional amenorrhea mentions the athletic triad and Youngwomenshealth.org has patient information on this condition at http://youngwomenshealth.org/2010/05/21/female-athlete-triad/.

Polycystic Ovarian Syndrome

It is now well recognized that PCOS occurs in adolescents, and may begin during childhood or earlier. Typical features/stigmata (not all present in all patients) include obesity, menstrual disturbances, hyperandrogenism, insulin resistance, metabolic syndrome, and polycystic/enlarged ovaries.[24–27] There is a familial tendency that probably results from both genetic and environmental influences. Because puberty, and specifically the first couple of years after menarche, can be a time of hyperestrogenism, hyperandrogenism, and oligo-ovulation, manifesting as irregular menses and acne, the subgroup of adolescent girls who will ultimately be diagnosed with PCOS can be difficult to identify (without incorrectly diagnosing some girls who are merely peripubertal and perimenarchal). Complicating matters is the current epidemic of childhood and adolescent obesity. Although obesity is not a mandatory feature of PCOS, it is present in a significant percentage of girls with PCOS, but this feature has become less discerning as average body weight and BMI has increased alarmingly in North America. Several groups have tried to create and impose diagnostic criteria to unify researchers and the literature for a better understanding of PCOS and to try to validate diagnoses. The most rigorous and selective of the diagnostic criteria schemes specific to adolescents is that put forth by Carmina and colleagues.[28] This definition requires that the teen be at least 2 years postmenarche and have both hyperandrogenism (as shown by acne, hirsutism, alopecia) and oligo-ovulation (<6 cycles per year). In this situation, PCOS is highly likely but, with these criteria, diagnosis is considered absolute if ovaries on ultrasonography show the classic polycystic look or increased ovarian volume. Carmina and colleagues'[28] criteria take into account the normal physiologic changes of early adolescence and the significant overlap between normal peripubertal (perimenarchal) ovaries and classic PCOS ovaries. In contrast, by insisting on 2 years postmenarche, diagnosis could be delayed for some teens, and not all experts support the requirement of ultrasonography features.

A subset of patients with PCOS have metabolic syndrome, which usually involves obesity but specifically refers to hypertension, insulin resistance, glucose intolerance/type II diabetes mellitus, and dyslipidemia. Another subset of patients with PCOS present with primary amenorrhea but these teens tend to be hyperandrogenized and more investigations may be indicated to rule out other conditions.

Consider referral to either a multidisciplinary team or a pediatric endocrinologist and a cardiologist if metabolic syndrome is suspected. Consider referral to a subspecialist if the teen presents with primary amenorrhea and presumed PCOS.

Clues on history that corroborate polycystic ovarian syndrome

Patients often report that cycles are irregular (frequent or infrequent), heavy, and seldom painful (except when there are large clots or occasionally when the patient is ovulatory). She could also be amenorrheic. Inquiry might identify unexplained excess weight gain at puberty, acne, and hirsutism.

Clues on physical examination that corroborate polycystic ovarian syndrome BMI tends to be high, and there could be increased blood pressure, acne, hirsutism (consider Ferriman-Gallwey score for charting hirsutism). There should not be true virilization. There may be dark, velvety, dirty-looking skin in creases (acanthosis nigricans) and boils in vulva/groin or axilla (hidradenitis suppurativa). Be sure to rule out signs of other endocrinopathies or syndromes (see **Figs. 1** and **2**) such as hypothyroidism, Cushing syndrome, or another androgen disorders causing marked virilization.

Clues from investigations that corroborate polycystic ovarian syndrome, and investigations to consider Normal FSH and LH levels, but possibly LH/FSH ratio greater than 2; normal TSH and prolactin levels; high fasting insulin level; fasting glucose/fasting insulin ratio less than 4.5; high 2-hour sample after 75-g glucose challenge (to be preceded by 12-hour fast and to include fasting glucose and fasting insulin); abnormal fasting lipid profile (high triglyceride level, low HDL level), and mild increase of total testosterone level (discussed later).

Comment It is this author's opinion (shared by some invesigators[29,30] but not by others[25,28]) that serum androgens are not often indicated in the diagnosis of PCOS or the setting of typical hirsutism. If there is marked hyperandrogenism or true virilization (and/or rapid onset/progression), then serum androgens (fasting 17-OH progesterone, plus or minus ACTH stimulation, testosterone (total and free), dehydroepiandrosterone sulfate, androstenedione, and imaging of ovaries and adrenal glands may be indicated, but this is in the extreme and rare setting and warrants referral.

Management of polycystic ovarian syndrome
Readers are also reminded to focus on the menstrual complaints and symptoms, to use **Table 1**, and to refer to this article's discussion of treatment options in general. For example, if the teen has heavy menses, she could use antifibrinolytics, but if she also has unpredictable menses and acne/hirsutism she may want to choose CCs; however, this does not address the need for healthy diet and exercise and achieving or maintaining ideal body weight. For an adolescent girl with PCOS, the agenda is more likely to be to gain control of acne, hirsutism, menstrual irregularity, or flow, and the girl's weight. The patient (or their parents) may also be concerned about future fertility. Ideally the health care provider educates and motivates the teen and her parents in order to avoid the recognized comorbidities and future health issues that patients with PCOS can experience: obesity and type II diabetes (and their sequelae, such as heart disease and sleep apnea), endometrial hyperplasia or malignancy, and psychological distress/poor self-esteem.

First and foremost, healthy diet and exercise need to be achieved. This goal is easier said than done, especially for teens. Teens may be more motivated if they are aware that even modest weight loss can be associated with improvement in their PCOS symptoms, such as menstrual disruption, acne, and hirsutism. While maximizing results through lifestyle, CCs (oral, transdermal, or vaginal) tend to be one of the main therapeutic modalities to achieve both menstrual management and reduced hyperandrogenism (plus pregnancy prevention where necessary). The role of insulin sensitizers in these teens is still a topic of intense debate and controversy, but this author has yet to be convinced they have a role in nondiabetic teens with PCOS.

Polycystic ovarian syndrome, combined contraceptives and venous thromboembolism in adolescents

It is generally accepted that the likelihood of experiencing a VTE event on CC (as an independent risk factor), is increased 2-fold to 3-fold. However, for most teens without an inherited tendency or thrombophilia such as factor V Leiden deficiency, the baseline absolute risk is extremely low (in the order of 1 to 2 per 10,000 woman-years), but hyperandrogenism and obesity (and smoking) are also independent risk factors. However, it is important to recognize that, without an inherited thrombophilia, the likelihood of a VTE event on a CC, regardless of progestin, even in an obese teen with PCOS, is not likely to be much higher than 1 in 1000 and is far lower than the risk associated with pregnancy/postpartum in that same teen.[31–37]

Key points/pearls

- Suspect PCOS if there is irregular (often infrequent) menses, hirsutism/acne, and tendency to easy weight gain.
- It can be difficult to select out patients with PCOS from those who are merely manifesting perimenarchal adolescent physiology.
- Diet, exercise, and maintenance of healthy body weight are paramount.
- CCs often address the adolescent's agenda (menstrual regularity, acne, and hirsutism).
- Risk of VTE on CCs is higher in teens with PCOS and obesity, but VTE is still a rare event unless there is a coexistent inherited thrombophilia.

Dysmenorrhea (Menstrual Cramps)

Primary dysmenorrhea is physiologic prostaglandin-mediated menstrual cramping. It tends to be midline and low pelvic, and sometimes radiates down legs or around to the low back. It is not usually present with the menarchal bleed. Gradually, over the months or few years postmenarche, as the HPO axis matures, cycles become ovulatory and more regular and with this comes primary dysmenorrhea of variable severity. Sometimes adolescents report that NSAIDs failed, but they were waiting too long. Other causes of menstrual cramping include (but are not limited to) endometriosis and cyclic constipation. Endometriosis most definitely does occur in adolescents and has been reviewed by several investigators recently.[38–42] There can be a family history, but the most common manifestations are intractable dysmenorrhea that eventually fails to respond to usual treatment strategies (discussed later), chronic pelvic pain, or deep dyspareunia. When the teen fails to respond adequately to NSAIDs (plus or minus acetaminophen) or when the teen also needs reliable family planning, hormonal contraception is the next strategy, along with a discussion of healthy sexual choices and dual protection. See this article's discussion of treatment options in general and **Table 1**.

Caution

When menarche is accompanied by severe pain, suspect a menstrual outflow obstruction. The most likely obstructive müllerian anomaly that would still allow menarchal flow is a noncommunicating uterine horn (see **Fig. 3**). In addition, be aware of teens who seemingly are premenarchal but have well-developed secondary sexual characteristics and are experiencing episodes of severe pelvic pain. An obstructive anomaly such as transverse vaginal septum, imperforate hymen (see **Fig. 3**), or vaginal agenesis (with uterine remnant) must be ruled out. For a detailed description of both obstructive and nonobstructive müllerian anomalies, consult the North American Society of Pediatric and Adolescent Gynecology (NASPAG) 2014 clinical recommendations.[18,19]

Refer to pediatric adolescent gynecology (or gynecology) when anything other than primary physiologic dysmenorrhea is suspected or when treatments are failing to control the menstrual pain.

Key points/pearls
- Be proactive with cramp medications. Combine acetaminophen with NSAIDs.
- Be suspicious if properly administered proactive NSAIDs (plus or minus acetaminophen) in combination with CCs fail to control dysmenorrhea.
- Consider endometriosis if there are other features of pelvic pain and dyspareunia.
- Be suspicious if there is significant pubertal progress but no menarche, especially if there is recurrent pelvic pain (müllerian anomaly).
- Be suspicious if the menarchal bleed is very painful (consider obstructive müllerian anomaly).

Inherited Bleeding Disorder

The most common inherited bleeding disorders in women include von Willebrand disease (VWD), symptomatic hemophilia (type A is factor VIII deficiency and type B is factor IX deficiency), platelet dysfunction, and other factor deficiencies (eg, VII and XI). It is estimated that up to 1 in every 5 women and girls with true menorrhagia (abnormally heavy flow) have an inherited bleeding disorder and most have VWD. Many of these bleeding diatheses have well-known inheritance patterns and ideally the diagnosis is made before menarche. However, this is not often the scenario. Menarche is often a time when the diagnosis is made after the girl has suffered psychologically, socially, and physically while trying to contend with her first menstrual cycle (or the first several). It is important to determine whether the girl has had other challenges with hemostasis, such as nose bleeds, gum bleeds, joint bleeds and bruising, excess bleeding with wisdom teeth extraction, or tonsillectomies, and this is the time to actively seek out the mother's menstrual and obstetric history and the family history of bleeding (eg, postpartum hemorrhages, anemia and heavy menses, the need for early hysterectomies). However, an absent family history does not exclude the diagnosis. For more information about abnormal menstruation caused by bleeding diatheses, the reader is referred to several outstanding reviews.[2,43–52]

Much effort has gone into trying to develop tools that will assist clinicians in selecting out those women and girls who warrant investigations for a bleeding disorder. These tools have included pictorial blood assessment charts (which are not always on hand and practical) and bleeding scores or questionnaires, and some have specifically examined children and teens.[53–56]

Key points/pearls
- Take bleeding history from teen and her family.
- Consider screening for inherited bleeding disorder if the patient reports one of the following:
  - A duration of menses greater than or equal to 7 days plus flooding or impairment of daily activities with menses
  - A history of treatment of anemia
  - A family history of a diagnosed bleeding disorder
  - A history of excessive surgical bleeding or obstetric (and gynecological) bleeding complications in teen or parent (ask specifically about tonsils/adenoids and dental extraction)

Investigations to be considered (in addition to those listed earlier)

- Peripheral blood smear
- Prothrombin time (PT), activated partial thromboplastin time (aPTT)
- International Normalized Ratio (INR) and thrombin time (TT)
- Renal and liver function tests
- ABO blood group
- VWF:Ag, VWF:RCo, FVIII*

However, there are many conditions and situational factors that can affect the test results, such as stress, acute bleeding, blood type O, and hyperthyroidism, so consultation with a hematologist is recommended to assist with making the diagnosis, interpretation of results, and/or additional testing. Be aware that many patients with an inherited bleeding disorder have normal PT, PTT, INR, and TT.

Treatment strategies for nonacute heavy menstrual flow in adolescents with an inherited bleeding disorder are identical to those described for treatment options in general and in **Table 1**. For example, heavy flow but migraines with focal neurologic features in a teen who has an inherited bleeding disorder but also needs reliable birth control might warrant a long-acting progestin. If intramuscular injections are used, prolonged pressure on the injection site may be needed. If an LIUS is inserted, the expulsion rate may be higher than usual.[57] If NSAIDs are to be used for dysmenorrhea, the hematologist should know and they should be used for only a couple of days each month to avoid aggravating hemostasis with platelet dysfunction. Sometimes hematologists prescribe desmopressin acetate (DDAVP) if the teen is a DDAVP responder.

PREGNANCY

Whenever a teen presents with a change in her menses, absent or atypical, astute clinicians always take a sexual history and have a low threshold for pregnancy testing. Pregnancy may be intrauterine or ectopic and viable or nonviable.

SUMMARY

Teens present with a variety of menstrual complaints, including heavy, irregular, painful, or absent flow. Using the hypothalamic, pituitary, ovarian, and outflow tract axis as a guide, most underlying conditions are identified and can easily be managed. Sometimes reassurance is all that is necessary but treatment is indicated if/when the symptoms are causing distress or dysfunction. NSAIDs and CCs tend to be first-line modalities. Immaturity of the HPO axis, hypothalamic factors (diet, stress, and exercise), functional amenorrhea, idiopathic anovulation, and PCOS are the most common causes, but astute clinicians never overlook inherited bleeding disorders or the possibility of pregnancy.

REFERENCES

1. American College Obstetricians and Gynecologists Committee on Adolescent Health Care. Menstruation in girls and adolescents: using the menstrual cycle as a vital sign. Pediatrics 2006;118(5):2245–50.
2. Wilkinson JP, Kadir RA. Management of abnormal uterine bleeding in adolescents. J Pediatr Adolesc Gynecol 2010;23(Suppl 6):S22–30.
3. NASPAG. North American Society of Pediatric and Adolescent Gynecology online Patient/Parent information handouts. Available at: http://www.naspag.org/index.php/patients2014. Accessed May, 2015.

4. SOGC. SexualityandU Canadian Web site online parent education. Available at: http://www.sexualityandu.ca/parents/discussing-menstruation. Accessed May, 2015.
5. Boston Children's Hospital. Available at: www.youngwomenshealth.org. Accessed May, 2015.
6. Kaplowitz PB. Delayed puberty. Pediatr Rev 2010;31(5):189–95.
7. Palmert MR, Dunkel L. Clinical practice. Delayed puberty. N Engl J Med 2012; 366(5):443–53.
8. Welt CK. Primary ovarian insufficiency: a more accurate term for premature ovarian failure. Clin Endocrinol (Oxf) 2008;68(4):499–509.
9. Rebar RW. Premature ovarian failure. Obstet Gynecol 2009;113(6):1355–63.
10. Panay N, Kalu E. Management of premature ovarian failure. Best Pract Res Clin Obstet Gynaecol 2009;23(1):129–40.
11. Nelson LM. Clinical practice. Primary ovarian insufficiency. N Engl J Med 2009; 360(6):606–14.
12. Naiditch JA, Milad MP, Rowell EE. Uterine leiomyoma causing menometrorrhagia with a concomitant mature teratoma in a 15-year-old child: a case report and review of the literature. J Pediatr Surg 2011;46(10):E33–6.
13. Diesen DL, Price TM, Skinner MA. Uterine leiomyoma in a 14-year-old girl. Eur J Pediatr Surg 2008;18(1):53–5.
14. Grapsa D, Smymiotis V, Hasiakos D, et al. A giant uterine leiomyoma simulating an ovarian mass in a 16-year-old girl: a case report and review of the literature. Eur J Gynaecol Oncol 2006;27(3):294–6.
15. Gallo MF, Grimes DA, Schulz KF, et al. Combination estrogen-progestin contraceptives and body weight: systematic review of randomized controlled trials. Obstet Gynecol 2004;103(2):359–73.
16. Lalonde A, Reid R. SOGC position statement – the birth control pill and cancer. Available at: http://www.sogc.org/media/guidelines-oc_e.asp. Accessed November 6, 2007.
17. Gordon CM. Clinical practice. Functional hypothalamic amenorrhea. N Engl J Med 2010;363(4):365–71.
18. Dietrich JE. Obstructive mullerian anomalies. (A NASPAG clinical recommendation). J Pediatr Adolesc Gynecol 2014;27(6):396–402.
19. Dietrich JE. Non-obstructive mullerian anomalies (A NASPAG clinical recommendation). J Pediatr Adolesc Gynecol 2014;27(6):386–95.
20. Koslowsky M. The factor structure and criterion validity of the short form of the Eating Attitudes Test. J Pers Assess 1992;58:27–35.
21. Clinical report - identification and management of eating disorders in children and adolescents. Pediatrics 2010;126(6):1240–53.
22. Auron M, Rome E. Anorexia nervosa and bulimia nervosa. What the hospitalist needs to know about CPT 269.9, or nutritional insufficiency. ACP Hospitalist; 2011. 38-39-45.
23. Findlay S. Family-based treatment of children and adolescents with anorexia nervosa: guidelines for the community physician. Paediatr Child Health 2010; 15(1):31–5.
24. Berlan ED, Emans SJ. Managing polycystic ovary syndrome in adolescent patients. J Pediatr Adolesc Gynecol 2009;22(2):137–40.
25. Connor EL. Adolescent polycystic ovary syndrome. Adolesc Med State Art Rev 2012;23(1):164–77.
26. Oberfield S. Treatment of polycystic ovary syndrome in adolescence. Semin Reprod Med 2014;32(3):214–21.

27. Pfeifer SM, Kives S. Polycystic ovary syndrome in the adolescent. Obstet Gynecol Clin North Am 2009;36(1):129–52.
28. Carmina E, Oberfield SE, Lobo RA. The diagnosis of polycystic ovary syndrome in adolescents. Am J Obstet Gynecol 2010;203(3):201.e1–5.
29. Franks S. The investigation and management of hirsutism. J Fam Plann Reprod Health Care 2012;38:182–6.
30. Jamieson MA. Hirsutism investigations–what is appropriate? J Pediatr Adolesc Gynecol 2001;14(2):95–7.
31. Reid R. Oral contraceptives and venous thromboembolism. Consensus opinion from an international workshop held in Berlin, Germany in December 2009. J Fam Plann Reprod Health Care 2010;36(3):117–22.
32. Jensen JT, Trussell J. Communicating risk: does scientific debate compromise safety? Contraception 2012;86:327–9.
33. Dinger J. Cardiovascular and general safety of a 24-day regimen of drospirenone-containing combined oral contraceptives: final results from the international active surveillance study of women taking oral contraceptives. Contraception 2014;89:253–63.
34. Mills A. Combined oral contraception and the risk of venous thromboembolism. Hum Reprod 1997;12(12):2595–8.
35. Reid R. Combined hormonal contraception and venous thromboembolism (VTE). Contraception 2014;89:235–6.
36. Reid R. Oral contraceptives and venous thromboembolism: pill scares and public health. J Obstet Gynaecol Can 2011;33(11):1150–5.
37. Reid RL. Oral hormonal contraception and venous thromboembolism (VTE). Contraception 2014;89:235–6.
38. Leyland N, Casper R, Laberge P. Endometriosis in the adolescent. J Obstet Gynaecol Can 2010;32(7 Suppl 2):S25–7.
39. Ballweg ML, Laufer MR. Adolescent endometriosis: improving the comfort level of health care providers treating adolescents with endometriosis. J Pediatr Adolesc Gynecol 2011;24(Suppl 5):S1.
40. Jamieson MA. Endometriosis. Chapter 49. In: Hillard P, editor. Hillard's practical pediatric and adolescent gynecology. 1st edition. Wiley-Blackwell; 2013. p. 351–4.
41. Laufer MR. Diagnosis and treatment of endometriosis in adolescents. www uptodate.
42. Laufer MR. Helping "adult gynecologists" diagnose and treat adolescent endometriosis: reflections on my 20 years of personal experience. J Pediatr Adolesc Gynecol 2011;24(Suppl 5):S13–7.
43. A pocket guide to the diagnosis, evaluation and management of von Willebrand disease. NIH; 2007. 08–5832.
44. ACOG Committee on Adolescent Health Care and Committee on Gynecologic Practice. Von Willebrand Disease in Women. The American College of Obstetricians and Gynecologists. 2013. p. 1–6.
45. Ahuja SP, Hertweck SP. Overview of bleeding disorders in adolescent females with menorrhagia. J Pediatr Adolesc Gynecol 2010;23(Suppl 6):S15–21.
46. Gringeri A. Quality of life assessment in clinical practice in haemophilia treatment. Haemophilia 2006;12(Suppl 3):22–9.
47. National Heart, Lung and Blood Institute VWD Expert Panel. A pocket guide to the diagnosis, evaluation and management of von Willebrand disease. NIH; 2008. 08–5833.
48. Rydz N, Jamieson MA. Managing heavy menstrual bleeding in adolescents. Contemp OB/Gyn 2013;58(7).

49. Rydz N, James PD. Approach to the diagnosis and management of common bleeding disorders. Semin Thromb Hemost 2012;38(7):711–9.
50. Society of Obstetricians and Gynaecologists of Canada. Gynaecologic and obstetrics management of women with inherited bleeding disorders. J Obstet Gynaecol Can 2005;27(7):707–32.
51. Tantawy A. Health-related quality of life in Egyptian children and adolescents with hemophilia A. Pediatr Hematol Oncol 2011;28:222–9.
52. Dietrich JE. Abnormal uterine bleeding supplement. J Pediatr Adolesc Gynecol 2010;23(6 Supp 1):S1–47.
53. Bowman M, Riddel J, Rand ML, et al. Evaluation of the diagnostic utility for von Willebrand disease of a pediatric bleeding questionnaire. J Thromb Haemost 2009;7(8):1418–21.
54. Higham JM, O'Brien PM, Shaw RW. Assessment of menstrual blood loss using a pictorial chart. Br J Obstet Gynaecol 1990;97(8):734–9.
55. Philipp CS, Faiz A, Dowling NF, et al. Development of a screening tool for identifying women with menorrhagia for hemostatic evaluation. Am J Obstet Gynecol 2008;198(2):163.e1–8.
56. Sanchez J, Andrabi S, Bercaw JL, et al. Quantifying the PBAC in a pediatric and adolescent gynecology population. Pediatr Hematol Oncol 2012;29(5):479–84.
57. Rimmer E, Jamieson MA, James P. Malposition and expulsion of the levonorgestrel intrauterine system among women with inherited bleeding disorders. Haemophilia 2013;19(6):933–8.

Short Stature
Is It a Psychosocial Problem and Does Changing Height Matter?

David E. Sandberg, PhD*, Melissa Gardner, MA

KEYWORDS

- Short stature • Psychosocial adaptation • Growth hormone • Height

KEY POINTS

- Beliefs about the psychosocial liabilities associated with short stature and the ability of recombinant human growth hormone (rhGH)-mediated increases in height to remedy quality-of-life problems are abundant; however, research provides little support for either.
- Health care providers must work with families to fully examine and weigh potential risks and benefits of using rhGH to address the perceived associations between short stature and psychosocial problems.
- Recent findings on the long-term safety of rhGH treatment, particularly those of the Safety and Appropriateness of Growth hormone treatments in Europe (SAGhE) study, although controversial, underscore the importance of defining safety for families beyond the period of active treatment.
- The authors recommend conducting a psychosocial screening assessment, in addition to physical, laboratory, and radiological evaluations, to learn about (and discuss) the factors parents and patients are using to make decisions, and working with them to evaluate the full range of strategies available to address their concerns about the child's height, including endocrinologic, psychological, educational, and others, as applicable.

INTRODUCTION

Short stature (SS) is conventionally defined as height 2 standard deviations (SDs) (approximately the second percentile) or more below the mean for age- and gender-specific norms[1]; however, growth charts that adopt the fifth percentile (-1.6 SDs) to demarcate the lower limit of the normal range remain commonly available.[2] Although SS frequently represents healthy variation in height, it may reflect

Disclosure: The authors have no disclosures.

The authors contributed equally to this article.

Child Health Evaluation & Research (CHEAR) Unit, Division of Child Behavioral Health, Department of Pediatrics, University of Michigan, 300 North Ingalls Street, Ann Arbor, MI 48109, USA

* Corresponding author. University of Michigan, 300 North Ingalls Street, Room 6C23, Ann Arbor, MI 48109-5456.

E-mail address: dsandber@med.umich.edu

pediatric.theclinics.com

consequences of a wide range of pathologic states, including growth hormone (GH) deficiency (GHD). Even without evidence of pathologic cause, SS is considered by some to constitute a disability requiring medical intervention: recombinant human GH (rhGH) therapy, first introduced in 1985, has been approved by the US Food and Drug Administration (FDA) to accelerate growth and increase adult height in several conditions not characteristically associated with GHD, including chronic renal insufficiency (1992),[3] Turner syndrome (TS) (1996),[4] Prader-Willi syndrome (2000),[5] children born small for gestational age (SGA) (2001),[6] idiopathic SS (ISS) (2003),[7,8] SHOX deficiency (2006),[9] and Noonan syndrome (2007).[10]

Proponents of rhGH treatment in non-GHD children assert height, as an isolated physical characteristic, is associated with psychosocial morbidity and a justification for treatment. Others note controversy about such treatment[11] and question the evidence underpinning this quality-of-life rationale.[12,13] The objective of this article is to address the following questions: (1) Is SS an obstacle to positive psychosocial adjustment? and (2) Does increasing height through rhGH treatment make a difference to the person's psychosocial adaptation and quality of life?

This article begins with case examples, explores the beliefs, stereotypes, and assumptions regarding SS as well as the status of research evidence, and concludes with recommendations.

Cases and Clinical Management Considerations

Case 1

A 9-year-old boy growing below the first percentile for height was referred for ongoing management of SS attributable to being born small for gestational age (SGA) following a move from a different state where he recently started rhGH treatment. A routine psychosocial screening during the initial growth evaluation visit collected information from both parents and child. The screening revealed the boy is teased, exhibits behavioral problems, and does poorly at school. History, physical examination, and review of earlier testing confirmed the SGA diagnosis; the psychosocial evaluation suggested a learning disability and the presence of attention deficit hyperactivity disorder (ADHD) symptoms.[14,15]

Case 2

A 10-year-old boy, growing steadily at the third percentile for height, was referred to pediatric endocrinology by his pediatrician to evaluate unexplained SS. No current concerns about his height were noted, but his parents wondered if SS will make their son's life difficult in the future. History, physical examination, and laboratory results led to a diagnosis of ISS. Psychosocial screening findings corroborated a positive psychosocial adaptation.

Case 3

A 10-year-old girl growing at the fifth percentile for height was referred to pediatric endocrinology by her family doctor for a growth evaluation. Referral paperwork noted recurrent otitis media and possible developmental delay that has not been formally evaluated. At clinic, her parents reported she is doing poorly at school, where she is teased by children who call her "shrimptard" (a portmanteau of 2 popular insults at her school). Her parents hold SS responsible for the teasing, and the teasing responsible for her academic difficulties; they reason rhGH will increase their daughter's height, eliminate teasing, and allow her to have friends and to succeed at school. Physical examination revealed cubitus valgus, short neck with a slight webbed appearance, low-set ears, and a low posterior hairline; genetics workup indicated a 45,X/46,XX karyotype. She was diagnosed with TS.

Each of these 3 cases is based on the 30-year clinical experiences of one of the authors (D.E.S.) and represents common presentations reported in the literature: physiologically, psychosocially, and educationally. Case 1 highlights issues common to endocrine management of SS: consider what both patient and parent think rhGH has accomplished to this point or what it will deliver in the future; how might the parent and child expectations be assessed before simply continuing with the established treatment plan? Case 2 highlights issues common to generally well-functioning healthy youth with SS; note the parents voiced concerns about their son's future adjustment, not his current psychosocial adaptation. Case 3 highlights issues common to girls with TS: consider the physical characteristics, potential hearing impairment, social skills deficits, academic difficulties, and SS. Also note the parental focus on stature as the proximal cause of their daughter's difficulties and intuition that increased height through rhGH will bring about a resolution of social and academic difficulties.

IS SHORT STATURE AN IMPEDIMENT TO PSYCHOSOCIAL ADJUSTMENT?
Beliefs, Stereotypes, and Assumptions

Negative stereotypes about the social adjustment of those with SS are plentiful and have been reviewed extensively.[16] As children, those with SS are thought to face more negative social experiences, including teasing, being less accepted, and having fewer friends.[16,17] As adults, those with SS are thought to experience difficulties driving a car, to hold less prestigious jobs, to earn less, to hold fewer high-level academic degrees, and to have problems with dating and marriage (particularly short men).[13,16] Pervasive cultural "truths" characterize assertive short people as having a "Napoleon complex" or "short-man syndrome"; there is a long tradition of perceiving those with SS as overcompensating for their size.[12,18] In general, children's and adults' beliefs about height demonstrate a bias toward the notion that "taller is better." With few exceptions, people attribute significantly less favorable characteristics to short people compared with those of tall or average height.[18–20] In this context, it is not surprising that youths and adults of both genders desire to be taller.[21–23] These beliefs are not limited to the general public, but extend to physicians. In a national census study of pediatric endocrinologists' recommendations regarding initiating and discontinuing rhGH (n = 727), more than 50% reported the emotional well-being of children and adults with heights less than the third percentile is "sometimes" impaired, and more than 25% responded it was "often" or "always" impaired.[24]

Evidence

Taken together, well-documented beliefs and assumptions about those with SS directly associate SS with dysfunction (ie, **Fig. 1**, path "A"). It also implies SS leads to dysfunction as a consequence of experiencing psychosocial stress arising from being shorter than average (eg, teasing as a child, being too short to drive a car as an adolescent, or being rejected by potential romantic partners as an adult) (ie, **Fig. 2**, paths "B" and "C" illustrate stressful experiences mediating the relationship between SS and dysfunction).[25] Research on the relationship between SS and psychosocial dysfunction examines both direct and mediated relationships. Because of space limitations, this review is selective. Priority was given to studies with stronger research designs and those more frequently cited.

Teasing and Juvenilization

Chronic psychosocial stress is a risk factor for poor psychosocial adjustment. Indeed, early research on the psychosocial aspects of SS showed it was associated

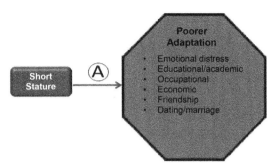

Fig. 1. Hypothesized relationship between SS and poorer psychological adaptation. Pathway (A) illustrates a direct effects model wherein short stature is posited to directly result in poorer adaptation.

with teasing and juvenilization (ie, treating people as if they were younger due to misperceiving chronologic age, thus potentially delaying social maturity).[17] These early reports were generally restricted to patients with complex medical conditions, and it is unclear if the findings are generalizable to the larger population of youth with SS seen by endocrinologists since the advent of rhGH in 1985. Studies of consecutively referred patients (some with normal growth pattern variants; others with pathologic growth) showed slightly more than half were regularly teased about being short; roughly the same proportion experienced juvenilization.[26,27] These studies corroborate anecdotal reports that SS is associated with childhood and adolescent psychosocial stress. However, not all short children in these studies shared these experiences; furthermore, stressors were not related to the degree of SS in either study.

Psychosocial Stress and Adaptation

A large, longitudinal, noninterventional community-based study conducted in a single UK region (ie, the Wessex Growth Study) found no evidence that SS (defined as height less than the third percentile) is associated with significant psychosocial or academic disadvantages.[28–31] Although shorter children preferred to be taller and reported more

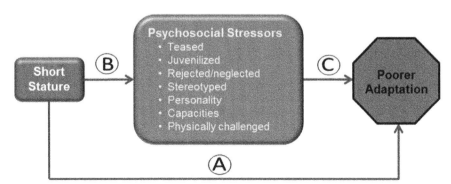

Fig. 2. Stressful psychosocial experiences mediating hypothesized relationship between SS and poorer psychological adaptation. Pathway (A) illustrates a direct effects model wherein short stature is posited to directly result in poorer adaptation. Pathways (B) and (C) illustrate a mediational effects model wherein psychosocial stressors mediate the effects of stature on adaptation.

"bullying" (the paper does not provide details for "bullying" in terms of either form or chronicity) when compared with their taller peers,[21] neither bullying, nor the desire to be taller, had measurable effects on self-esteem or school performance.[28,29,31] Similarly, a school-based study conducted in the United States (n = 956; 11–18 years old) assessed the influence of height on students' peer status (ie, popularity, friendships, and reputation) using peer nomination techniques.[32] Height was unrelated to popularity, total number of friends, or whether friendships were reciprocated. In terms of reputation among peers, short youths were distinguished from classmates on only one item ("looking younger"); but even here, being judged as younger was unrelated to social acceptance among peers.[32] Short students were not more likely to have the reputation of being someone who "gets picked on," "is often left out," or "is a class clown." Findings did not vary by gender, peer-report, or self-report, or whether data from the entire sample were used (ie, full range of heights) nor when very short ($\leq$ −2.25 height SD; first percentile) or very tall ($\geq$ +2.25 height SD; 99th percentile) students were contrasted with classmates of average height (25th to 75th percentile for norms). An interesting finding was that, just as marked SS was not associated with the predicted liabilities, marked tall stature was not associated with social advantages. It might be speculated that this study's findings would have conformed to predictions based on societal stereotypes if students had been informed at the outset that the association between "height" and peer relations was a focus (see Focusing Illusion in later discussion).[33]

How does one make sense of the reports that teasing and juvenilization related to SS are commonly experienced,[21,27] yet dysfunction does not necessarily follow? It is known that teasing and bullying are relatively common developmental phenomena that change in form and frequency with children's age.[34,35] A US study found approximately 30% reported some type of involvement in moderate or frequent bullying: 13% as a bully, 11% as a target of bullying, and 6% involved in both; both perpetrating and experiencing bullying were associated with poorer psychosocial adjustment.[36] Does this finding then amount to smoking-gun evidence that SS-related psychosocial stress is a predictor of dysfunction? To directly examine this question, the association between reported SS-related stressors and psychosocial adaptation was tested using data from the psychosocial screening of consecutively referred patients with SS being evaluated by pediatric endocrinology. The patient population was partitioned into 3 groups: (1) those experiencing neither teasing nor juvenilization; (2) those experiencing one, but not both, stressor; and (3) those concomitantly experiencing both stressors. Analyses revealed 2 patterns: stature-related stressors had a statistically significant negative effect on psychosocial adaptation and self-esteem only when more than one class of stressor was present (ie, a threshold effect), and the negative effects of stressors increased with their number (ie, a combination of teasing and juvenilization had a more negative influence on adjustment than either alone).[37] Of equal importance is the overall level of psychosocial adaptation of the patient sample: by parent report, there were limited differences between the clinic-referred group of short youths and questionnaire norms, and these typically were categorized into the small effect-size range.[38] By patient self-report, significantly higher behavior problems or lower social competencies were not observed. In sum, psychosocial stress does not imply dysfunction.[27,37]

Certainly, it does not follow from this interpretation that individual experiences of stature-related stresses should be ignored.[39] For example, for the 10-year-old girl with TS whose classmates tease her (case 3), the authors would not discount her experience as normative; rather, they advise interventions such as individual counseling to promote adaptive strategies for responding to name-calling that leaves self-image and body image intact and for working with her school or teachers.[40] To avoid the likelihood of unintended negative consequences, the reflex to intervene must be balanced against the evidence that parental intercession can exacerbate school-based stressors via unintentionally labeling the child as "overprotected."[37]

Educational Achievement

In the largest study of its type, and the only one based on a national probability sample of the US population (6–17 years), the relationship between stature and intellectual function (intelligence quotient [IQ] and academic achievement) was assessed.[41] Statistically controlling for potentially confounding socioeconomic characteristics, height contributed significantly (approximately 2%) to predicting both indices. The Wessex Growth Study replicated this general finding but identified socioeconomic factors, rather than stature, as best predicting psychosocial and academic outcomes.[29,42]

A difficulty in interpreting the literature on stature and intelligence or academic performance is that potential causal relationships cannot be fully determined. It may be that low socioeconomic status, associated with poor prenatal care, inadequate postnatal health care, or nutrition, contributes to poor growth velocity, reduced IQ, and reduced academic performance. Conversely, social or psychological burdens associated with SS contribute to downward socioeconomic mobility. The latter possibility becomes viable only with evidence that SS is, in fact, associated with stressors that result in dysfunction. However, the preponderance of evidence reviewed here suggests that, at a minimum, children and adolescents with SS do not differ significantly from their taller peers in terms of their psychosocial or educational adjustment.

Applied to these cases, evidence suggesting the presence of a learning disability and ADHD in the 9-year-old boy with SGA (case 1) and possible developmental delay and hearing loss in the 10-year-old girl with TS (case 3) should prompt additional evaluations (neuropsychological, otological) that can inform interventions including school-based individual educational plans.

Adult Educational Attainment and Economic Status

Turning from research on children to studies of adults, several investigations have explored the association between adult height, educational attainment, type of employment, and income.[43–48] Indeed, studies of stature and income often report taller men and women earn more than their shorter peers.[44,46–49] Such findings are commonly interpreted as reflecting influences of lowered self-esteem, social dominance, and height-based discrimination. An alternative conceptualization accounting for observed associations between height and psychosocial outcomes derives from extrapolations of the "thrifty phenotype" hypothesis (also known as the "fetal origins" or "Barker hypothesis," named for the clinical epidemiologist, David Barker). This hypothesis proposes that conditions early in life (ie, intrauterine malnutrition marked by low birth weight, poor postnatal growth, and SS) predispose individuals to health problems in adulthood.[50] In the context of the Barker hypothesis, SS is not viewed as directly causing differences in adaptation and achievement. Rather, both growth velocity and psychological adaptation are viewed as consequences of early events, such as those occurring during fetal development (**Fig. 3**). Research by Barker and other research groups that examine the relationship between stature and cognitive ability, employment, income, and even marital status provide support for the hypothesis.[51–53] A case in point comes from analyses conducted by Case and Paxson,[53] who suggested that, on average, taller people earn more because they possess stronger cognitive abilities throughout their lives. In secondary analyses of epidemiologic data sets from the

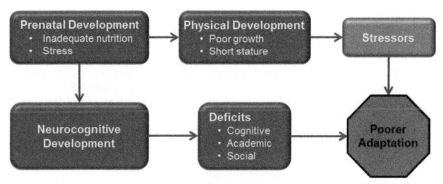

Fig. 3. Relationship between SS and psychosocial adaptation: a modified version of the Barker hypothesis.

United States and United Kingdom, they found support for the hypothesis that superior cognitive ability (which covaries with the timing of the adolescent growth spurt and adult height) accounted for differences in occupational status and income. They suggested that height only served as a proxy measure for an attribute of far greater importance in predicting occupational status and income: cognitive ability. This study is in line with a report by Barker and colleagues[51] suggesting that prenatal and early postnatal developmental factors exert lasting effects on health, educational, and occupational (including income) outcomes. An additional population-based study in Sweden leads one to similar conclusions.[54,55]

Adult Height and Quality of Life

Two population-based studies examined the relationship between adult height and health-related quality of life (HRQoL). The first study,[56] a secondary data analysis of the Health Survey for England, reported SS was associated with reduced HRQoL. Affected domains included "mobility," "usual activities," and "pain/discomfort." Emotional state ("anxiety/depression") domain scores did not show a relationship with height.[56] The second study, using a nationally representative sample of households in France, reported adult height was a very weak predictor of HRQoL in both men and women (adjusted R^2 always <0.2%).[57] Similar to the UK study,[56] the HRQoL dimension most consistently associated with height was "physical functioning." However, it was only height less than 149.2 cm (ie, -3.8 SD) and 136.0 cm (ie, -4.2 SD) or higher than 203.6 cm (ie, 3.8 SD) and 188.7 cm (ie, 3.9 SD) in men and women, respectively, which was associated with a lower physical functioning score. To note, these z scores reflect percentile scores less than the first and greater than the 99th percentile. The other HRQoL dimensions tapped (pain, role physical, role emotional, and social functioning) were either not significantly associated with height or the effects were not clinically meaningful. Finally, no interaction was detected between height and age.[57] The authors reconciled their findings with those of Christensen and colleagues[56] by pointing out that participants in the French study were approximately 15 years younger than those in the UK sample. They concluded that the findings of the Christensen and colleagues study were "heavily confounded by chronic conditions that were neither adequately controlled for nor even analyzed in relation to height."

Notwithstanding substantial clinical and population-based evidence that SS is not an independent psychosocial risk factor, one can certainly point to instances (real or imagined) wherein SS can limit activities or serve as a disadvantage. However, many of these suspected disadvantages prove to be false dilemmas; for example, not being able to play in the National Basketball Association (NBA). First, consider, tall or short, how likely it is for one to become a professional basketball player; then consider the examples of Muggsy Bogues (5'3") and Spud Webb (5'6"), who each had multiple-year careers in the NBA. Although these are exceptional examples, they point out that relative SS does not serve as a barrier to inclusion in any absolute sense. In clinical interactions with short youth, one of the authors (D.E.S.) never recommends against participation in a sport that selects for tall stature if the person expresses a passion for that sport. Instead, the author prepares them for the predictable challenges (competitive or bias), but points out that they would not be the first to succeed against the odds. He counsels that athleticism is often generalizable (ie, if gifted in one sport, they very likely would be above average in another in which SS may not be a disadvantage or, potentially, an asset).

Turning to activities of daily living, one issue that repeatedly surfaces concerns barriers SS is thought to represent to safe driving, particularly pedal access and air bag deployment. In 1997, the National Highway Traffic Safety Administration (NHTSA) reported a safe distance between the steering wheel (ie, from where the air bag deploys) is 10".[58] NHTSA investigated the degree to which this distance is achievable in a small study of 21 drivers whose heights ranged from 4'9" to 5'5". One person measured under a 10" distance (and another of the same height had a 13" distance); in several cases, shorter people had greater distance measurements. NHTSA underscored the importance of considering a vehicle's interior design, steering wheel position, driver's seat position, seat back angle, relative proportion of height to arm length, and driving habits.[58] Frontal air bags underwent a redesign in 1998/1999; a 2006 NHTSA technical report on the evaluation of this redesign showed no significant differences in fatality risk between the first- and second-generation air bags involving adult drivers and adolescent passengers.[59] Focusing only on severe frontal collisions in which the driver is unrestrained, both small drivers (women; height up to 5'3"; weight up to 125 lbs) and taller drivers (over 6') were "worse off" with the redesigned air bags. NHTSA concluded: "There is an exceedingly simple and increasingly popular way for drivers to avoid any of these problems: BUCKLE UP" (emphasis in original document).[59(p51)]

There are other ways around this and related issues. For instance, one can select a car in which height, either short or tall, is not a barrier to either comfort or safety.[60] Adaptive driving aids exist and can be found online with relative ease. Similarly, adaptive devices for one's home and office are available.[61] However, this is not to say that, once identified as an issue for a person, it should be brushed off as "not a real problem." Rather, it is to say that challenges in a person's environment should be identified and one should work with them to achieve a positive adaptation.[17]

DOES CHANGING HEIGHT MATTER?
Beliefs, Stereotypes, and Assumptions

In light of salient beliefs and cultural stereotypes, including evidence that primary care pediatricians endorse, to varying degrees, the notion that SS is associated with problems of psychosocial adaptation, it is not surprising that there is a public demand that is reciprocated by a willingness to refer young patients for evaluation and potential rhGH treatment. In a national study of US pediatricians, 39.2%, 46.6%, and 9.2%, respectively, thought that height less than the third percentile "sometimes," "often," or "always" impairs the emotional well-being of children. The parallel proportion thinking that height less than the third percentile in adulthood "sometimes," "often," or "always" impairs emotional being was 37.7%, 43.3%, and 12.3%, respectively.[62]

Even before examining the relevant evidence, it seems important to ask what the expectations of rhGH treatment are beyond increased measured height. The literature reviewed above challenges many of the beliefs and assumptions leading to predictions of psychosocial problems, and systematic reviews have failed to show that functional impairment is associated with isolated SS.[63,64] Of course, if one believes that taller stature is associated with higher quality of life, it is intuitively appealing to conclude that adding additional height with rhGH will deliver greater well-being. One industry-sponsored study reporting a correlation between height and quality of life suggested the finding, "may indicate that improving final height in children with growth disorders who are receiving rhGH treatment should result in positive HRQoL outcomes."[56] Such statements contribute to the common error of inferring causality from correlational data. Another example makes this point nicely: in a study of the relationship between height and income, the authors write, "prior research has estimated that an additional inch of height is associated with a 0.025 to 5.5 percent increase in predicted wages" and "we find that among white British men every additional inch of adult height is associated with a 2.2 percent increase in wages … we find that among adult white males in the US, every additional inch of height as an adult is associated with a 1.8 percent increase in wages."[44] The use of the word "increase" can easily be misunderstood as implying that doing X (ie, promoting additional inches of growth) will result in Y (ie, higher wages), which would be an example of the causal fallacy.

In an earlier section of this article (section entitled, Adult educational attainment and economic status), the thrifty phenotype (Barker) hypothesis was used to provide an alternate developmental pathway to account for the association between adult height and income (see **Fig. 3**). The Barker hypothesis emphasizes the role of nutrition (prenatal and during infancy) apparent in varying patterns of fetal and infant growth, in programming the person's physiology making it more prone to illness, in particular, cardiovascular disease.[50] Reports stemming from this line of research show that low birth weight and poor growth in infancy predict income at age 50 after adjusting for socioeconomic factors.[51] Other reports also suggest the relationship between adult height and income is best understood by viewing height as a proxy of early health and cognitive development.[53,65]

In brief, by interpreting correlations as evidence of causality, one risks promoting unrealistic expectations of outcomes by both patients and parents. One may also act out the idiom of closing the stable door after the horse has bolted: to the extent that growth and height are indices of healthy early development, strategic public health opportunities are missed by focusing on pharmacologically modifying visible consequences rather than proactively addressing cause.

Evidence

Physiologic response: height gain attributable to recombinant human growth hormone

Height gains from rhGH treatment in children with chronic renal insufficiency are approximately 3 to 9 cm[3]; 5 to 8 cm in TS[4]; 18 to 24 cm in Prader-Willi syndrome[5]; 6 cm in SGA[6]; 3 to 7 cm in ISS[7,8,66]; 8 cm in SHOX deficiency[9]; and 4–14 cm in Noonan syndrome.[10] Considering the 3 cases, height gained higher than expected through rhGH might raise the child's relative height in adulthood from the first to the 6.6th percentile (ie, −1.5 SD) in case 1 (SGA), from the third to between the seventh and 18th percentile (ie, between −1.5 and −0.9 SD) in case 2 (ISS), and from the fifth to between the 19th and 34th percentile (ie, between −0.9 and −0.4 SD) in case 3 (TS). Although all of these height outcomes for rhGH therapy have met the criterion of efficacious for FDA approval, all 3 cases are expected to remain below "average" height compared with their peers. Will these changes in height be judged "good enough" by the children and their parents? What is the likelihood that the children described in cases 1 and 3 will start performing better academically because of rhGH treatment? Should it be expected that rhGH will reduce teasing associated with signs of TS other than SS? Finally, as with case 2, is it possible that focusing on growth and stature, a consequence of daily injections and quarterly visits to the endocrinologist and associated laboratory tests, bone-age radiographs, height measurement, and comparison with norms, could be harmful (ie, a source of nosocomial distress brought on by focusing on growth)?[67,68]

Psychosocial consequences of increased growth velocity and height induced by recombinant human growth hormone therapy

Three randomized controlled trials of rhGH treatment in ISS were designed to investigate psychological outcomes. In the aforementioned Wessex Growth Study, children who were treated with rhGH were compared with those in an untreated control group at recruitment and after 3 and 5 years.[69] Despite significant increases in height in the treatment group, no differences existed between groups on behavioral measures at any of the 3 assessments. Comparable results were found in a prospective randomized controlled rhGH dose-response study in which no improvement on self-reported or parent-reported psychosocial adaptation and self-esteem measures were found, despite increases in height.[70] In the only randomized, double-blind, placebo-controlled study of the psychological effects of rhGH treatment in ISS, psychosocial adaptation and self-esteem of youths in both treated and placebo groups were comparable to the general population before treatment initiation.[71] Significant between-group differences in psychosocial adaptation were not detected in the first 2 years of treatment; parent- (but not patient-) reported behavior problems for the placebo-treated group were significantly higher than the rhGH-treated group after 4 years, and self-esteem scores did not differ between groups at any time point. Interpretation of the apparent benefit of rhGH on behavioral functioning (but not self-esteem) reported by parents is complicated by the fact that no systematic relationship was observed between participants' attained height (or change in height) and annual changes in psychosocial adjustment. Methodological issues, notably substantial participant attrition by year 4 in which only 3 participants remained in the placebo control group, limit conclusions based on this dataset.

In a retrospective study of young adults who either had or had not been treated with rhGH therapy for ISS, no differences in educational attainment or HRQoL were detected; however, treated patients had a romantic partner less often than those who did not receive rhGH in childhood.[23]

Factors accounting for inconsistencies in reports of the psychological effects of recombinant human growth hormone

Not all research studies are created equal. "Bias" refers to systematic error in results or inferences. Biases can lead to either underestimation or overestimation of the actual intervention effects. The dependability of randomized trial results depends on the extent to which potential sources of bias have been avoided. Accordingly, differences in risks of bias can help explain variation in the results of studies.

In an ongoing systematic review of studies examining the effects of rhGH following the procedures specified in the *Cochrane Handbook for Systematic Reviews of Interventions* for assessing risk of bias,[72] 47 studies were identified in which GH, either cadaveric human GH, biosynthetic/recombinant growth hormone (rhGH), or a combination of these, was administered to youth with SS (not attributable to GHD) for the purpose of increasing growth velocity and adult height in which HRQoL, psycho-social adaptation, or cognitive/academic outcomes were evaluated in non-GHD conditions (Sandberg and Gardner, 2014, unpublished findings). Study methods included both group (ie, experimental, quasi-experimental, and observational) and single-subject (ie, case study, case-control, and case-series) designs. Studies using random assignment to condition (eg, rhGH treatment vs no treatment) and nonrandom assignment (eg, pre-/postdesign within one group) were assessed for the presence or absence of bias in selection, performance, detection, attrition, and reporting.[72]

Results of the review revealed the vast majority of studies included features that present a high risk of bias in either their design or their execution (**Table 1**). A near-universal weakness, introducing the risk of bias and seriously weakening confidence in results, is the failure to blind study participants or research personnel from the knowledge of whether the participant received rhGH (ie, studies lacked a placebo control group). Placebo effects are most evident in studies assessing outcomes measured continuously (vs binary/dichotomous coding) and subjectively (eg, from the patient's perspective).[73] Continuous subjective variables characterize much of what has been studied regarding psychosocial outcomes in rhGH treatment trials.

Risks/ethical issues associated with recombinant human growth hormone treatment to increase adult height in non-growth hormone deficient youth
In prescribing rhGH to GH-sufficient children, potential benefits must be carefully weighed against the risks, known and unknown.[74] Regarding benefits, rhGH accelerates growth velocity during treatment and increases adult height, although adult height often remains substantially less than average. Nevertheless, patients overwhelmingly express satisfaction with height gained: at least one study has shown formerly treated patients and their parents greatly overestimated the additive growth benefit of rhGH.[23] Satisfaction, however, is not accompanied by demonstrable changes in short- or long-term psychosocial adaptation. Related to this, the Endocrinologic and Metabolic Drugs Advisory Committee of the FDA, responsible for approving rhGH in 2003 for ISS, expressed concern about the absence of data supporting purported psychological and psychosocial benefits, particularly quality-of-life data, and questioned the long-term safety of rhGH.[75] Although "many members of the committee were unsure … as to whether there was a reasonable risk-benefit profile," rhGH was approved for children with ISS, as "the majority of the committee … felt fairly secure that the drug is reasonably safe." Nine of the 10 committee members recommended mandatory surveillance of treated patients.[75]

The use of rhGH in non-GHD children and adolescents has been viewed as "safe," but that presumption has been questioned, in particular, with regard to safety

Table 1
Risk of bias in studies examining the effects of recombinant human growth hormone on psychological outcomes in growth hormone–sufficient youth

Study Design[a]	Risk of Bias		
	High	Unclear	Low
Random assignment	23	2	0
Nonrandom assignment	23	1	1

[a] n = 47 studies: risk of bias was assessed for each psychological endpoint. Ratings were performed separately for each psychological endpoint measured within a study (psychosocial, cognitive, or academic) because risk of bias varied by outcome. The 47 studies included 50 outcomes.

beyond the period of treatment.[66,76–78] In December 2010, the FDA posted a warning about the long-term safety of rhGH, referencing prepublication findings from the French component of the Safety and Appropriateness of GH treatments in Europe (SAGhE) study. SAGhE is an 8-country observational prospective epidemiologic study on the long-term effects of childhood rhGH treatment. Reports from the French cohort suggested that children treated with rhGH and followed for years after discontinuing treatment faced an increased risk of death when compared with the general population.[79] There was, and continues to be, disagreement about the veracity of the SAGhE findings. Indeed, in August 2011, the FDA updated the safety communication noting concerns over design weaknesses that limited interpretability and recommended physicians continue to prescribe according to labeled recommendations.[80] In a 2012 special feature commentary in the *Journal of Clinical Endocrinology and Metabolism*, opinion leaders in pediatric endocrinology from North America and Europe responded to preliminary reports by calling for the establishment of lifespan cohorts of patients treated with either rhGH or insulin-like growth factor 1 (IGF-1) during childhood, adolescence, and adult life.[81] The French study that prompted safety concerns was published later the same year.[82] Most recently, the same investigators of the same French cohort, using registry data (n = 6874) of those prescribed rhGH during childhood to treat idiopathic GHD, ISS, or SGA and comparing them to population-based registries, demonstrated a "strong relationship between hemorrhagic stroke and GH treatment in childhood."[83(p6)] The investigators encouraged that patients treated with rhGH should be informed of the risk of stroke. These findings and recommendations continue to be a source of debate (see replies to the 2014 article in *Neurology*).[84]

As clinicians, what is the right course of action when confronted with controversy about long-term safety? It is evident that parents want to know the relative risks and benefits of decisions they make on behalf of their children: in a study of parent attitudes and preferences regarding rhGH treatment for their children, researchers found that the most important attribute was "long-term side effects (risk)" followed by cost, child's attitude, the likelihood and magnitude of height increase, and route of treatment (in that order).[85] However, here, clear data are not presented to be able to speak with certainty about long-term risk. In the midst of controversy, and in the absence of evidence, using a shared decision-making paradigm in which clinicians, parents, and patients (inasmuch as their cognitive development allows) make decisions based on the best available evidence with full knowledge about evolving scientific controversies is recommended.[74]

WHY DO BELIEFS AND STEREOTYPES PERSIST DESPITE CONTRADICTORY EVIDENCE?

Contrary to popular beliefs and stereotypes that SS is an impediment to positive psychosocial adjustment and that rhGH-induced growth acts as remedy, the evidence reviewed here suggests that height, as an isolated physical characteristic, does not pose a threat to positive psychosocial adaptation, nor does rhGH treatment enhance psychological outcomes. Why, then, do these stereotypes and beliefs persist? First, consider that young children will ascribe positive attributes to tall silhouettes and negative attributes to short silhouettes.[19] What are the origins of such attitudes? One possibility explored is that the disposition to view taller people more positively than shorter ones is due to an evolutionary-based perceptual bias favoring phenotypic markers of good health.[86] Regardless of their origins, if negative perceptions of SS are focused on, there is a strong likelihood that will be overweighted relative to other characteristics, as predicted by the "focusing illusion."

The Focusing Illusion

A focusing illusion occurs "when a judgment about an entire object or category is made with attention focused on a subset of that category… whereby the attended subset is overweighted relative to the unattended subset."[67,68] In other words, if there is the stereotype that most people believe that SS is associated with less positive characteristics, it follows that quality-of-life evaluations that focus on this isolated trait would be negative. For example, in a study involving college students and dating, investigators asked 2 questions: "How happy are you?" and "How many dates did you have last month?"[87] Results demonstrated that the correlation between responses depended on which question was asked first. When the happiness question came first, the correlation was −0.12 (not statistically significant); when the dating question came first, the correlation increased to 0.66 (P<.001). Thus, focusing on one aspect of life (in this case, dating frequency) to the exclusion of others results in overweighting of that factor in the experience of well-being. In a different study, participants with Parkinson syndrome were randomly assigned to 2 conditions, differing only in the introductions, which were then followed by the same questions, including, "How satisfied are you with your life as a whole these days?," and next, "How satisfied are you with your current health?" Respondents in the *general public condition* were told the study was "being conducted by researchers at the University of Pennsylvania and is an attempt to better understand the quality of life of people who live in the eastern United States." In the *Parkinson condition*, they were told the study was "being conducted by researchers at the University of Pennsylvania Movement Disorders Clinic, and is an attempt to better understand the quality of life people who have Parkinson's disease."[33] Conforming to the predictions of the focusing illusion, reports of general life satisfaction correlated to a lower degree (r = 0.34) with their subsequent reports of health satisfaction when the study was introduced as a general population survey than when the study was introduced as a survey of the well-being of patients with Parkinson (r = 0.63). The introductions differentially primed respondents in the 2 conditions to consider their health status when responding to the items.

In light of the findings on the focusing illusion, might the clinical management of SS (eg, regular visits to measure height, blood draws for laboratory studies, bone-age radiographs, and, for some, daily rhGH injections) inadvertently prime both the parents and the affected child to focus on SS and overvalue taller stature compared with those in which the child is not medically followed or treated? Ironically, rhGH treatment of children who are destined to be shorter than average as adults, and the attendant focusing of attention on height over the years, may amplify the negative influence of this cognitive phenomenon. Of note, in the Wessex Growth Study, many parents of children with SS reported they were not aware that their children were short for their age until entering the study; nor had parents considered height to be a developmental issue.[88]

Height as a Proxy for Health

A large body of research in evolutionary biology suggests that somatic characteristics that are correlated with physical health serve as "signals" of such and are perceived as attractive.[89] For example, body symmetry, which refers to the extent to which one-half of the body mirrors the other half, is correlated with physical health and ratings of physical attractiveness. Similarly, taller stature is an index of physical health[50] and is viewed as a physically attractive characteristic.[90,91] Biological signals do not need to be perfectly predictive to add value in partner selection; they only need to enhance accuracy to be useful. In a recent analysis of a nationally representative dataset of American youth (National Longitudinal Study for Adolescent Health; $n \approx$ 15,000; 25–34 years), the more attractive a respondent was rated, the less likely he or she reported a history of chronic disease or neuropsychological disorders, a finding observed for both sexes.[86]

Perhaps theories in evolutionary biology provide the causal links between physical health, somatic phenotypes considered attractive, and the "taller is better" bias.[86,92] A strongly conserved biological mechanism influencing perceptions of physical attractiveness would account for its presence even in young children (eg, Ref.[19]) as well as its resistance to conflicting empirical evidence. In this context, the desire to manipulate any physical characteristic thought to be associated with mate selection is perfectly understandable. In fact, cosmetic procedures could be interpreted as an effort at uncoupling physical health from appearance.[89] Studies conducted in nonhuman species have allowed researchers to experimentally manipulate physical characteristics associated with mate selection; for example, lengthening the tail feathers of male birds, in a species in which the female mate preference is for male birds with long tail feathers, results in a compromised response to a novel immune system challenge when compared with male birds with naturally occurring long feathers.[93] The lesson here is attempts at decoupling appearance from naturally occurring biological mechanisms responsible for them can be associated with unintended and negative consequences.

SUMMARY AND RECOMMENDATIONS

Beliefs about the psychosocial liabilities of SS are common, but research provides variable support. SS is predictably associated with teasing and juvenilization, but these experiences do not translate to problems of psychosocial adaptation. This apparent paradox is potentially reconciled by understanding that psychosocial stressors, of one sort or another, are normative experiences and that children, adolescents, and adults are generally equipped to manage these without expressing signs of dysfunction.

In light of repeated observations that SS, as an isolated physical characteristic (ie, not confounded by underlying pathologic abnormality), is not associated with psychological dysfunction, it is not surprising that rhGH-potentiated growth has not been reliably demonstrated to evoke positive change in HRQoL. Beyond the need to first demonstrate a "problem" that rhGH then ameliorates, clinical trials investigating the effects of rhGH on psychological endpoints need to address threats of bias that permeate this literature. At this time, other than unequivocal evidence that rhGH yields taller stature than predicted without it, there is little to no evidence indicating that rhGH treatment alters HRQoL.

Recent reports from the European long-term health surveillance of people treated with rhGH in childhood or adolescence (SAGhE) have raised the specter of mortality in otherwise low-risk individuals. Findings from the French cohort have, as yet, not been replicated by other participating countries in the SAGhE network and controversies over the investigators' stated conclusions and recommendations exist.[84] Parents' desire to incorporate findings on long-term side effects (risks) of rhGH into their decision-making, juxtaposed with the evolving scientific controversy about safety, serve as a trigger to inform patients and parents of this controversy as part of a shared decision-making process [that there is a theoretic and, now, an evidentiary basis for concern about the long-term safety of rhGH, notwithstanding rhGH's "enviable track record of safety"[81(p81)]].

> **Box 1**
> **Clinical management recommendations**
>
> *Recommendations*
>
> • Conduct a psychosocial screening assessment
>
> • Learn about, and discuss, factors parents and patients are using to make treatment decisions (eg, do they think rhGH will "fix" problems at school? help find friends?)
>
> • Discuss rhGH treatment efficacy in terms of the degree of certainty and magnitude of effects
>
>   ○ Discuss what treatment is expected to accomplish
>
>   ○ Discuss what treatment is NOT expected to accomplish
>
> • Discuss the known and suspected benefits and risks of rhGH treatment in terms of actual height gain, what it will or will not do to address issues related to psychosocial adaptation, and the potential for long-term health risks associated with its use
>
> • Recommend psychosocial, educational, and other strategies known to directly address challenges associated with SS (whether it is the height itself or sequelae of the condition underlying the SS; eg, hearing loss associated with otitis media in TS)

For each of the 3 patient cases described earlier, it is recommended that psychosocial screening assessments be conducted in addition to physical, laboratory, and radiological evaluations to learn about (and discuss) the factors parents and patients are using to make decisions regarding treatment options, and working with families to consider the full range of services available to address their concerns, including endocrinologic (rhGH), psychological (psychosocial counseling), educational, and others as applicable (**Box 1**).

REFERENCES

1. Tanner JM, Whitehouse RH. Clinical longitudinal standards for height, weight, height velocity, weight velocity, and stages of puberty. Arch Dis Child 1976; 51(3):170–9.
2. Centers for Disease Control and Prevention. Clinical growth charts. Available at: http://www.cdc.gov/growthcharts/clinical_charts.htm. Accessed August 16, 2014.
3. Vimalachandra D, Craig JC, Cowell CT, et al. Growth hormone treatment in children with chronic renal failure: a meta-analysis of randomized controlled trials. J Pediatr 2001;139(4):560–7.
4. Baxter L, Bryant J, Cave Carolyn B, et al. Recombinant growth hormone for children and adolescents with Turner syndrome. Cochrane Database Syst Rev 2007;(1):CD003887. Available at: http://onlinelibrary.wiley.com.
5. Sipilä I, Sintonen H, Hietanen H, et al. Long-term effects of growth hormone therapy on patients with Prader–Willi syndrome. Acta Pædiatrica 2010;99(11):1712–8.
6. Rogol AD. Growth hormone treatment for children born small for gestational age. UpToDate 2014. Available at: http://www.uptodate.com/contents/growth-hormone-treatment-for-children-born-small-for-gestational-age. Accessed August 29, 2014.
7. Finkelstein BS, Imperiale TF, Speroff T, et al. Effect of growth hormone therapy on height in children with idiopathic short stature: a meta-analysis. Arch Pediatr Adolesc Med 2002;156(3):230–40.
8. Bryant J, Baxter L, Cave C, et al. Recombinant growth hormone for idiopathic short stature in children and adolescents. Cochrane Database Syst Rev 2007;(3):CD004440. Available at: http://onlinelibrary.wiley.com.

9. Blum WF, Cao D, Hesse V, et al. Height gains in response to growth hormone treatment to final height are similar in patients with SHOX deficiency and Turner syndrome. Horm Res Paediatr 2009;71(3):167–72.

10. Dahlgren J. GH Therapy in Noonan syndrome: review of final height data. Horm Res Paediatr 2009;72(Suppl 2):46–8.

11. Allen DB, Fost N. hGH for short stature: ethical issues raised by expanded access. J Pediatr 2004;144:648–52.

12. Voss LD. Is short stature a problem? The psychological view. Eur J Endocrinol 2006;155(Suppl 1):S39–45.

13. Sandberg DE, Colsman M. Growth hormone treatment of short stature: status of the quality of life rationale. Horm Res 2005;63(6):275–83.

14. Nomura Y, Halperin JM, Newcorn JH, et al. The risk for impaired learning-related abilities in childhood and educational attainment among adults born near-term. J Pediatr Psychol 2009;34(4):406–18.

15. Heinonen K, Raikkonen K, Pesonen AK, et al. Behavioural symptoms of attention deficit/hyperactivity disorder in preterm and term children born small and appropriate for gestational age: a longitudinal study. BMC Pediatr 2010;10(1):91.

16. Sandberg DE, Colsman M, Voss LD. Short stature and quality of life: a review of assumptions and evidence. In: Pescovitz OH, Eugster E, editors. Pediatric endocrinology: mechanisms, manifestations, and management. Philadelphia: Lippincourt, Williams & Wilkins; 2004. p. 191–202.

17. Meyer-Bahlburg HF. Short stature: psychological issues. In: Lifshitz F, editor. Pediatric endocrinology, vol. 2. New York: Marcel Dekker; 1990. p. 173–96.

18. Martel LF, Biller H. Stature and stigma: the biopsychosocial development of short males. Lexington (MA): Lexington Books; 1987.

19. Clopper R, Mazur T, Ellis A, et al. Height and children's stereotypes. In: Stabler B, Underwood L, editors. Growth, stature, and adaptation. Chapel Hill (NC): University of North Carolina at Chapel Hill; 1994. p. 7–18.

20. Gacsaly SA, Borges CA. The male physique and behavioral expectancies. J Psychol 1979;101:97–102.

21. Voss LD, Mulligan J. Bullying in school: are short pupils at risk? Questionnaire study in a cohort. BMJ 2000;320(7235):612–3.

22. Arkoff A, Weaver HB. Body image and body dissatisfaction in Japanese-Americans. J Soc Psychol 1966;68:323–30.

23. Rekers-Mombarg LT, Busschbach JJ, Massa GG, et al. Quality of life of young adults with idiopathic short stature: effect of growth hormone treatment. Acta Pædiatrica 1998;87(8):865–70.

24. Silvers JB, Marinova D, Mercer MB, et al. A national study of physician recommendations to initiate and discontinue growth hormone for short stature. Pediatrics 2010;126(3):468–76.

25. Rose BM, Holmbeck GN, Coakley RM, et al. Mediator and moderator effects in developmental and behavioral pediatric research. J Dev Behav Pediatr 2004;26:58–67.

26. Zimet GD, Powell SS, Farley GK, et al. Psychometric characteristics of the multidimensional scale of perceived social support. J Pers Assess 1990;55(3):610–7.

27. Sandberg D, Michael P. Psychosocial stresses related to short stature: does their presence imply psychiatric dysfunction?. In: Drotar D, editor. Assessing pediatric health-related quality of life and functional status: implications for research. Mahwah (NJ): Lawrence Erlbaum Associates; 1998. p. 287–312.

28. Voss LD, Mulligan J, Stabler B, et al. The short 'normal' child in school: self-esteem, behavior and attainment before puberty (The Wessex Growth Study).

In: Stabler B, Underwood LE, editors. Growth, stature and adaptation. Chapel Hill (NC): University of North Carolina at Chapel Hill Press; 1994. p. 47–64.

29. Downie AB, Mulligan J, Stratford RJ, et al. Are short normal children at a disadvantage? The Wessex growth study. BMJ 1997;314(7074):97–100.

30. Voss LD. Short but normal. Arch Dis Child 1999;81(4):370–1.

31. Ulph F, Betts P, Mulligan J, et al. Personality functioning: the influence of stature. Arch Dis Child 2004;89:17–21.

32. Sandberg DE, Bukowski WM, Fung CM, et al. Height and social adjustment: are extremes a cause for concern and action? Pediatrics 2004;114(3):744–50.

33. Smith D, Schwarz N, Roberts T, et al. Why are you calling me? how study introductions change response patterns. Qual Life Res 2006;15(4):621–30.

34. Keltner D, Capps L, Kring AM, et al. Just teasing: a conceptual analysis and empirical review. Psychol Bull 2001;127:229–48.

35. Warm TR. The role of teasing in development and vice versa. J Dev Behav Pediatr 1997;18(2):97–101.

36. Nansel TR, Overpeck M, Pilla RS, et al. Bullying behaviors among US youth: prevalence and association with psychosocial adjustment. JAMA 2001;285(16): 2094–100.

37. Sandberg DE. Short stature: psychosocial interventions. Horm Res Paediatr 2011;76(Suppl 3):29–32.

38. Cohen J. Statistical power for the behavioral sciences. Hillsdale (NJ): Lawrence Erlbaum Associates; 1988.

39. Horowitz JA, Vessey JA, Carlson KL, et al. Teasing and bullying experiences of middle school students. J Am Psychiatr Nurses Assoc 2004;10(4):165–72.

40. DeRosier ME. Building relationships and combating bullying: effectiveness of a school-based social skills group intervention. J Clin Child Adolesc Psychol 2004;33(1):196–201.

41. Wilson DM, Hammer LD, Duncan PM, et al. Growth and intellectual development. Pediatrics 1986;78(4):646–50.

42. Voss LD, Mulligan J, Betts PR. Short stature at school entry — an index of social deprivation? (The Wessex Growth Study). Child Care Health Dev 1998;24(2): 145–56.

43. Schultz TP. Wage gains associated with height as a form of health human capital. Am Econ Rev 2002;92(2):349–53.

44. Persico N, Postlewaite RJ, Silverman D. The effect of adolescent experience on labor market outcomes: the case of height. J Polit Econ 2004;112:1019–53.

45. Heineck G. Up in the skies? The relationship between body height and earnings in Germany. Labour 2005;19(3):469–89.

46. Ekwo E, Gosselink C, Roizen N, et al. The effect of height on family income. Am J Hum Biol 1991;3:181–8.

47. Harper B. Beauty, stature and the labour market: a British cohort study. Oxf Bull Econ Stat 2000;62:771–800.

48. Judge TA, Cable DM. The effect of physical height on workplace success and income: preliminary test of a theoretical model. J Appl Psychol 2004;89:428–41.

49. Sargent JD, Blanchflower DG. Obesity and stature in adolescence and earnings in young adulthood. Analysis of a British birth cohort. Arch Pediatr Adolesc Med 1994;148(7):681–7.

50. Barker DJ. The developmental origins of well-being. Philos Trans R Soc Lond B Biol Sci 2004;359:1359–66.

51. Barker DJ, Eriksson JG, Forsen T, et al. Infant growth and income 50 years later. Arch Dis Child 2005;90:272–3.

52. Phillips DI, Handelsman DJ, Eriksson JG, et al. Prenatal growth and subsequent marital status: longitudinal study. BMJ 2001;322(7289):771.
53. Case A, Paxson C. Height, health, and cognitive function at older ages. Am Econ Rev 2008;98(2):463–7.
54. Lundgren EM, Tuvemo T, Gustafsson J. Short adult stature and overweight are associated with poor intellectual performance in subjects born preterm. Horm Res Paediatr 2011;75(2):138–45.
55. Sandberg DE. Comments on 'Short adult stature and overweight are associated with poor intellectual performance in subjects born preterm' by Lundgren et al., Horm Res Paediatr 2011;75:138–145. Horm Res Paediatr 2011;75(2):146–7.
56. Christensen TL, Djurhuus CB, Clayton P, et al. An evaluation of the relationship between adult height and health-related quality of life in the general UK population. Clin Endocrinol (oxf) 2007;67(3):407–12.
57. Coste J, Pouchot J, Carel JC. Height and health-related quality of life: a nationwide population study. J Clin Endocrinol Metab 2012;97(9):3231–9.
58. National Highway Traffic Safety Administration, Office of Regulatory Analysis and Evaluation, Plans and Policy. FMVSS NO. 208: Air bag on-off switches. November, 1997. Available at: http://autopedia.com/html/Airbag/RegEval/. Accessed October 12, 2014.
59. Department of Transportation, National Highway Traffic Safety Administration. NHTSA technical report (DOT HS 810 685): an evaluation of the 1998-1999 redesign of frontal air bags August 2006. Available at: http://www-nrd.nhtsa.dot.gov/Pubs/810685.pdf. Accessed October 12, 2014.
60. Best cars for tall or short drivers. Consumer reports May 2014. Available at: http://www.consumerreports.org/cro/2012/02/best-cars-for-tall-or-short-drivers/index.htm. Accessed October 12, 2014.
61. Little People of America. Adaptive products. Available at: http://www.lpaonline.org/index.php?option=com_content&view=article&id=24. Accessed October 12, 2014.
62. Cuttler L, Marinova D, Mercer MB, et al. Patient, physician, and consumer drivers: referrals for short stature and access to specialty drugs. Med Care 2009;47(8):858–65.
63. Wheeler PG, Bresnahan K, Shephard BA, et al. Short stature and functional impairment: a systematic review. Arch Pediatr Adolesc Med 2004;158(3):236–43.
64. Agency for Healthcare Research and Quality. Criteria for determining disability in infants and children: short stature. Evidence report/technology assessment: number 732003. Available at: http://www.ahrq.gov/clinic/tp/shorttp.htm. Accessed October 12, 2014.
65. Heineck G. Too tall to be smart? The relationship between height and cognitive abilities. Econ Lett 2009;105(1):78–80.
66. Watson SE, Rogol AD. Recent updates on recombinant human growth hormone outcomes and adverse events. Curr Opin Endocrinol Diabetes Obes 2013;20(1):39–43.
67. Kahneman D, Krueger AB, Schkade D, et al. Would you be happier if you were richer? A focusing illusion. Science 2006;312(5782):1908–10.
68. Schkade DA, Kahneman D. Does living in California make people happy? A focusing illusion in judgments of life satisfaction. Psychol Sci 1998;9(5):340–6.
69. Downie AB, Mulligan J, McCaughey ES, et al. Psychological response to growth hormone treatment in short normal children. Arch Dis Child 1996;75(1):32–5.
70. Theunissen NC, Kamp GA, Koopman HM, et al. Quality of life and self-esteem in children treated for idiopathic short stature. J Pediatr 2002;140:507–15.

71. Ross JL, Sandberg DE, Rose SR, et al. Psychological adaptation in children with idiopathic short stature treated with growth hormone or placebo. J Clin Endocrinol Metab 2004;89(10):4873–8.

72. Higgins JPT, Green S, editors. Cochrane Handbook for Systematic Reviews of Interventions Version 5.1.0 [updated March 2011]. The Cochrane Collaboration, 2011. Available at: www.cochrane-handbook.org. Accessed March 21, 2011.

73. Hrobjartsson A, Gotzsche PC. Is the placebo powerless? An analysis of clinical trials comparing placebo with no treatment. N Engl J Med 2001;344:1594–602.

74. Laventhal NT, Shuchman M, Sandberg DE. Warning about warnings: weighing risk and benefit when information is in a state of flux. Horm Res Paediatr 2013; 79(1):4–8.

75. Department of Health and Human Services, Food and Drug Administration, Center for Drug Evaluation and Research (CDER). Endocrinologic and metabolic drugs advisory committee meeting. June 10, 2003; Available at: http://www.fda.gov/ohrms/dockets/ac/03/transcripts/3957T1.htm. Accessed October 12, 2014.

76. Cuttler L. Editorial: safety and efficacy of growth hormone treatment for idiopathic short stature. J Clin Endocrinol Metab 2005;90(9):5502–4.

77. Quigley CA, Gill AM, Crowe BJ, et al. Safety of growth hormone treatment in pediatric patients with idiopathic short stature. J Clin Endocrinol Metab 2005; 90(9):5188–96.

78. Kemp SF, Kuntze J, Attie KM, et al. Efficacy and safety results of long-term growth hormone treatment of idiopathic short stature. J Clin Endocrinol Metab 2005; 90(9):5247–53.

79. Food and Drug Administration. Drug safety communication. Recombinant human growth hormone (somatropin): ongoing safety review—possible increased risk of death. December 22, 2010. Available at: www.fda.gov/Safety/MedWatch/SafetyInformation/SafetyAlertsforHumanMedicalProducts/ucm237969.htm. Accessed October 12, 2014.

80. U.S. Food and Drug Administration. FDA Drug Safety Communication: Safety review update of recombinant human growth hormone (somatropin) and possible increased risk of death. August 4, 2011. Available at: http://www.fda.gov/Drugs/DrugSafety/ucm265865.htm. Accessed October 12, 2014.

81. Rosenfeld RG, Cohen P, Robison LL, et al. Long-term surveillance of growth hormone therapy. J Clin Endocrinol Metab 2012;97(1):68–72.

82. Carel JC, Ecosse E, Landier F, et al. Long-term mortality after recombinant growth hormone treatment for isolated growth hormone deficiency or childhood short stature: preliminary report of the French SAGhE Study. J Clin Endocrinol Metab 2012;97(2):416–25.

83. Poidvin A, Touzé E, Ecosse E, et al. Growth hormone treatment for childhood short stature and risk of stroke in early adulthood. Neurology 2014;83(9):780–6.

84. Coste J, Touzé E, Carel JC. Should learned societies be blind to new safety evidence? Response to letters to the editor re "Growth hormone treatment for childhood short stature and risk of stroke in early adulthood". Neurology 2014, September 18. Available at: http://www.neurology.org/content/83/9/780/reply#neurology_el_61719. Accessed October 12, 2014.

85. Finkelstein BS, Singh J, Silvers JB, et al. Patient attitudes and preferences regarding treatment: GH therapy for childhood short stature. Horm Res 1999; 51(Suppl 1):67–72.

86. Nedelec JL, Beaver KM. Physical attractiveness as a phenotypic marker of health: an assessment using a nationally representative sample of American adults. Evol Hum Behav 2014;35(6):456–63.

87. Strack F, Martin LL, Schwarz N. Priming and communication: social determinants of information use in judgments of life satisfaction. Eur J Soc Psychol 1988;18(5): 429–42.
88. Stratford R, Mulligan J, Downie B, et al. Threats to validity in the longitudinal study of psychological effects: the case of short stature. Child Care Health Dev 1999; 25(6):401–21.
89. Gangestad SW, Scheyd GJ. The evolution of human physical attractiveness. Annu Rev Anthropol 2005;34(1):523–48.
90. Jackson LA, Ervin KS. Height stereotypes of women and men: the liabilities of shortness for both sexes. J Soc Psychol 1992;132(4):433–45.
91. Pawlowski B, Koziel S. The impact of traits offered in personal advertisements on response rates. Evol Hum Behav 2002;23(2):139–49.
92. Gallup GG Jr, Frederick DA. The science of sex appeal: an evolutionary perspective. Rev Gen Psychol 2010;14(3):240–50.
93. Saino N, Møller AP. Sexual ornamentation and immunocompetence in the barn swallow. Behav Ecol 1996;7(2):227–32.

Approach to the Infant with a Suspected Disorder of Sex Development

Diane K. Wherrett, MD, FRCPC

KEYWORDS

- Disorders of sex development • Genital ambiguity • Sexual differentiation
- Congenital adrenal hyperplasia • Androgen insensitivity syndrome • Family support
- Gender assignment

KEY POINTS

- A thoughtful approach to the diagnostic evaluation of infants with a suspected disorder of sex development can optimize the process of reaching a diagnosis and assigning a gender.
- Psychosocial support to families is a critical aspect of comprehensive care.
- Referral to a multidisciplinary team with expertise in the care of disorders of sex development is recommended.

INTRODUCTION

A request to see a newborn with genital ambiguity is an uncommon experience in the career of most pediatricians. However, when including the full range of disorders of sex development (DSD), the prevalence is approximately 1 in 1500 births with significant genital ambiguity found in about 1 in 5000 births.[1] The pediatrician is faced with the clinical concerns of acute threats to the infant's clinical status, establishing a differential diagnosis, determining appropriate investigations and, importantly, providing explanation and support to the parents in an honest and sensitive way. This article reviews normal sexual differentiation, highlights key points in the medical history and physical examination noting normal findings, suggests a rational approach to investigation, and provides guidance on support for parents and families.

SEXUAL DIFFERENTIATION

The components of physical sexual differentiation include chromosomes, gonads, and internal and external genitalia. Other important concepts include gender identity,

Division of Endocrinology, Department of Pediatrics, Hospital for Sick Children, University of Toronto, 555 University Avenue, Toronto, Ontario M5G 1X8, Canada
E-mail address: diane.wherrett@sickkids.ca

Pediatr Clin N Am 62 (2015) 983–999
http://dx.doi.org/10.1016/j.pcl.2015.04.011   **pediatric.theclinics.com**
0031-3955/15/$ – see front matter © 2015 Elsevier Inc. All rights reserved.

one's internal sense of gender, and gender role, one's gender-related behavior and interests in society. The recognition that all infants begin sexual differentiation with the same bipotential structures and that the expression of many genes, transcription factors, enzymes, and receptors leads to typical male and female development is critical (**Fig. 1**). Explanation of these concepts to parents is helpful in describing how atypical sexual differentiation occurs.

Development occurs in 2 phases, first "sex determination", the development of the undifferentiated gonad into a testis or ovary and then, "sexual differentiation", where phenotypic sex develops through the action of gonadal and other hormones. In typical male development, action of the SRY gene (which resides on the Y chromosome) and many other genes lead to the development of testes at around 6 weeks of gestation. Primordial germ cells then migrate to the gonad. In early pregnancy human chorionic gonadotropin (hCG) stimulates the Leydig cells of the testes to produce androgens. Luteinizing hormone (LH) from the pituitary gland takes over this function during the second and third trimesters. Signaling through the androgen receptor then leads to the development of the Wolffian ducts to form the internal genital structures of vas deferens, seminal vesicles, and epididymis during the first trimester. Anti-Müllerian hormone (AMH) production by the Sertoli cells of the testes leads to regression of the Müllerian ducts. Androgens and AMH act on the internal genitalia in a local fashion. Testosterone converted in the external genital structures to dihydrotestosterone (DHT) by the enzyme, 5α-reductase, leads to pigmentation, rugation, and fusion of the labioscrotal folds, growth of the phallic structure to form the penis, and migration of the urethra to the tip of the penis. The majority of these events occur in the first

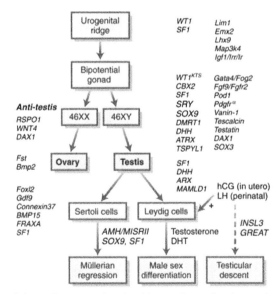

Fig. 1. Overview of the major events involved in sex determination and sex differentiation. Mutations or deletions in the genes shown in upper case letters have been reported or proposed as causes of disorders of sex development or gonadal failure in humans. The genes and factors shown in lower case letters have been proposed to play an important role in sex development, largely from studies of mice. DHT, dihydrotestosterone; hCG, human chorionic gonadotropin; LH, luteinizing hormone. (*From* Kronenberg HM, Melmed S, Polonsky KS, et al. Textbook of Endocrinology, 12th edition. Philadelphia: Elsevier; 2011. p. 868–934; with permission.)

trimester with ongoing growth of the penis throughout gestation and descent of the testes in the last half of the third trimester.

In typical female development, actions of genes on the X chromosome and other autosomal genes such as WNT4, R-spondin 1, and FOXL2 lead to ovarian development. Estrogen secretion by the ovary is not required for female internal or external genital development. The WNT4 gene is also required for formation of the Müllerian structures of the uterus, fallopian tubes, and upper third of the vagina. Without testis, the lack of AMH allows the Müllerian structures to persist, whereas lack of androgen leads to regression of the Wolffian ducts and allows typical female external genitalia to develop.

NOMENCLATURE

Terms used in this area such as "hermaphrodite," "pseudohermaphrodite," and "sex reversal" have been confusing to many and have been experienced as stigmatizing by patients. A consensus conference was held in 2005 that led to the development of new terminology that has been widely adopted. This terminology is based on the sex chromosomal constitution and uses the term "disorders of sex development" (DSD) to describe the wide range of conditions involved. Some criticism of this nomenclature has been presented, but overall it has been helpful.[2] See **Table 1** for details.

CARE OF THE INFANT

Infants with genital ambiguity benefit from assessment and care by a specialized team with expertise in DSD.[3–5] Subspecialty telephone consultation with the local team can help to determine the immediate plan of action, particularly when the distance to an experienced team is great or travel is difficult. Those babies with severe genital ambiguity need a rapid assessment by an expert team to facilitate efficient access to the appropriate consultations and investigations while providing support to the family. This goal can be accomplished by transferring the infant to the team's site or by a timely outpatient multidisciplinary assessment.

The majority of infants with genital ambiguity are otherwise healthy. Concern about the possibility of an adrenal crisis in healthy full-term infants often leads to admission to a neonatal intensive care unit. Because clinically significant salt wasting is extremely uncommon until the second week of life, full-term infants without other health issues can stay in their mother's room at the birthing hospital or, if transferred to a tertiary care hospital, be admitted to a ward competent in newborn care with the parents staying with the infant. This approach supports bonding with the infant and may reduce the trauma that some parents experience. It is also important that the baby undergo a careful physical examination by those involved in the infant's care, but not be subjected to multiple examinations by junior learners, because parents may experience that the infant is "on display." Care should be taken to use gender neutral terms such as "your baby," avoiding the use of he or she and definitely not "it." The role of the nursing staff caring for the infant is integral in ensuring sensitive care for the family. Establishing a single common person to communicate with the family can help to avoid confusion before being seen by the specialized team.

HISTORY

A thorough history can provide important clinical clues. Maternal virilization during pregnancy can point to an androgen-secreting tumor or placental aromatase deficiency. Maternal progestin use can lead to undervirilization of a genetically male infant.

Table 1
Nomenclature for DSD

Sex Chromosome DSD	46, XY DSD	46,XX DSD
A. 47,XXY (Klinefelter syndrome and variants)	A. Disorders of gonadal (testicular) development	A. Disorders of gonadal (ovarian) development
B. 45,X (Turner syndrome and variants)	1. Complete or partial gonadal dysgenesis (eg, SRY, SOX9, SFI, WT1, DHH, etc)	1. Gonadal dysgenesis
C. 45,X/46,XY (mixed gonadal dysgenesis)	2. Ovotesticular DSD	2. Ovotesticular DSD
D. 46,XX/46,XY (chimerism)	3. Testis regression	3. Testicular DSD (eg, SRY+, dup SOX9, RSP01)
	B. Disorders in androgen synthesis or action	B. Androgen excess
	1. Disorders of androgen synthesis	1. Fetal
	a. LH receptor mutations	a. 3 β-hydroxysteroid dehydrogenase 2 (HSD3B2)
	b. Smith–Lemli–Opitz syndrome	b. 21-hydroxylase (CYP21A2)
	c. Steroidogenic acute regulatory protein mutations	c. P450 oxidoreductase (POR)
	d. Cholesterol side-chain cleavage (CYP11A1)	d. 11 β-hydroxylase (CYP11B1)
	e. 3 β-hydroxysteroid dehydrogenase 2 (HSD3B2)	e. Glucocorticoid receptor mutations
	f. 17 β-hydroxysteroid dehydrogenase (HSD17B3)	2. Fetoplacental
	g. 5 α-reductase 2 (SRD5A2)	a. Aromatase deficiency (CYP19)
	2. Disorders of androgen action	b. Oxidoreductase deficiency (POR)
	a. Androgen insensitivity syndrome	3. Maternal
	b. Drugs and environmental modulators	a. Maternal virilizing tumors (eg, luteomas)
	C. Other	b. Androgenic drugs
	1. Syndromic associations of male genital development (eg, cloacal anomalies; Robinow, Aarskog, hand–foot–genital pterygium)	C. Other
	2. Persistent Müllerian duct syndrome	1. Syndromic associations (eg, doacal anomalies)
	3. Vanishing testis syndrome	2. Müllerian agenesis/hypoplasia (eg, MURCS)
	4. Isolated hypospadias (CXorf6)	3. Uterine abnormalities (eg, MODY5)
	5. Congenital hypogonadotropic hypogonadism	4. Vaginal atresis (eg, KcKusick-Kaufman)
	6. Cryptorchidism (INSL3, GREAT)	5. Labial adhesions
	7. Environmental influences	

Abbreviations: DSD, disorders of sex development; LH, luteinizing hormone.

From Pasterski V, Prentice P, Hughes IA. Impact of the consensus statement and the new DSD classification system. Best Pract Res Clin Endocrinol Metab 2010;24:187–95.

Other health issues in the infant can point to syndromes such as Smith–Lemli–Optiz or Denys–Drash syndromes. Consanguinity is important to ascertain, because many defects in androgen and/or adrenal hormone production are autosomal recessive. A family history of unexplained early infant death suggests congenital adrenal hyperplasia (CAH), and a history of hypospadias, primary amenorrhea, or infertility in the mother's family raises the possibility of an androgen receptor mutation, because this is an X-linked condition. A family history of infants with genital ambiguity is frequently not known to the extended family, but infertility, hypospadias, and amenorrhea are known more commonly to family members. It is also important to ask parents what investigations were done during the pregnancy, whether the infant's karyotype is known from prenatal testing, and what prenatal ultrasounds have shown. Finally, it is very helpful to understand what parents have been told by other health professionals.

PHYSICAL EXAMINATION

A careful general physical examination is essential, because the presence of other anomalies may lead to the diagnosis of a syndrome associated with genital anomalies. Assessment of growth parameters is important because hypospadias and undervirilization are more common in 46 XY infants born small for gestational age.[6] Examination of the genitalia should involve a careful assessment of each component—the gonads, labioscrotal folds, phallus, and urogenital openings. If gonads are not palpable in the labioscrotal folds, gentle downward palpation of the inguinal canals, using a lubricant, may demonstrate a palpable structure slipping under the fingers. The size of the palpable gonad should be measured. A palpable gonad is almost always a testicle, although rarely it can be an ovotestes. A normal, full-term infant's testicle has a mean volume of 1.1 mL.[7] The labioscrotal folds should be assessed for rugation, pigmentation, degree of fusion, and symmetry. Fusion begins posteriorly. The phallus should be assessed for size, the presence of chordee and the location of the urethra. The stretched phallic length (without foreskin) should be measured using a flexible ruler to allow for more accurate measurement in infants with chordee. The mean phallic length in a full-term boy is 3.5 cm with less than 2.0 to 2.5 cm being considered as micropenis.[8] Detailed references for phallic length can be found in the Consensus Statement on Management of Disorders of Sex Development.[5] An assessment of the phallic breadth and amount of corporal tissue is also important. A phallus that is of a normal breadth for a male infant but seems to be short may be a "buried" phallus that is partially hidden in the suprapubic fat pad rather than a microphallus. The normal clitoral size in a full term newborn is 2 to 6 mm in breadth and 2 to 8.5 mm in length.[9,10] The perineum should be examined for the number of orifices. A grading scale, the Prader scale, is used commonly to describe the degree of virilization in the external genitalia (**Fig. 2**). Some newborns with a disorder of sex development have very subtle findings on physical examination. **Table 2** outlines features that may alert to the possible presence of a DSD.

INVESTIGATIONS
Which Infants Need Investigation?

In many cases, it is clear that an infant needs investigation, such as when overt genital ambiguity exists. However, other infants with more mild clinical presentations should also be investigated, such as an apparently female infant with clitoromegaly with posterior labial fusion or an apparently male infant with bilateral undescended testes. There is debate around whether male infants with hypospadias need investigation. Most studies have found a very low rate of chromosomal or hormonal

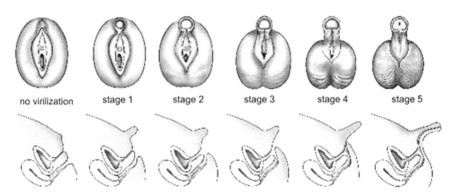

Fig. 2. Prader Scale. Prader scale reflecting the degree of virilization of the external genitalia. The internal genitalia reflect the changes in the urogenital sinus that may be seen with a 46XX disorders of sex development, such as congenital adrenal hyperplasia. (*From* Allen L. Disorders of sexual development. Obstet Gynecol Clin North Am 2009;36(1):25–45; with permission.)

abnormalities.[11–13] Only those infants with more severe hypospadias, most often when found with other issues such as micropenis or undescended testes, have a significant rate of clinically important hormonal abnormalities. Therefore, in most cases of isolated hypospadias with bilaterally descended testes and no other features of undervirilization, no investigations are warranted. Infants with isolated clitoromegaly merit investigation because there are many reports of the discovery of a 46XY disorder of sex development such as 5-α reductase deficiency, gonadal dysgenesis, or a disorder of androgen synthesis. Premature infants have a greater frequency of isolated clitoromegaly that does not typically have a pathogenic cause.[14,15] A family history suggestive of a previous DSD lowers the threshold for investigation. **Table 3** outlines clinical "pearls and pitfalls" in assessment of these infants.

Initial Investigations

Initial investigations may be undertaken by the general pediatrician if access to appropriate laboratory measurements with age-appropriate reference ranges and diagnostic imaging are available. In the setting where access to these investigations performed through facilities with the necessary expertise is not easily available, referral to a pediatric endocrinologist or specialized team before embarking on investigations is indicated.

Traditionally, the approach to initial investigations has been based on the presence or absence of palpable gonads. Palpable gonads are almost always testes and lead to investigations to elucidate the cause of undervirilization. Now, given the current rapid availability of detection, usually within 48 hours, of X and Y chromosomal markers by fluorescence in situ hybridization (FISH) or polymerase chain reaction, investigations can be guided by the preliminary indication of karyotype. Full karyotyping should

| Table 2 |
| Red flags for possible DSD in apparent male or female infants |

Apparent "Male Infant"	Apparent "Female Infant"
Bilateral undescended testes	Clitoromegaly
Bifid scrotum	Single genitourinary opening
Hypospadias with one other abnormal finding (undescended testis/micropenis)	Inguinal hernia

Table 3 Clinical "pearls and pitfalls"	
Clinical Assessment	**Pearls and Pitfalls**
Family history	Ask about hypospadias, early infant death, amenorrhea, infertility
Physical examination	Examine inguinal canals for gonads Assess girth of phallus, measurement of phallic length can be difficult with significant chordee A blind ending dimple at the tip of the phallus can be mistaken for the urethral opening in severe hypospadias Urinary flow can track along midline raphe and give appearance of a stream from the end of the phallus in hypospadias
Electrolytes	Salt wasting is rare before the second week of life
Hormonal	Measurement of androgens and adrenal hormones can be misleading, optimal assay techniques with age-appropriate reference ranges are required Adrenal hormones best measured after 48 h
Imaging	Abnormal adrenal appearance on ultrasonography can indicate CAH[24] Lack of visualization of uterus and/or ovaries on ultrasonography does not mean they are not present

Abbreviation: CAH, congenital adrenal hypoplasia.

always be obtained for confirmation and to detect mosaicism. These results, in concert with assessment of the internal genitalia by ultrasonography, allow a more streamlined approach to investigations (outlined in **Fig. 3**). If FISH results indicate the presence of 2 X chromosomes, therefore, an infant with 46XX DSD, CAH must be ruled out because it is the most common cause of 46XX DSD. Measurement of 17-hydroxyprogesterone (17-OHP) and renin at 48 hours of age (one must wait until after the surge of adrenal hormone production at birth) to diagnose CAH owing to 21-hydroxylase deficiency. Serum should be saved before initiating treatment for CAH to allow further hormonal assessment to be done if results point to other forms of CAH or alternate diagnoses. Newborn screening for CAH is done in many jurisdictions. Electrolytes can become abnormal toward the end of the first week of life in infants with salt wasting CAH, but the decrease in sodium and increase in potassium typically begin during the second week.

If FISH results indicate the presence of a Y chromosome, LH, follicle-stimulating hormone (FSH), and testosterone should be measured to assess testicular function. Increased LH and FSH indicates gonadal dysfunction. Testosterone and other androgen assays in the newborn period can be inaccurate, so an assay known to be accurate in newborns should be used. In addition, testicular production of testosterone varies with age with greater production at 12 to 36 hours, decreasing over the first week, and beginning to increase at 2 weeks with peak levels at approximately 6 weeks of life.[16] Again, serum should be saved for analysis of other androgens, such as androstenedione and DHT as needed. Testosterone is also elevated in most forms of CAH.

Ultrasonography can detect inguinal gonads, some intraabdominal gonads, uterus, and adrenal abnormalities such as enlargement, abnormal echotexture, or borders that are found in CAH.[17] Ultrasonography has limited ability to locate ovaries and intraabdominal testes. If a structure is demonstrated clearly, it is helpful, but lack of detection of a structure is not definitive. The quality and sensitivity of ultrasonography can vary, so review with a skilled pediatric radiologist may help when findings are not clear.

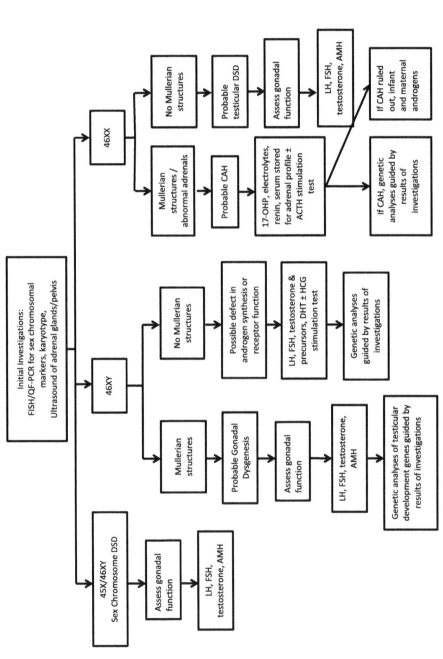

Fig. 3. Approach to investigations of infant with genital ambiguity. Flow of investigations based on results of initial assessment of sex chromosomes and ultrasound appearance of internal genitalia and adrenal glands. 17OHP, 17-hydroxy-progesterone; ACTH, adrenocorticotrophic hormone; AMH, anti-Müllerian hormone; CAH, congenital adrenal hyperplasia; DSD, disorder of sex development; FISH, fluorescence in situ hybridization; FSH, follicle-stimulating hormone; LH, luteinizing hormone; QF-PCR, quantitative fluorescent-polymerase chain reaction.

Secondary Investigations

Second-line investigations are often needed in the more rare forms of CAH, many cases of 46XY DSD and in sex chromosome DSDs. These investigations are best performed in a center with expertise in care of children with DSDs and are rarely undertaken by general pediatricians.

Assessment of adrenal function

Steroid profiling in serum or urine by mass spectrometry is done in some centers. Detection of elevated levels of steroid precursors and use of ratios of precursors to products allows identification of enzyme defects in CAH. An adrenocorticotrophic hormone (ACTH) stimulation (35 μg/kg) test can also be used to identify enzyme defects. Mineralocorticoid deficiency is detected by an increase in renin.

Assessment of testicular function

Leydig cell function and androgen production can be determined by an hCG stimulation test. hCG binds to the gonadotropin receptor and stimulates androgen production. Elevation of androgen precursors can indicate a defect of enzymes required for androgen production. It is also useful to measure DHT production to allow identification of 5-α reductase deficiency. Many protocols for hCG stimulation testing exist. Measurement of AMH allows assessment of Sertoli cell function. AMH levels are significantly higher in those with normal Sertoli cell function than in those with gonadal dysgenesis and those with ovaries.[18] Because AMH is now being used in assessment of ovarian reserve in adult women, this assay is available more widely. Use of age appropriate reference intervals is important in interpreting results. Inhibin B is also produced by Sertoli cells and has shown value in determining testicular function in DSD.[19]

Assessment of internal anatomy

The anatomy of the urethra and vagina can be defined with a genitogram. Radiopaque dye injected into the urethra can outline where the urogenital sinus separates into the vagina and urethra. Intraabdominal gonads may be located on MRI. In rare cases, laparoscopy with gonadal biopsy may be needed to reach a diagnosis.

Genetic testing

Molecular analysis is available in many forms of DSD, particularly CAH and complete androgen insensitivity. This analysis allows confirmation of clinical diagnosis and genetic counseling. Infants with syndromic forms of DSD may benefit from microarray analysis to detect chromosomal deletions. Newer genetic techniques, such as whole genome and exome sequencing, are beginning to be used and have shown to be promising.[20,21] These techniques will be particularly helpful in reaching a diagnosis for infants with 46XY DSD, because a definitive diagnosis is currently not found in many.

INTERPRETATION OF RESULTS
46XY Disorders of Sex Development

The causes of 46XY DSD in a newborn with genital ambiguity are disorders of testicular (gonadal) development, disorders of androgen synthesis or action and other causes, most commonly syndromic causes of abnormalities of genital development (see **Fig. 3**).

Low testosterone and low precursors (dehydroepiandrosterone sulfate, androstenedione)

Disorders of gonadal development Disorders of testicular development are characterized by the presence of Müllerian structures owing to lack of AMH production.

LH and FSH are elevated and androgen levels low, but this can be variable if the testicular dysgenesis is partial. The degree of dysgenesis generally correlates with the severity of the genital ambiguity. Those with complete gonadal dysgenesis have a female phenotype.

Defects in androgen production These conditions are characterized by lack of Müllerian structures because AMH production by the testes is normal. Enzyme defects high in the steroidogenic pathway (**Fig. 4**) result in significantly reduced androgen production. These disorders include deficiencies of steroid acute regulatory protein and p450 side chain cleavage enzyme. Both conditions result in severe adrenal insufficiency with salt wasting and most often female external genitalia or more rarely genital ambiguity. Very rare forms of defects in androgen production include 17α-hydroxylase/17,20 lyase deficiency and p450 oxidoreductase deficiency. Stimulation testing with ACTH, hCG, or both is often required to establish these diagnoses. These conditions are autosomal recessive.

Luteinizing hormone receptor defects (Leydig cell hypoplasia) Infants with LH receptor defects have elevated levels of LH, normal levels of FSH, low levels of all androgens, and poor response to hCG stimulation. They have no Müllerian structures because AMH production by the Sertoli cells is normal. The phenotype varies from female to male with micropenis, severe hypospadias, or cryptorchidism.[22] This is an autosomal recessive condition.

Hypogonadotrophic hypogonadism 46XY infants with severe deficiency of gonadotropins often present with micropenis and undescended testes. They have low levels of LH, FSH, and all androgens. There are no Müllerian structures.

Low testosterone and elevated precursors
Defects in enzymes required to make testosterone such as 17α-hydroxylase, 3ß-hydroxysteroid dehydrogenase (3ß-HSD), and 17ß-hydroxysteroid dehydrogenase result in low levels of testosterone and elevated levels of hormones proximal to the deficient enzyme. 3ß-HSD deficiency also results in adrenal insufficiency. Phenotype varies from female external genitalia to genital ambiguity. These enzyme defects are inherited in an autosomal-recessive manner and identified by ACTH and/or hCG stimulation tests. Müllerian structures are absent.

Normal/Increased testosterone and normal precursors and low dihydrotestosterone
5α-Reductase converts testosterone to the more active DHT, which is required for complete masculinization of the external genitalia. Defects in 5α-reductase activity result in normal or elevated basal and hCG-stimulated testosterone levels and a high ratio of testosterone to DHT. Affected newborns have variable phenotypes ranging from typical female appearance to small phallus with severe hypospadias. There are no Müllerian structures. This is an autosomal-recessive condition.

Normal/Increased testosterone, precursors, and dihydrotestosterone
Normal androgen production with lack of effects of androgen on genital development point to a defect in the androgen receptor. Both LH and testosterone can be mildly elevated due to lack of negative feedback at the LH receptor. There are no Müllerian structures. Those infants with complete androgen insensitivity have typical female genitalia and can be identified at birth when there is discordance between an XY prenatal karyotype and the genitalia. They can sometimes present with palpable gonads in the labia or in an inguinal hernia, or later in life owing to lack of pubic hair and

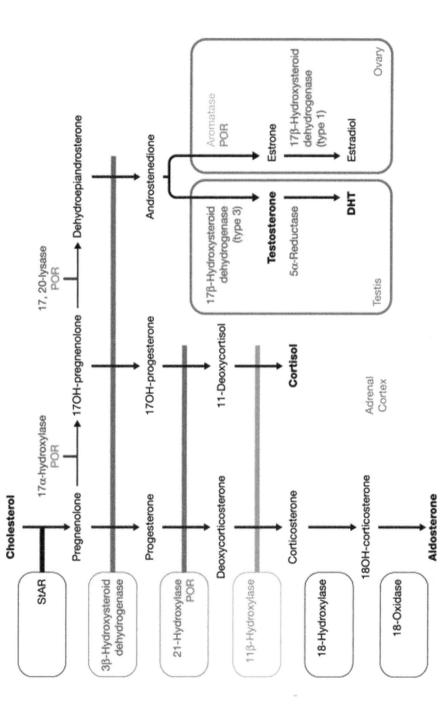

Fig. 4. Steroidogenesis pathway. DHT, dihydrotestosterone; POR, P450 oxioreductase; StAr, steroid acute regulatory protein. (*From* Murphy C, Allen L, Jamieson MA. Ambiguous genitalia in the newborn: an overview and teaching tool. J Pediatr Adolesc Gynecol 2011;24(5):236–50; with permission.)

menses. Those with partial receptor function present with genital ambiguity. Müllerian structures are absent. Androgen receptor defects are X-linked recessive.

46XX DISORDERS OF SEX DEVELOPMENT
Androgen Excess

Congenital adrenal hyperplasia
This is the most common cause of 46XX DSD. It is caused by 21-hydroxylase deficiency in more than 90% of infants with about 70% having salt wasting. Infants have high 17-OHP, androstenedione, and testosterone levels (see **Fig. 4**). The 17-OHP levels are higher in the first 48 hours of life and in premature and sick infants so caution is needed in interpretation of results in these settings. Cortisol levels can be relatively well-preserved, so they are often not helpful in making a diagnosis. Those infants with salt wasting begin to have low sodium and high potassium at the end of the first week. Renin is elevated in these infants. The degree of virilization varies from mild clitoromegaly to complete masculinization of the external genitalia but, importantly, without palpable gonads. Müllerian structures are normal. A genitogram is helpful in determining the relative length of the vagina and urogenital sinus (see **Fig. 2**). More rare forms of CAH are 11ß-hydroxylase deficiency and 3ß-hydroxysteroid dehydrogenase deficiency. These are diagnosed by identification of elevated levels of 11-deoxycortisol and 17-hydroxypregeneolone, respectively. ACTH stimulation testing may be helpful in clarifying the diagnosis.

Maternal/Fetoplacental causes
Rarely, pregnant mothers develop androgen-secreting tumors, such as a luteoma of pregnancy. The androgen secretion results in virilization of the female external genitalia. Testosterone is elevated in both mother and baby with normal 17-OHP levels in the baby. There is often a history of maternal virilization during pregnancy. Another uncommon cause of virilization in a female infant and mother is placental aromatase deficiency that results from a defect in the enzyme that converts androgen to estrogen. Drugs with androgenic activity taken during pregnancy can also cause virilization of a female fetus.

Gonadal causes
Ovotesticular DSD is most commonly associated with a 46XX karyotype, but is found with mosaic and XY karyotypes. Gonads containing both normal ovarian and testicular tissue or the presence of a normal ovary on 1 side and normal testes on the other side characterize this condition.[23] Infants can have ovotestes bilaterally or unilaterally with ovaries or testes on the opposite side. Internal genital development varies, as does external masculinization, although genital ambiguity is common. Asymmetry of the external genitalia often occurs. Testosterone levels are not helpful in reaching a diagnosis. Müllerian structures are often present, although they may be unilateral. A definitive diagnosis is reached most frequently on gonadal biopsy.

Testicular DSD can be found in those with 46XX karyotypes. This most often occurs in those with a translocation of the SRY gene to the X chromosome.[24] These infants usually have normal male genital development, so infants are identified when there is discordance between the phenotype and antenatal karyotype. Genital ambiguity can occur in other causes of 46XX testicular DSD, such as duplications of the SOX9 or SOX3 genes.[25] Müllerian structures are absent due to gonadal production of AMH.

SEX CHROMOSOME DISORDERS OF SEX DEVELOPMENT

Infants with mosaic karyotypes including 45X/46XY and 46XX/46XY may present with genital ambiguity. Asymmetry is often present in both the external and internal genitalia. Many of these infants have mixed gonadal dysgenesis with a streak gonad on 1 side and an ovary or testes on the other side. A smaller number have ovotesticular DSD. The most common phenotype in those with 45X/46XY detected antenatally is typical male. Testicular hormone levels correlate with the amount of normal testicular tissue present, so it is common to see levels of testosterone and AMH that are lower than the reference range for boys but higher than that for girls. Because the effects of androgens and AMH are local, Müllerian structures are found on the side of the pelvis where an ovary or streak gonad is present (due to lack of AMH production on that side) and Wolffian structures are absent (due to lack of testosterone production on that side).

SEX OF REARING DECISIONS

In many infants, the physical examination and investigations will allow a quick and easily made sex of rearing decision. In those with significant ambiguity, particularly in mixed gonadal dysgenesis, ovotesticular DSD, partial androgen insensitivity, and the most virilized infants with CAH, the decision is much more difficult. This decision needs to be made after careful review of the infant by an expert multidisciplinary team including endocrinology, urology, genetics, gynecology, and mental health professionals. Extensive discussion with the family to explain the underlying condition and treatment options must take place. Factors that are considered include the diagnosis, external genital appearance, internal genitalia, gonadal function, surgical options and outcomes, need for hormonal replacement therapy, potential for fertility, knowledge of gender identity based on the diagnosis, and wishes of the family. It is essential that the team works with the family to help them to understand the medical information and listens carefully to the aspects of the sex of rearing decisions that are most important to them.[26] The decision must be made jointly with the family and health professionals. The current approach is to assign a social sex, although there are some who advocate for delaying this decision until the child's gender identity is established.[5] German law now allows birth registration without indication of a gender.

NORMAL VARIANTS THAT CAN SEEM TO BE A DISORDER OF SEX DEVELOPMENT

Newborns girls can have prominent clitoris and/or enlarged labia owing to swelling associated with labor and delivery. This typically resolves over days to weeks. Lack of posterior labial fusion, and a normally placed urethra and vagina along with normal ultrasonography and 17-OHP levels indicate that this is a normal variant. Similarly, some infant boys have a full suprapubic fat pad that makes the penis appear to be very small. The presence of normal penile breadth, normally formed scrotum with 2 descended testicles, and the lack of hypospadias all point to this as a normal variant.

CURRENT CONTROVERSIES

There have been a number of controversial areas in care of patients with DSD over the past 20 years. Concerns began to be expressed by patients and patient advocacy and support groups in the early 1990s about a number of aspects of care. One concern was lack of patient-centered care, including the practice of not fully explaining medical information to patients and parents or giving inaccurate information, lack of psychosocial support for patients and their families, and the negative experience of having repeated genital examinations. The validity of these concerns has been recognized by the medical community and recommendations to address these issues exist and have become the standard of care.[5]

A second area of controversy is centered in surgery for DSDs. A number of publications have noted poor outcomes of surgery.[27-29] A lack of comprehensive follow-up of DSD surgery is also noted, with recognition of the obstacles in collecting such information given that surgery is typically done in infancy and results are not fully known until adulthood, and that surgical techniques continue to evolve. Furthermore, surgery done in infancy is before the time that the gender identity of the child is clear and is long before the child is able to consent for surgery. These concerns have led to recommendations by some in the field to delay surgery until the child's gender identity is clear and the child is able to give informed consent. This point of view is not held by all in the field, but there is uniform strong recognition of the need for detailed discussion and fully informed parental consent, including careful consideration of delayed surgery.[30,31] Because of implications for future fertility, these considerations are important when surgery to remove gonadal tissue is being considered.

PSYCHOSOCIAL CARE AND COMMUNICATION WITH THE PARENTS AND FAMILY

As the newborn with a disorder of sex development is assessed by the multidisciplinary team, it is important that the team's mental health professional does a careful assessment of the family to better gain insight into pertinent factors that will require exploration and support. Factors to consider include financial or social concerns, previous health care experiences, comprehension of medical information, family functioning and communication, coping skills, and perceptions of the impact of gender. The mental health professional often assists the family in articulating their questions and concerns. Helpful suggestions to families include the use of a journal to record the names and roles of health care team members, the family's questions, and results of tests. Audio recordings of important discussions with health professionals, particularly if 1 parent is not able to take part in the discussion, can be helpful. Many parents find the support of another family who has shared their experience is very valuable, as is referral to a DSD support group.

Sensitive communication is critical. Use of inappropriate terms and lack of open communication can be very psychologically damaging for families. Similar care needs to be taken in avoiding examinations by large groups of professionals. Suggestions for answers to common questions posed by families are described in the "Clinical Guidelines for the Management of Disorders of Sex Development in Childhood" published by Accord Alliance[32] such as:

Q: Is my child a boy or a girl?

A: Your question is very important. We wish we could tell you right this minute, but we really can't tell yet. We will have more information after we conduct some tests. It's hard for parents to wait for these test results so we will try to update you every day, and you can call [give contact person's name] at anytime. Although your baby has a condition you probably haven't heard much about, it isn't that uncommon. We've encountered this before, and we'll help you through this time of confusion. As soon as the tests are completed, we will be able to talk with you about the gender in which it makes most sense to raise your child, and we'll give you a lot more information, too, since quite a lot is known about these variations and we are learning more each day. We want to reassure you that our focus is on supporting you and your child in this time of uncertainty.

Web-based educational resources for families include:

www.aboutkidshealth.ca/En/HowTheBodyWorks/SexDevelopmentAnOverview
This website provides detailed graphically illustrated explanations of sex development and DSDs that health professionals can use when working with families.

www.accordalliance.org. This group provides advocacy and education to families and health care teams. Their website contains "Clinical Guidelines for the Management of Disorders of Sex Development in Childhood" for health professionals and "Handbook for Parents."

Support Groups
Androgen Insensitivity Syndrome: Differences of Sex Development Support Group; http://aisdsd.org/
CARES foundation: Congenital Adrenal Hyperplasia Research, Education and Support; http://www.caresfoundation.org
Hypospadias and Epispadias Association http://heainfo.org/

SUMMARY

DSD resulting in ambiguity of the genitalia are rare but significant. Newborns with these conditions require care by a multidisciplinary team that provides medical, surgical, and mental health expertise. Sensitive and supportive communication is important in helping parents and family to manage decisions and discussions. Psychosocial care for parents and the family is particularly important. Careful investigations typically allow a clear cause of the DSD to be ascertained, but a specific genetic diagnosis is not reached in many infants with 46XY currently. Sex of rearing decisions need to be made jointly with parents. Surgical decisions need to be made with full disclosure of the potential risks and benefits of any procedure, including the possibility of delay of surgery until the child is old enough to be part of decision making.

REFERENCES

1. Thyen U, Lanz K, Holterhus PM, et al. Epidemiology and initial management of ambiguous genitalia at birth in Germany. Horm Res 2006;66(4):195–203.
2. Pasterski V, Prentice P, Hughes IA. Impact of the consensus statement and the new DSD classification system. Baillieres Best Pract Res Clin Endocrinol Metab 2010;24(2):187–95.
3. Ahmed SF, Rodie M. Investigation and initial management of ambiguous genitalia. Baillieres Best Pract Res Clin Endocrinol Metab 2010;24(2):197–218.
4. Hiort O, Birnbaum W, Marshall L, et al. Management of disorders of sex development. Nat Rev Endocrinol 2014;10(9):520–9.
5. Lee PA, Houk CP, Ahmed SF, et al. International Consensus Conference on Intersex organized by the Lawson Wilkins Pediatric Endocrine S, the European Society for Paediatric E. Consensus statement on management of intersex disorders. International Consensus Conference on Intersex. Pediatrics 2006;118(2): e488–500.
6. Jensen MS, Wilcox AJ, Olsen J, et al. Cryptorchidism and hypospadias in a cohort of 934,538 Danish boys: the role of birth weight, gestational age, body dimensions, and fetal growth. Am J Epidemiol 2012;175(9):917–25.
7. Cassorla FG, Golden SM, Johnsonbaugh RE, et al. Testicular volume during early infancy. J Pediatr 1981;99(5):742–3.
8. Feldman KW, Smith DW. Fetal phallic growth and penile standards for newborn male infants. J Pediatr 1975;86(3):395–8.
9. Oberfield SE, Mondok A, Shahrivar F, et al. Clitoral size in full-term infants. Am J Perinatol 1989;6(4):453–4.
10. Riley WJ, Rosenbloom AL. Clitoral size in infancy. J Pediatr 1980;96(5):918–9.

11. Feyaerts A, Forest MG, Morel Y, et al. Endocrine screening in 32 consecutive patients with hypospadias. J Urol 2002;168(2):720–5 [discussion: 725].

12. Holmes NM, Miller WL, Baskin LS, et al. Lack of defects in androgen production in children with hypospadias. J Clin Endocrinol Metab 2004;89(6): 2811–6.

13. Moreno-Garcia M, Miranda EB. Chromosomal anomalies in cryptorchidism and hypospadias. J Urol 2002;168(5):2170–2 [discussion: 2172].

14. Couch R, Girgis R. Postnatal virilization mimicking 21-hydroxylase deficiency in 3 very premature infants. Pediatrics 2012;129(5):e1364–7.

15. Williams CE, Nakhal RS, Achermann JC, et al. Persistent unexplained congenital clitoromegaly in females born extremely prematurely. J Pediatr Urol 2013; 9(6 Pt A):962–5.

16. Tomlinson C, Macintyre H, Dorrian CA, et al. Testosterone measurements in early infancy. Arch Dis Child Fetal Neonatal Ed 2004;89(6):F558–9.

17. Al-Alwan I, Navarro O, Daneman D, et al. Clinical utility of adrenal ultrasonography in the diagnosis of congenital adrenal hyperplasia. J Pediatr 1999;135(1): 71–5.

18. Hagen CP, Aksglaede L, Sorensen K, et al. Clinical use of anti-Mullerian hormone (AMH) determinations in patients with disorders of sex development: importance of sex- and age-specific reference ranges. Pediatr Endocrinol Rev 2011;9(Suppl 1):525–8.

19. Valeri C, Schteingart HF, Rey RA, et al. The prepubertal testis: biomarkers and functions. Curr Opin Endocrinol Diabetes Obes 2013;20(3):224–33.

20. Tobias ES, McElreavey K. Next generation sequencing for disorders of sex development. Endocr Dev 2014;27:53–62.

21. Baxter RM, Vilain E. Translational genetics for diagnosis of human disorders of sex development. Annu Rev Genomics Hum Genet 2013;14:371–92.

22. Latronico AC, Arnhold IJ, Latronico AC, et al. Inactivating mutations of the human luteinizing hormone receptor in both sexes. Semin Reprod Med 2012; 30(5):382–6.

23. Sircili MH, Denes FT, Costa EM, et al. Long-term followup of a large cohort of patients with ovotesticular disorder of sex development. J Urol 2014;191(5 Suppl): 1532–6.

24. Wu QY, Li N, Li WW, et al. Clinical, molecular and cytogenetic analysis of 46, XX testicular disorder of sex development with SRY-positive. BMC Urol 2014; 14:70.

25. Eggers S, Sinclair A. Mammalian sex determination-insights from humans and mice. Chromosome Res 2012;20(1):215–38.

26. Magritte E, Magritte E. Working together in placing the long term interests of the child at the heart of the DSD evaluation. J Pediatr Urol 2012;8(6):571–5.

27. Creighton SM, Minto CL, Steele SJ. Objective cosmetic and anatomical outcomes at adolescence of feminising surgery for ambiguous genitalia done in childhood. Lancet 2001;358(9276):124–5.

28. Minto CL, Liao LM, Woodhouse CR, et al. The effect of clitoral surgery on sexual outcome in individuals who have intersex conditions with ambiguous genitalia: a cross-sectional study. Lancet 2003;361(9365):1252–7.

29. Creighton S, Chernausek SD, Romao R, et al. Timing and nature of reconstructive surgery for disorders of sex development - introduction. J Pediatr Urol 2012;8(6):602–10.

30. Warne GL, Mann A. Ethical and legal aspects of management for disorders of sex development. J Paediatr Child Health 2011;47(9):661–3.

31. Karkazis K, Tamar-Mattis A, Kon AA, et al. Genital surgery for disorders of sex development: implementing a shared decision-making approach. J Pediatr Endocrinol 2010;23(8):789–805.

32. Consortium on the Management of Disorders of Sex Development. Clinical guidelines for the management of disorders of sex development in childhood. 2006. Available at: http://www.accordalliance.org/dsdguidelines/htdocs/clinical/index.html. Accessed November 24, 2014.

Gender Variance and Dysphoria in Children and Adolescents

Herbert J. Bonifacio, MD, MSc, MPH, MA[a],*,
Stephen M. Rosenthal, MD[b]

KEYWORDS

- Gender dysphoria • Gender identity • Gender variance • Cross-sex hormones
- Pubertal blockers • Transgender youth

KEY POINTS

- Gender nonconforming and transgender youth are seeking medical care at younger ages.
- Youth with gender variance are often marginalized and misunderstood by their health care providers.
- Mental health comorbidities in youth with gender dysphoria significantly diminish when receiving gender-affirming care.
- Providers should understand the use of hormone blockers and cross-sex hormones as a strategy in addressing gender dysphoria.
- Prompt referrals by medical professionals should be made to an interdisciplinary team experienced in addressing the unique challenges faced by transgender youth and their families.

Over the past decade, there has been an increase in the number of gender variant children and adolescents seeking care at gender clinics and centers around the world.[1] Many of these gender variant youth are seeking care at younger ages for many reasons, including greater access to information about transgender or gender variant youth via the Internet, more exposure to gender variant or transgender characters in the media, and greater openness toward dialogue concerning one's gender with his or her peers and family members.

Disclosure Statement: The authors have nothing to disclose.
[a] Division of Adolescent Medicine, Department of Pediatrics, Transgender Youth Clinic, The Hospital for Sick Children, University of Toronto, 555 University Avenue, Toronto, Ontario M5G 1X8, Canada; [b] Pediatric Endocrine Outpatient Services, Pediatric Endocrinology, Child and Adolescent Gender Center, University of California, San Francisco, 513 Parnassus Avenue, Room S-672, Box 0434, San Francisco, CA 94143-0434, USA
* Corresponding author.
E-mail address: joey.bonifacio@sickkids.ca

Pediatr Clin N Am 62 (2015) 1001–1016
http://dx.doi.org/10.1016/j.pcl.2015.04.013
0031-3955/15/$ – see front matter © 2015 Elsevier Inc. All rights reserved.

Gender variance is an umbrella term used to describe the behaviors, interests, appearance, expression, or an identity of persons who do not conform to culturally defined norms expected of their natal gender.[2] Related terms include *gender nonconforming, gender creative, transgender*, and, in Aboriginal culture, *two-spirited*. To meet the needs of such youth, there has been an increase in the number of pediatric clinics in Canada, the United States, and Europe that specialize in the care of gender variant children and adolescents.[3]

For most youth, the natal gender (ie, the gender assumed based on the physical sex characteristics present at birth) is consistent with their gender identity (a person's intrinsic sense of self as male, female, or an alternative gender). In a small minority, however, there is a discrepancy between assigned (or natal) gender and gender identity. The distress that is caused by this discrepancy is called *gender dysphoria* (GD).[4] This article reviews the epidemiology of youth with gender variance and GD and the models of care used to manage youth with GD.

TERMINOLOGY

When working with youth and their families, medical professionals should be inclusive, sensitive, and respectful regarding the use of preferred names and gender pronouns. There is an abundance of gender-related terms that may be used by youth, their families, and health care professionals.

Biological/Anatomic Sex

Biological/anatomic sex are the physical attributes that characterize maleness or femaleness (eg, the genitalia).

Cisgender

Cisgender refers to individuals whose affirmed gender matches their physical sex characteristics.

Gender Dysphoria

GD is distress that is caused by a discrepancy between a person's gender identity and that person's natal gender (ie, the gender that is assumed based on the physical sex characteristics present at birth). Not all gender-variant individuals experience GD.[2]

Gender Identity (or Affirmed Gender)

Gender identity is a person's intrinsic sense of self as male, female, or an alternate gender. Gender identity likely reflects a complex interplay of biological, environmental, and cultural factors.[2,5,6]

Gender Nonconforming

Gender nonconforming is an adjective used to describe individuals whose gender identity, role, or expression differs from what is normative for their assigned sex in a given culture and historical period.

Gender Role or Expression

Gender role or expression refers to characteristics in personality, appearance, and behavior that, in a given culture and historical period, are designated as masculine or feminine (that is, more typical of the male or female social role).[7] Although most individuals present socially in clearly masculine or feminine gender roles, some people present in an alternative gender role. Gender expression does not always correlate with gender identity or physical sex characteristics.

Gender Variance

The term *gender variance* refers to the behaviors, appearance, or identity of people who do not conform to culturally defined norms for their assigned gender.[2]

Female-to-Male

Female-to-male (FTM) refers to assigned female persons who identify as male.

Male-to-Female

Male-to-female (MTF) refers to assigned male persons who identify as female.

Transgender

Transgender is an adjective to describe individuals with an affirmed gender identity different than their physical sex characteristics. *Transgender* can also be used to describe people whose gender identity, expression, or behaviors cross or transcend culturally defined categories of gender.[2]

Transitioning

Transitioning is a process whereby individuals change their social and/or physical characteristics for the purpose of living in their desired gender role. Transitioning may or may not include hormonal and/or surgical procedures.[2]

Sexual Orientation

Sexual orientation is the personal quality inclining persons to be romantically or physically attracted to persons of the same sex, opposite sex, both sexes, or neither sex. Sexual orientation is distinct from gender identity and gender expression.[2]

EPIDEMIOLOGY

The prevalence of gender variant behavior and GD in childhood and adolescence are largely unknown. One study investigating gender variant behavior found that 2% to 4% of boys and 5% to 10% of girls behaved as the opposite sex from time to time.[8,9] Another study found that 22.8% of boys and 38.6% of girls exhibited 10 or more different "gender atypical behaviors."[9]

As opposed to studies of gender variant behavior, other studies have attempted to investigate the prevalence of GD, a psychiatric diagnosis present in the *Diagnostic and Statistical Manual of Mental Disorders* (Fifth Edition) (*DSM-5*). Using such criteria in adults, the prevalence of GD ranges from 0.005% to 0.014% for assigned men and 0.002% to 0.003% for assigned women.[4] Such numbers are based on referrals to medical and surgical reassignment clinics and are likely modest underestimates. Sex differences are also noted in referrals to pediatric specialty clinics focused on gender variant youth. In children, sex ratios from natal boys to girls range from 2:1 to 4.5:1, whereas in adolescents the sex ratio is close to parity.[4]

In May 2013, the *DSM-5* replaced the term *gender identity disorder* (GID) previously found in the *Diagnostic and Statistical Manual of Mental Disorders* (Fourth Edition) (*DSM-IV*) with the term *GD* after much complex debate. Many view the replacement as a paradigmatic shift toward depathologizing gender variant identity and behavior. The criteria for GD (with or without a disorder of sex development) are detailed in the DSM-5. No studies have thus far used these newer criteria to determine the prevalence of GD in children and adolescents.

GENDER IDENTITY DEVELOPMENT

Gender identity development begins around 2 to 3 years of age. At this age, children have a general sense of what is male or female and identify their own gender soon after. At 6 to 7 years of age, a child realizes that one's gender is likely to remain constant.[10,11]

The findings from studies investigating the trajectory of gender variant children who meet the criteria for GID or GD as an adult are inconsistent. The percentage of children initially diagnosed with GID who display persistence of GID range from 12% to 27%.[12,13] Such studies suggest most children who meet the criteria for GD do not have persistence of GD by the time they have initiated puberty. There is research to suggest, however, that this may be caused, in part, by an internalizing pressure to conform rather than a natural progression to non–gender variance.[14,15] Studies have also indicated that a significant percent of prepubertal gender-nonconforming youth eventually identify as gay at puberty and may not have been on a transgender trajectory in the first place, as discussed later. Studies have been carried out to identify predictors of persistence of GD. Factors that increase the likelihood of persistence of GD in adulthood include more gender-variant behavior in childhood, greater intensity of GD in childhood, and persistence of GD during adolescence. Qualitative research also found that cognitive statements were predictive of gender identity outcome (eg, I *am* of the other gender.) versus affective statements (eg, I *wish* to be of the other gender.).[12,16–18] There are also many individuals whose GD emerged in adolescence and adulthood.

Sexual orientation is often confused with gender identity. Just as cisgender individuals can have any sexual orientation, the same holds true for transgender individuals.

ISSUES FACED BY GENDER VARIANT AND TRANSGENDER YOUTH AND THEIR FAMILIES

Although gender variance is not a disorder, many gender variant youth face a variety of issues that affect emotional and psychological wellbeing. Very often, gender variant youth experience levels of stigma, social ostracizing, and verbal and physical violence so great that their psychological well-being is compromised, potentially leading to depression and/or anxiety.[19] A recent study found that gender variance during childhood was a risk factor for experiencing childhood physical, psychological, and sexual abuse.[20] Moreover, gender nonconformity predicted an increased risk of lifetime posttraumatic stress disorder. A recent study investigating transgender-identified youth and younger adults found very high rates of suicidal ideation and suicide attempts.[21,22] These studies suggest that such rates increase as youth reach adulthood.

Gender variant children experience a higher level of social rejection from their peers, and this may increase through their years in school. A study examining transphobia in the education system found that 56% of gender variant students were called names, made fun of, or bullied compared with only 33% of their cisgender peers.[23] A Canadian survey found that 90% of trans youth heard transphobic comments daily or weekly from other students. Moreover, the rates of verbal and physical harassment of transgender students because of their gender expression were 74% and 37%, respectively.[24] More than three-quarters (78%) of transgender students indicated feeling unsafe in some way at school. For such reasons, the truancy rates were also much higher in lesbian, gay, bisexual, transgender, and questioning (LGBTQ) teens than non-LGTBQ teens.

Some parents continue to have intolerant views toward their child's gender expression. Studies have found that gender variant children have poorer relationships with their parents. Another study found that gender variant youth were more likely than nongender variant children to experience abuse and violence from their own family members.[20] A recent report from Ontario, Canada found greater satisfaction with life and self-esteem in transgender youth whose parents were "very supportive" versus those whose parents were "somewhat to not at all supportive."[25] At the same time, depression and suicide attempts were significantly decreased in transgender youth whose parents were supportive in comparison with those whose parents were not supportive.[25] Unfortunately, many youth feel unsafe at home and leave their homes, being rejected or forced out by their families because of their sexual orientation or gender identity.[26] LGBTQ youth are also overrepresented in youth accessing housing programs, such as shelters.

Just as gender variant youth may face rejection from their peers, some families may face rejection from friends and family members who do not accept their child's gender expression and behavior or the parent's decision to affirm their child's gender expression and behavior.[14,27] Although many are well intentioned, some parents may also have conflict with each other in deciding how to support their child. Lastly, various professionals and child welfare authorities may incorrectly seek reparative approaches and apprehend gender variant children from their parents out of concern that support of gender variant expression and behavior constitutes child abuse.

EVOLVING APPROACH TO PREPUBERTAL GENDER VARIANT CHILDREN

In the 1960s, children with gender variance began to be viewed through a disease medical model whereby such behaviors, expression, and identity were pathologic and needed correction.[28,29] Such children and adolescents were subjected to psychological interventions to attempt to redirect behaviors, expression, and identity so they were consistent with social norms. The main goal of this reparative approach was to prevent children and adolescents from identifying as transgender. The inclusion of GID in children in the *DSM-IV* in 1980 was seen by many to further pathologize nonconforming gender identity and expression and reinforce gender stereotypes.

There has been a steady shift from the reparative approach in gender variance in childhood and adolescence toward an affirmative model that validates and encourages parents supporting their gender variant children and adolescents.[5] The major premises of the gender affirmative model are as follows: (1) Gender variations are not disorders. (2) Gender presentations are diverse and varied across cultures and, therefore, require our cultural sensitivity. (3) To the best of the authors' knowledge at present, gender involves an interweaving of biology, development and socialization, and culture and context, with all of these factors influencing an individual's gender self. (4) Gender may be fluid and is often not binary, both at a particular time and, if and when it changes within an individual, across time. (5) If there are mental health or behavioral concerns, it more often stems from negative cultural reactions (eg, transphobia) rather than from within the child. In this approach, the goals are not to pathologize the child or adolescent's behavior or identity but to destigmatize gender variance, promote the child's self-worth, allow for opportunities to access peer support, and enable parents and other community members to create safer spaces for such children in day care, schools, and other social environments. Although a gender-affirmative model encourages parents of gender variant children to follow their child's lead, parents should be careful to avoid imposing their own preferences on their children.

Many parents who favor the gender affirmative approach will support their child's social transition. A social transition consists of a change in social role to their affirmed gender and may include a change of name, clothing, appearance, and gender pronoun.[30] Parent and clinician reports suggest that children's happiness may vastly improve after socially transitioning.[19,31] Because the approach is completely reversible, proponents of social transition argue that children can be reminded that they may return to their natal gender at any time and another transition is possible.[32] Those who oppose social transitioning in prepubertal children argue that it may contribute to GD persistence and increase one's likelihood of identifying as transgender in adolescence.[16,33] The decision for a child to socially transition is not a simple one and should be made jointly among the child, the parents, and supportive professionals if available.

Many prepubertal gender variant children do not seek help from medical centers. In these cases, parents and the adults surrounding such gender variant children are able to create safe environments where these youth are able to explore their gender and are supported in living in a gender role that corresponds to their internal gender identity. Other prepubertal gender variant children and their parents may present to medical centers seeking guidance and resources. These parents may be either supportive or not supportive of their child's gender expression and/or identity. These children and their families may benefit from validation of their gender concerns and learning about puberty and the physical changes that may occur in the upcoming years. Meetings at earlier ages may also facilitate greater comfort with medical professionals, as many youth may not want their parents to address or monitor pubertal development. Lastly, medical clinics may coordinate or facilitate access to individual or group therapy to provide greater insight and understanding of their gender identity, screen and monitor for mental health concerns, and improve resiliency through peer support. Recent evidence indicates that youth in gender clinics incorporating an affirmative model have experienced significantly fewer behavioral problems.[32]

APPROACH TO PUBERTAL YOUTH

Many gender variant youth may experience discomfort during puberty. For assigned females, the first sign of puberty is usually breast budding, whereas, for assigned males, the first sign is an increase in testicular volume. Gender variant youth who may identify as male may experience significant distress as breast development occurs. For many gender variant youth, such changes may cause much discomfort and, for some, even represent a traumatic experience. Increasing GD during puberty may also result in many negative psychosocial outcomes, such as depression, anxiety, social withdrawal, cutting and other self-harming behavior, suicidal ideation, suicide attempts, sexual behavioral risks, and substance use.

Youth with GD may not directly present with gender concerns. Instead, such youth may present with declining academic performance, behavioral problems at home and/ or school, or drug use.[34,35] Other gender dysphoric youth may present with disordered eating, for example, male-affirmed natal females may restrict food intake to avoid a more feminine body type. Many youth may have been diagnosed and may be currently treated for depression, anxiety, and/or other mood disorders.

Even if a provider asks, many youth may deny gender concerns. Clinicians should, therefore, incorporate gender inclusive questions as part of their adolescent screen to facilitate future disclosure of such gender issues and concerns. A more gender-inclusive environment can also be created with the presence of LGBTQ posters, brochures, and/or other media and a visible nondiscrimination statement stating that equal care will be provided to all patients, regardless of age, race, ethnicity, physical ability or attributes, religion, sexual identity, and gender identity.

If available, referrals should be made to a qualified mental health professional who specializes in gender concerns and who is also able to assess for the presence of other concurrent mental health issues. The following section addresses the use of puberty suppression and cross-sex hormones in pubertal youth with GD.

PUBERTY SUPPRESSION

There are many reasons to suppress puberty in youth with GD. First and foremost, pubertal suppression allows youth to explore their gender identity and expression without having to worry about impending pubertal changes and undesired secondary sexual characteristics. Youth have more time to access appropriate resources and support, such as individual or group therapy. Depending on when youth share their gender concerns with their families, some parents may need more time to process and incorporate such information, find community support and resources for their child and themselves, and provides more time to make future decisions. Lastly, puberty suppression likely prevents surgical procedures that might otherwise be sought in adulthood in an attempt to undue physical characteristics of the undesired puberty.[36] Puberty suppression entails the use of medications for the purpose of suppressing endogenous hormones that lead to the development of secondary sexual characteristics during puberty, such as laryngeal prominence, increased muscle development, deepening voice in natal boys, and breast development and menstruation in natal girls.

PUBERTY-SUPPRESSING MEDICATIONS

The initiation of puberty begins when gonadotropin-releasing hormone (GnRH) is secreted in a pulsatile manner from the hypothalamus and triggers the pituitary gland to release luteinizing hormone (LH) and follicle-stimulating hormone (FSH). These pituitary hormones act on the gonads to release sex steroids that either feminize or masculinize the body. GnRH agonists put puberty on hold by providing a nonpulsatile, continuous release of a GnRH analogue that desensitizes the GnRH receptors on the pituitary gland and inhibits the secretion of LH and FSH.[37] With markedly reduced LH and FSH, the ovaries and testes, in turn, reduce secretion of gonadal sex steroids leading, in a short period of time, to a prepubertal physiologic state. Pubertal suppression with GnRH agonists is completely reversible, as pubertal development will resume if and when the GnRH agonist is discontinued. **Table 1** lists different medical options for pubertal suppression. Some clinics will start with a monthly GnRH analogue formulation (such as leuprolide acetate depot) for several months before switching to a longer-acting formulation.

TIMING OF PUBERTY SUPPRESSION

Pioneering studies from the Netherlands among adolescents with GD endorsed the use of GnRH agonists to induce pubertal suppression at Tanner stage II to III if those youth were at least 12 years of age.[36] The US Endocrine Society released their clinical practice guidelines in 2009.[38] These guidelines recommend that adolescents who maintain a strong and consistent cross-gender identification should be considered for GnRH agonists at Tanner stage II to III, independent of chronologic age. The World Professional Association for Transgender Health (WPATH) Standards of Care Version 7, released in 2011, also endorsed this approach.[2]

Table 1
Inhibitors of gonadal sex steroid secretion or action

Type	Dose	Frequency
GnRH analogues: inhibition of the HPG axis (FTM and MTF)		
Leuprolide acetate	7.5 mg SC	Monthly
	22.5 mg SC	Every 3 mo
	40 mg SC	Every 4 mo
	45 mg SC	Every 6 mo
Leuprolide acetate	7.5 mg IM	Monthly
	11.25 mg IM	Every 3 mo
Histrelin SC implant (50 mg)	65 mcg/d	Every 12 mo (may have longer duration of action)
Alternative approaches		
Medroxyprogesterone acetate (FTM and MTF)	150 mg IM	Every 3 mo
Spironolactone (MTF)	100–300 mg/d oral	Twice daily
Finasteride (FTM)	2.5–5.0 mg/d oral	Once daily

Abbreviations: HPG, hypothalamic-pituitary-gonadal; IM, intramuscular; SC, subcutaneous.

There are several reasons why older transgender adolescents who have already developed undesirable secondary sexual characteristics may still benefit from GnRH agonists. First, the administration of puberty blockers is useful in preventing further progression of puberty and giving time to youth to consolidate their gender identity. Second, some parents may disagree with their child's desire for cross-sex hormones. The use of puberty blockers may allow for more time to reach consensus among youth, families, and their medical team. Third, the administration of GnRH agonists for both transgender male and female youth effectively ceases the production of gonadal sex steroids, thereby potentially lowering the doses of cross-sex hormones needed for future feminization or masculinization.

MONITORING AND SIDE EFFECTS

Puberty suppression should be assessed both clinically and biochemically through measurements of LH, FSH, estradiol, and/or testosterone 1 to 3 months following administration of the puberty blocker. Recommendations for surveillance (as per the current Endocrine Society's clinical practice guidelines) during pubertal suppression are summarized in **Table 2**. Utility, need, and the cost-effectiveness of several of these measures need to be studied and established.

Because of their agonist effects, GnRH analogues may temporarily increase pubertal signs in the first few weeks after initiation of GnRH agonist (eg, increased moodiness, increased breast development, hot flashes, and vaginal bleeding in natal females; increased aggressiveness in natal males). Such effects will reverse once secretion of LH, FSH, and the gonadal sex steroids are reduced. Other side effects may depend on the type of administration. If given intramuscularly, youth may experience pain and swelling at the injection site and a small chance of developing a sterile abscess. GnRH agonists are also commonly given by subcutaneous implants that can be effective for 1 to 2 years.

Many youth who are administered puberty blockers for GD may go on to use cross-sex hormones for phenotypic transition (see later discussion). Under such circumstances, fertility will likely be compromised, particularly if pubertal blockers are

Table 2 Follow-up protocol during suppression of puberty		
	Every 3 mo	Yearly
Anthropometry	Height Weight Sitting height Tanner stages	—
Laboratory	LH FSH Estradiol Testosterone	Renal function Liver function Lipids Glucose Insulin HbA$_{1c}$
Imaging	—	Bone density Bone age

Abbreviation: HbA$_{1c}$, hemoglobin A$_{1c}$.
Data from Hembree WC, Cohen-Kettenis P, Delemarre-van de Waal HA, et al. Endocrine treatment of transsexual persons: an Endocrine Society clinical practice guideline. J Clin Endocrinol Metab 2009;94(9):3142.

initiated at the earliest stages of puberty. For such reasons, issues regarding future fertility should be addressed before consent and the commencement of pubertal blockers and potential subsequent use of cross-sex hormones. Gender dysphoric youth who have gone through significant pubertal maturation may choose to cryopreserve gametes through sperm banking or egg preservation before any hormonal treatments are initiated. Once testosterone is administered in transgender men, the ovaries will release fewer eggs. There are cases, however, in which transgender men (who have not had sex reassignment surgery) have interrupted their testosterone therapy to allow their ovarian function to recover and some have even chosen to carry pregnancy. Estrogen administration decreases sperm count, although it may increase if estrogen therapy is interrupted.

PHYSIOLOGIC AND MEDICAL OUTCOMES

A principal concern of GnRH agonist treatment is decreased bone mineral density. The lack of endogenous sex steroid hormones in youth administered GnRH agonists results in slower accrual of bone mineral density compared with those whose puberty is not blocked. The bone density of youth on puberty blockers remained unchanged during GnRH agonist administration.[36] When cross-sex hormones were administered, however, bone density significantly increased and reached age-appropriate levels in both affirmed males and females.[36] The same study also found that the percentage of fat mass increased and stabilized and lean body mass decreased and stabilized over the 2-year follow-up. There were also no changes in lipid or carbohydrate metabolism.[36]

PSYCHOLOGICAL AND MENTAL HEALTH OUTCOMES

There have been few studies investigating the mental health effects of puberty blockers. One Dutch study measured psychological outcomes before and during puberty suppression in 70 youth diagnosed with GID according to *DSM-IV* criteria.[39] After pubertal suppression, most behavioral and emotional problems and depressive symptoms decreased and general functioning improved significantly; however, feelings of anxiety and anger persisted, and GD did not change. Of note, no adolescent discontinued puberty suppression, and all eventually started cross-sex hormone treatment.[39]

CROSS-SEX HORMONES

Many youth who identify as transgender in adolescence will continue to identify as transgender into adulthood and would benefit from cross-sex hormones during adolescence. Cross-sex hormones allow the youth to either physically masculinize or feminize their body in alignment with their affirmed gender. Ideally a multidisciplinary team composed of both mental and medical professionals will help youth and their families.[2]

The cornerstone of hormonal treatment of FTM transgender adolescents who wish to undergo physical transition is testosterone. As per the Endocrine Society's clinical practice guidelines, puberty would have been previously suppressed at Tanner stage II (or later depending on when the youth sought medical care) with GnRH agonists, with testosterone subsequently administered to induce masculinization.[38] Desired effects of testosterone therapy include deepened voice, facial hair, cessation of regular menses, increased muscle mass, and fat distribution leading to a more masculine body habitus. Although breast tissue may lose glandularity, the amount of breast tissue will not decrease. Voice changes, clitoral growth, and fat redistribution are irreversible changes. Coarsening of body and facial hair begins soon after initiation of testosterone but will take several years to reach full growth. Clitoral growth usually begins in the first few months of therapy.

Testosterone is administered by either injectable or transdermal preparations (**Table 3**). Injectable intramuscular formulations of testosterone cypionate or enanthate are most commonly used, although subcutaneous routes may also be used. The advantage of transdermal preparations is the relatively steady state of

Table 3 Hormone regimens	
Medication	**Full Adult Dosage**
MTF Persons	
Estrogens 17-β estradiol	
17-β estradiol (oral)	2–6 mg daily
17-β estradiol (transdermal)	0.1–0.4 mg twice weekly
Estradiol cypionate (parenteral)	5–20 mg IM every 2 wk
Estradiol valerate	2–10 mg IM every wk
FTM Persons	
Testosterone	
Testosterone cypionate or enanthate (parenteral: IM or SC)	100–200 mg every 2 wk, 50–100 mg every wk
1% Gel (transdermal)	2.5–10.0 mg daily
Patch (transdermal)	2.5–7.5 mg daily

Note that induction of puberty with cross-sex hormones will start at one-quarter of adult dose and increased every 6 months until adult dose is reached. Induction of puberty may be administered over a shorter or longer period of time depending on the clinical situation.
Abbreviations: IM, intramuscular; SC, subcutaneous.

testosterone, as opposed to the fluctuations with injectables, although it may take longer for clinical changes to take place in transdermal preparations. Oral versions of testosterone are available but not in North America.

The cornerstone of cross-sex hormonal treatment for MTF transgender adolescents is estrogen with an antiandrogen. If used as a monotherapy, high doses of estrogen would be needed to adequately suppress androgens. Thus, estrogen is usually administered concurrently with another medication that lowers the levels of androgens or blocks their activity. The reduction of androgen action results in decreasing facial and body hair, whereas estrogen increases female secondary sex characteristics, such as breast and hip development. GnRH agonists or other puberty blockers decrease androgen levels or action and allow for lower doses of estrogen to be used. For youth who do not have access to GnRH agonists, antiandrogens, such as spironolactone or finasteride, are commonly prescribed.

The most common regimens for estrogen include oral estradiol, transdermal estrogens, and injectable estrogens (see **Table 3**). No studies have confirmed that one form of estrogen results in more desired physical effects. 17-β Estradiol is the preferred form of estrogen used for hormonal transition; it can be administered in oral or transdermal formulations, and serum levels can be monitored. Because transdermal formulations avoids first pass through the liver, they are thought to have fewer hepatic side effects. Injectable estrogens (in the form of estradiol valerate or cypionate) are also not subject to hepatic first pass metabolism and have the benefit of weekly or biweekly administration. Oral 17-β estradiol can also be given sublingually.

EVALUATING READINESS

Before the administration of cross-sex hormones, mental health professionals may reevaluate GD, screen for concurrent mental health disorders, provide individual psychotherapy for youth and counseling for families, and connect the youth and families with community resources to improve resiliency. Both mental and medical health professionals can also give information to adolescents about gender transition and cross-sex hormone therapy.

Both WPATH and the Endocrine Society advocate for a real-life experience or test (RLE or RLT, respectively) before cross-sex hormones. RLE is a period of time in which transgender individuals live full-time in their affirmed gender. The purpose of RLE is to help youth confirm their affirmed gender and evaluate their ability to function as a member of that gender before initiating cross-sex hormones. Some providers do not require RLE and may follow an individualized plan for transitioning as many youth may feel more comfortable in socially transitioning when cross-sex hormones have been started.

Fertility counseling, as noted earlier, should be rediscussed with the adolescent and family before cross-sex hormone therapy.[2]

MEDICAL EVALUATION

Before cross-sex hormone administration, the medical professional will screen for contraindications and other medical conditions that could be exacerbated by cross-sex hormones.[38] Contraindications to cross-sex hormone therapy may include ischemic cardiovascular disease, cerebrovascular disease, history of deep vein thrombosis or pulmonary embolus, marked hypertriglyceridemia, hyperprolactinemia, estrogen-dependent cancer, uncontrolled high blood pressure, pregnancy, or psychiatric conditions that limit the ability to provide informed consent. Such conditions will require referral to subspecialists for further evaluation and medical clearance. Other precautions include other cardiac disease, family history of abnormal clotting, smoking status, history of benign intracranial hypertension, metabolic syndrome, refractory migraine or focal migraine, seizure disorder, strong family of breast cancer, and/or family history of porphyria.

A physical examination should be performed including height, weight, and blood pressure. Genital and breast examinations for Tanner staging should be performed before the administration of cross-sex hormones but only after rapport has been developed between youth and the professional. Recommendations for laboratory surveillance based on the Endocrine Society's current clinical practice guidelines are summarized in **Boxes 1** and **2**.

Routine medical care and screening should continue to take place at follow-up visits and annual physical examinations if youth do not have a primary care provider. Even then, some transgender youth may feel more comfortable with the medical professional providing transgender care. For such reasons, medical care professionals should provide holistic comprehensive care that also includes sexual and reproductive care. Regardless of their affirmed gender, persons with a cervix and uterus should be provided gynecologic care. Screening for sexual and blood-borne infections, such as human immunodeficiency virus, gonorrhea, chlamydia, syphilis, and laboratory work for hepatitis A, B, and C, should be performed depending on risk factors. The use of tobacco and other substances should be addressed. Medical professionals should be able to use the HEADSS assessment (home, education, activities, drugs, sex, and suicide) to screen for other risk factors and tailor their care accordingly.

TIMING OF CROSS-SEX HORMONES

According to the Endocrine Society's clinical practice guidelines, transgender adolescents should have their endogenous puberty suppressed until 16 years of age, after which cross-sex hormones may be given. Delay of cross-sex hormone therapy may unnecessarily lead to negative mental health outcomes.[3] In some cases, a thoughtful decision among the youth, families, and care providers may suggest earlier administration of cross-sex hormones. With the use of puberty blockers, more youth without

---

Box 1
Monitoring of MTF persons on cross-sex hormone therapy

1. Evaluate patients every 2 to 3 months to monitor for appropriate signs of feminization and for development of adverse reactions.

2. Monitor complete blood count, liver function, renal function, lipids, glucose, insulin, and hemoglobin A_{1c} at the initial and annual visit.

3. Measure serum LH, FSH, testosterone, and estradiol every 3 months.

   a. Serum testosterone levels should not exceed the peak physiologic range for young healthy females.

   b. Serum estradiol should not exceed the peak physiologic range for young healthy females.

   c. Doses of estrogen should be adjusted according to the serum levels of estradiol.

4. For individuals on spironolactone, serum electrolytes, particularly potassium, should be monitored every 2 to 3 months initially in the first year.

5. Monitor bone density and bone age annually.

Box 2
Monitoring of FTM persons on cross-sex hormone therapy

1. Evaluate patients every 2 to 3 months to monitor for appropriate signs of virilization and for development of adverse reactions.

2. Monitor complete blood count, liver function, renal function, lipids, glucose, insulin, and hemoglobin A_{1c} at the initial and annual visit.

3. Measure serum testosterone every 2 to 3 months until levels are in the normal physiologic male range:

   a. For testosterone enanthate/cypionate injections, the testosterone level should be measured midway between injections. If the level is greater than 700 ng/dL or less than 350 ng/dL, adjust the dose accordingly.

   b. For transdermal testosterone, the testosterone level can be measured at any time after 1 week.

4. Monitor bone density and bone age annually.

---

exposure to cross-sex hormones may be at risk for bone mineral density loss; earlier administration of cross-sex hormones may decrease this risk.

Induction of puberty with cross-sex hormones (ie, testosterone or estradiol) may start with quarter doses of the adult dose and increased every 6 months until the adult dose is reached after 2 years. If phenotypic transition is started after endogenous puberty has been completed, sex steroids are typically increased to full adult doses more rapidly.

SIDE EFFECTS OF CROSS-SEX HORMONES

Unwanted side effects of testosterone include increased weight, acne, body odor, mood changes, and male-pattern balding as well as more serious side effects, such as increased risk for coronary artery disease and altered hematologic and lipid profiles that match genetic males. For such reasons, medical professionals should suggest affirmed males maintain an exercise program to avoid excess weight gain. Moreover, attempts to increase muscle mass through weightlifting should be done slowly as there has been evidence of tendon rupture with testosterone administration. Mood changes may occur with testosterone, with many affirmed males being aware of when testosterone levels have decreased between doses.

The negative side effects of estrogen therapy have been illustrated in both postmenopausal females and MTF individuals. The Women's Health Initiative, a study investigating the effect of estrogen in combination with a progestin on a large cohort of menopausal women, showed increased incidence of breast cancer, heart disease, and stroke.[40] Synthetic estrogen (eg, ethinyl estradiol), as compared with 17-β estradiol, is associated with higher rates of deep vein thrombosis and death from cardiovascular causes and should not be used.[41,42]

PROGESTERONE

Anecdotally, some individuals and clinicians think the administration of progesterone leads to better areolar growth, more natural appearance, and/or more breastlike tissue. The negative findings from the Women's Health Initiative have resulted in many protocols preferring estrogen-only therapy. Common side effects associated with progesterone are depression, weight gain, and edema.

CROSS-SEX HORMONES AND GENDER-AFFIRMING SURGERY

A recent study following 55 transgender youth found the use of puberty suppression, cross-sex hormones, and gender reassignment surgery alleviated GD and steadily improved psychological functioning.[43] Improvements in psychological functioning were positively correlated with postsurgical subjective well-being. Moreover, the well-being of these young adults was similar to or better than same-age young adults from the general population.[43]

Surgical options for FTM young adults may include mastectomy and male chest contouring, whereas MTF young adults may elect for breast augmentation; such surgeries are also known as *top surgeries*. FTM young adults may choose to have a hysterectomy and/or oophorectomy, and FTM or MTF adults may also consider genital reconstruction; such surgeries are also known as *bottom surgeries*. Current guidelines endorse the potential for sex-reassignment surgery at 18 years of age.

SUMMARY

Gender nonconforming and transgender youth are seeking medical care at younger ages, some even before the onset of puberty. Pediatricians and other primary care physicians are often the first professionals who encounter such youth and, therefore, have a responsibility to create inclusive spaces to raise potential issues concerning gender and educate these youth and their families that a gender variant identity is not considered pathologic but, rather, may be viewed as a normal variant of human development. Medical professionals should understand the rationale for both social and medical transitioning and the use of puberty suppression and cross-sex hormones to address GD. The best current evidence suggests that mental health comorbidities in youth with GD significantly diminish or resolve when such youth are subject to a gender-affirming model of care. Prompt referrals by medical professionals should be made to an interdisciplinary team that understands the unique challenges faced by transgender youth and their families. If such a clinic is not available, there are also many medical professionals who are able to provide care by comanaging with a specialized clinic. In doing so, medical professionals are able to advocate for the mental and physical health of this marginalized population and facilitate this much-needed access to care.

REFERENCES

1. de Vries AL, Cohen-Kettenis PT. Clinical management of gender dysphoria in children and adolescents: the Dutch approach. J Homosex 2012;59(3):301–20.
2. Coleman EB, Bockting WO, Botzer M, et al. Standards of care for the health of transsexual, transgender and gender non-conforming people, version 7. Int J Transgend 2011;13:165–232.
3. Spack NP, Edwards-Leeper L, Feldman HA, et al. Children and adolescents with gender identity disorder referred to a pediatric medical center. Pediatrics 2012; 129(3):418–25.
4. American Psychiatric Association. Diagnostic and statistical manual of mental disorders. 5th edition. Washington, DC: American Psychiatric Association; 2013.
5. Hidalgo M, Ehrensaft D, Tishelman AC, et al. The gender affirmative model: what we know and what we aim to learn. Hum Dev 2013;56:285–90.
6. Rosenthal S. Approach to the patient: transgender youth: endocrine considerations. J Clin Endocrinol Metab 2014;99(12):4379–89.

7. Ruble DN, Martin C, Berenbaum S. Gender development. In: Eisenberg N, editors. Handbook of child psychology: personality and social development, vol. 3. New York: Wiley; 2006.

8. Achenbach TM. Manual for behavioral behavior checklist 4-18 and 1991 profile. Burlington (VT): University of Vermont Department for Psychiatry; 1991.

9. Sandberg DE, Meyer-Bahlburg HF, Ehrhart AA, et al. The prevalence of gender atypical behaviour in elementary school children. J Am Acad Child Adolesc Psychiatry 1993;32:306–14.

10. Kohlberg L. A cognitive-developmental analysis of children's sex-role concepts and attitudes. In: Maccoby EE, editor. The development of sex differences. Stanford (CA): Stanford University Press; 1966. p. 82–172.

11. Slaby RG, Frey KS. Development of gender constancy and selective attention to same-sex models. Child Dev 1975;46:849–56.

12. Wallien MS, Cohen-Kettenis PT. Psychosexual outcome of gender-dysphoric children. J Am Acad Child Adolesc Psychiatry 2008;47(12):1413–23.

13. Zucker K, Bradley SJ. Gender identity disorder and psychosexual problems in children and adolescents. , New York: Guilford Press; 1995.

14. Menvielle E, Tuerk C, Perrin E. To the best of a different drummer: the gender-variant child. Contemp Pediatr 2005;22(2):38–45.

15. Gray SC, Carter AS, Levitt H. A critical review of assumptions about gender variant children in psychological research. J Gay Lesbian Ment Health 2012; 16:4–30.

16. Steensma TD, McGuire JK, Kreukels BP, et al. Factors associated with desistence and persistence of childhood gender dysphoria: a quantitative follow-up study. J Am Acad Child Adolesc Psychiatry 2013;52(6):582–90.

17. Steensma TD, Biemond R, de Boer F, et al. Desisting and persisting gender dysphoria after childhood: a qualitative follow-up study. Clin Child Psychol Psychiatry 2011;16(4):499–516.

18. Drummond KD, Bradley SJ, Peterson-Badali M, et al. A follow-up study of girls with gender identity disorder. Dev Psychol 2008;44(1):34–45.

19. Ehrensaft D. From gender identity disorder to gender identity creativity: true gender self child therapy. J Homosex 2012;59(3):337–56.

20. Roberts A, Rosario M, Corliss HL, et al. Childhood gender nonconformity: a risk indicator for childhood abuse and post-traumatic stress in youth. Pediatrics 2012; 129(3):410–7.

21. Scanlon K, Travers R, Coleman T, et al. Ontario's trans communities and suicide: transphobia is bad for our health. TransPULSE e-Bulletin; November 12, 2010.

22. Grossman AH, D'Augelli AR. Transgender youth and life-threatening behaviors. Suicide Life Threat Behav 2007;37(5):527–37.

23. GLSEN, Harris Interactive. Playgrounds and prejudice: elementary school climate in the United States, a survey of students and teachers. New York: GLSEN; 2012.

24. Taylor C, Peter T, Schachter K, et al. Youth speak up about homophobia and transphobia: the first national climate survey on homophobia in Canadian schools. Phase one report. Toronto: Egale Canada Human Rights Trust; 2008.

25. Travers R, Bauer G, Pyne J, et al. Impacts of strong parental support for trans youth: a report prepared for children's aid society of Toronto and Delisle youth services. Trans Pulse; 2012. p. 1–5.

26. Durso LE, Gates GJ. Serving our youth: findings from a national survey of service providers working with lesbian, gay, bisexual, and transgender youth who are homeless or at risk of becoming homeless. Los Angeles (CA): The Williams Institute with True Colors Fund and The Palette Fund; 2012.

27. Cohen-Kettenis PT, Owen A, Kaijser VG, et al. Demographic characteristics, social competence, and behavior problems in children with gender identity disorder: a cross-national, cross-clinic comparative analysis. J Abnorm Child Psychol 2003;31(1):41–53.
28. Green R. Diagnosis and treatment of gender identity disorders during childhood. Arch Sex Behav 1971;1(2):167–73.
29. Rekers G, Lovaas O. Behavioral treatment of deviant sex-role behaviors in a male child. J Appl Behav Anal 1974;7:173–90.
30. Brill S, Pepper R. The transgender child. San Francisco (CA): Cleis Press; 2008.
31. Ehrensaft D. Gender born, gender made. New York: The Experiment; 2011.
32. Menvielle EA. Comprehensive program for children with gender variant behaviors and gender identity disorders. J Homosex 2012;59:337–56.
33. Steensma T, Cohen-Kettenis P. Gender transitioning before puberty? Arch Sex Behav 2011;2011(40):649–50.
34. Olson J, Forbes C, Belzer M. Management of the transgender adolescent. Arch Pediatr Adolesc Med 2011;165(2):171–6.
35. Cohen-Kettenis P, Delemarre-van de Waal H, Gooren L. The treatment of adolescent transsexuals: changing insights. J Sex Med 2008;5(8):1892–7.
36. Delemarre-van de Waal HA, Cohen-Kettenis PT. Clinical management of gender identity disorder in adolescents: a protocol on psychological and paediatric endocrinology aspects. Eur J Endocrinol 2006;155:S131–7.
37. van Loenen A, Huirne JA, Schats R, et al. GnRH agonists, antagonists, and assisted conception. Semin Reprod Med 2002;20(4):349–64.
38. Hembree W, Cohen-Kettenis P, Delemarre-van de Waal HA, et al. Endocrine treatment of transsexual persons: an Endocrine Society clinical practice guideline. J Clin Endocrinol Metab 2009;94(9):3132–54.
39. de Vries AL, Steensma TD, Doreleijers TA, et al. Puberty suppression in adolescents with gender identity disorder: a prospective follow-up study. J Sex Med 2011;8(8):2276–83.
40. Writing Group for the Women's Health Initiative Investigators. Risks and benefits of estrogen plus progestin in healthy postmenopausal women: principal results from the Women's Health Initiative randomized controlled trial. JAMA 2002;288(3):321–33.
41. Asscheman H, Giltay EJ, Megens JA, et al. A long-term follow-up study of mortality in transsexuals receiving treatment with cross-sex hormones. Eur J Endocrinol 2011;164:635–42.
42. Toorians A, Thomassen MC, Zweegman S, et al. Venous thrombosis and changes of hemostatic variables during cross-sex hormone treatment in transsexual people. J Clin Endocrinol Metab 2003;88(12):5723–9.
43. de Vries AL, McGuire JK, Steensma TD, et al. Young adult psychological outcome after puberty suppression and gender reassignment. Pediatrics 2014;134(4):696–704.

Hyperinsulinemic Hypoglycemia

Maria Güemes, MD, Khalid Hussain, MD, PhD*

KEYWORDS

- Hyperinsulinism • Hypoglycemia
- 18F-ʟ-dihydroxyphenylalanine positron emission tomographic scan • Diazoxide
- Octreotide • Mammalian target of rapamycin (mTOR) inhibitor • Pancreatectomy

KEY POINTS

- Hyperinsulinemic hypoglycemia (HH) is characterized by the inappropriate secretion of insulin from pancreatic β-cells and is a major cause of hypoglycemic brain injury.
- It is recommended that blood glucose concentrations be maintained greater than 3.5 mmol/L in patients with HH because of the lack of alternative substrates for the brain to use.
- Genetic testing for mutations in the genes *ABCC8/KCNJ11* for congenital HH helps in determining if the child has focal or diffuse disease.
- The 18F-ʟ-3,4-dihydroxyphenylalanine ([18F]-DOPA)-PET/computed tomographic (CT) scan is now the gold standard for the accurate preoperative localization of the focal lesion.
- Novel therapeutic drugs such as mammalian target of rapamycin (mTOR) inhibitors (like sirolimus) and glucagon-like peptide-1 (GLP-1) receptor antagonist offer new medical treatment options for severe diffuse disease, decreasing the requirement for a near-total pancreatectomy.

INTRODUCTION

In HH there is dysregulation of insulin secretion so that insulin continues to be secreted despite blood glucose levels being in the hypoglycemic range. Typically HH occurs in the neonatal period, but it can also occur in the infancy and childhood periods. In the neonatal and infancy periods, it is a major cause of persistent and recurrent hypoglycemia associated with hypoglycemic brain injury.[1]

The biochemical basis of HH involves not only the dysregulation of insulin secretion but also defects in glucose counterregulatory hormones.[2,3] The unregulated insulin secretion drives glucose into the insulin-sensitive tissues especially skeletal muscle,

Disclosure: the authors have nothing to disclose.
Developmental Endocrinology Research Group, Molecular Genetics Unit, Institute of Child Health, University College London, 30 Guilford Street, London WC1N 1EH, UK
* Corresponding author.
E-mail address: Khalid.Hussain@ucl.ac.uk

adipose tissue, and liver causing profound hypoglycemia. This situation is compounded by the fact that insulin simultaneously inhibits glycogenolysis (glycogen breakdown), gluconeogenesis (glucose production from noncarbohydrate sources), lipolysis, and ketogenesis. The normal physiologic glucagon and cortisol counterregulatory hormonal response to hypoglycemia are blunted in the neonatal period, further exacerbating the hypoglycemia.[2,3] This biochemical milieu is a recipe for depriving the brain of its most important fuel, namely, glucose. This brain glucopenia is accompanied by the lack of alternative substrates such as ketone bodies and lactate. Under these conditions, the risk of brain damage is the highest.

HH can be either congenital or secondary to certain risk factors (such as intrauterine growth retardation [IUGR]). Congenital HH is caused by defects in key genes involved in regulating insulin secretion from pancreatic β-cells. The major causes of congenital HH involve defects in the genes *ABCC8* and *KCNJ11* (encoding the 2 proteins SUR1 and KIR6.2 of the pancreatic β-cell ATP-sensitive K^+ channel [K_{ATP} channel], respectively)[4,5] or abnormalities in the enzymes glucokinase (GCK), glutamate dehydrogenase (GDH), and short-chain acyl-coenzyme A (CoA) dehydrogenase.[6–8] Loss-of-function mutations in the genes *ABCC8* and *KCNJ11* cause the most severe forms of HH, which are usually medically unresponsive.

Histologically, HH can be classified into 2 broad categories: diffuse (affecting the whole pancreas) and focal (localized to a single region of the pancreas) disease. Recent developments in using 18F-DOPA-PET scanning help to differentiate focal from diffuse disease and accurately localize the focal lesion preoperatively. With the advent of 18F-DOPA-PET scan and laparoscopic surgery, the clinical approach has changed dramatically. This review provides an overview of HH by outlining the physiologic mechanisms of insulin secretion, discussing the genetic mechanisms of congenital HH, reviewing the histologic basis of HH, and finally, reviewing the latest advances in management.

DEFINITION OF HYPOGLYCEMIA

The definition of hypoglycemia remains one of the most contentious and confusing areas (especially in the newborn) in glucose physiology.[9] This confusion stems from the fact that there is poor correlation between plasma glucose concentrations, the onset of clinical symptoms, and the long-term neurologic sequelae. It is difficult to define a blood glucose level that requires intervention because there is uncertainty over the level and duration of hypoglycemia that can cause neurologic damage.

Several different approaches have been used to define hypoglycemia (based on clinical manifestations; epidemiology; acute changes in metabolic, endocrine responses; neurologic function; and long-term neurologic outcome), but none of these approaches are satisfactory.[10] The approach based on neurophysiological responses to falling blood glucose concentrations has led to the proposal that hypoglycemia should be defined as a blood glucose concentration less than 2.6 mmol/L as measured with a laboratory research method.[11] However, around 20% of entirely normal full-term infants have blood glucose concentrations less than this in the first 48 hours after delivery. These infants demonstrate concurrent hyperketonemia, and the assumption (which still needs to be proved) is that these babies will not demonstrate neural dysfunction at this time because of the protective effect of the alternative fuels available.

Recently, it has been recommended that operational thresholds be used when assessing an interventional response in a patient with hypoglycaemia.[9] An operational threshold is defined as the concentration of plasma or whole blood glucose at which clinicians should consider intervention, based on the evidence currently available in the literature. Operational thresholds for the management of hypoglycemia have been published.[12] For any baby with signs and symptoms of hypoglycemia, blood glucose should be maintained above 45 mg/dL (2.6 mmol/L) unless there is a suspicion of HH when a higher threshold (65 mg/dL or 3.5 mmol/L) should be used.[12] Similarly, the Canadian Paediatric Society guidelines also use the glucose cutoff of less than 2.6 mmol/L for at-risk newborns, particularly if the hypoglycemia is persistent or symptomatic.[13]

Significant hypoglycemia is not and can never be defined by a single number that can be applied universally to every individual patient. Rather, it is characterized by a value that is unique to each individual and varies with both the state of physiologic maturity and the influence of pathology. Significant hypoglycemia can be defined as the concentration of glucose in the blood or plasma at which the individual demonstrates a unique response to the abnormal milieu caused by the inadequate delivery of glucose to a target organ (eg, the brain). It is therefore clear that hypoglycemia is a continuum and that the blood glucose concentration should be interpreted in the context of the clinical presentation and counterregulatory hormonal responses and in relation to the intermediate metabolites.

METABOLIC AND ENDOCRINE CHANGES IN GLUCOSE PHYSIOLOGY AT THE TIME OF BIRTH

At birth, the healthy term newborn must adapt to an independent existence. The transplacental supply of nutrients including glucose is interrupted, and the newborn must now initiate metabolic and endocrine responses to maintain adequate circulating blood glucose concentrations. For extrauterine adaptation, there must be adequate glycogen stores; intact and functional glycogenolytic, gluconeogenic, and lipogenic mechanisms; and appropriate counterregulatory hormonal responses.

A normal infant at term shows an immediate postnatal decrease in blood glucose concentrations during the first 2 to 4 hours from values close to maternal levels to around 2.5 mmol/L.[14] The trigger for the metabolic and endocrine adaptation with reference to glucose control is unclear, but surges in catecholamine levels and glucagon secretion are thought to be important. The raised plasma insulin to glucagon ratio is reversed at birth, allowing glucagon to activate adenylate cyclase and increase the activity of cyclic AMP (cAMP)-dependent protein kinase A. This step in turn activates phosphorylase kinase, which facilitates glucose release. The catecholamine surge activates lipolysis and lipid oxidation resulting in increases in the levels of glycerol and free fatty acids. Free fatty acids are then used to generate ketone bodies, which are used as an alternative source of fuel. Healthy term breast-fed babies have significantly lower blood glucose concentrations than bottle-fed babies, but their ketone body concentrations are elevated in response to breast-feeding.

Major changes occur in the function of several physiologic systems after birth, which enables the neonate to adapt to postnatal nutrition.[15] Successful enteral feeding in healthy-term newborns triggers the secretion of gut peptides and plays a key role in triggering a cascade of developmental changes in gut structure and function, and in relating pancreatic endocrine secretion to intermediary metabolism.[15] Hence full-term infants are functionally and metabolically programmed to make the transition from their intrauterine-dependent environment to their extrauterine existence without the need for metabolic monitoring or interference with the natural breast-feeding process. This complex metabolic and endocrine adaptation process is incomplete and compromised when the infant is born prematurely or after IUGR.

MECHANISMS OF INSULIN SECRETION

Pancreatic β-cells produce and secrete insulin to keep the fasting blood glucose concentration between 3.5 and 5.5 mmol/L. This precise regulation of insulin secretion in the β-cell is mainly under the control of K_{ATP} channels.[16] These K_{ATP} channels play a key role in glucose homeostasis by linking glucose metabolism to electrical excitability of the β-cell membrane and subsequent insulin secretion.[17,18] The β-cell K_{ATP} channel is made up of 2 different types of subunits: 4 inward-rectifying potassium channel pore-forming (Kir6.2) subunits and 4 high-affinity sulfonylurea receptor 1 (SUR1) subunits.[19] SUR1 acts as a regulatory subunit, whereas Kir6.2 forms the core of the channel. The biophysical properties of this channel complex, such as K^+ selectivity, rectification, inhibition by ATP, and activation by acyl-CoAs are determined by the Kir6.2 subunit.[20] K_{ATP} channels only function if they are assembled and correctly transported to the cell membrane (trafficking). Kir6.2 is encoded by the gene *KCNJ11*, and SUR1, by gene *ABCC8*, both being genes localized in chromosome 11p15.1.

When glucose enters the β-cell, it is converted to glucose-6-phosphate by the enzyme GCK. GCK acts as a glucose sensor providing a link between the extracellular glucose concentration and the metabolism of glucose in the β-cell.[21] When the blood glucose concentration is increased, the activity of GCK is also increased. Glucose metabolism increases intracytosolic ATP:ADP ratio, which inhibits SUR1 and in turn results in the closure of the K_{ATP} channel. This closure causes β-cell membrane depolarization and calcium (Ca^{2+}) influx into the cell through voltage-gated calcium channels. The increase of intracellular calcium triggers the release of insulin. When the blood glucose concentrations drop below 3.5 mmol/L (65 mg/dL), the K_{ATP} channels open hyperpolarizing the β-cell membrane and inhibiting insulin secretion.[22,23] In patients with congenital HH, there is a disruption in the synchronized activity between glucose metabolism and insulin secretion, resulting in inappropriate secretion of insulin during hypoglycemia.

Although the K_{ATP} channel pathway of insulin secretion is pivotal in regulating insulin secretion, K_{ATP}-channel-independent pathways also operate.[24–26] In these pathways, the signals for insulin secretion generated by changes in the K_{ATP} channel pathway are amplified to augment insulin secretion further by modulators of protein kinases and phosphatases.[27] The changes in the intracellular Ca^{2+} concentration are important for the K_{ATP}-channel-independent pathways.[27]

TYPES OF HYPERINSULINEMIC HYPOGLYCEMIA
Transient Hyperinsulinism

This term is generally used to describe those patients in whom HH resolves spontaneously within a few days after birth. This condition is associated with perinatal conditions/maternal risk factors such as maternal diabetes mellitus (gestational or insulin dependent), IUGR, perinatal stress (birth asphyxia), erythroblastosis fetalis, maternal use of drugs such as sulfonylureas, and intravenous maternal glucose infusions during labor.[28] Occasionally, some patients with IUGR and perinatal asphyxia have a prolonged form of HH, which may require treatment with diazoxide but resolves after several months.[29] The mechanism of transient HH is not fully understood.

Persistent (Congenital) Forms of Hyperinsulinemic Hypoglycemia

The molecular basis of the congenital forms of HH involves defects in key genes regulating insulin secretion from pancreatic β-cells. So far mutations in 9 different genes have been described that lead to dysregulated insulin secretion. These mutations are briefly reviewed in the following sections. **Fig. 1** shows the different genetic mechanisms that lead to dysregulated insulin secretion.

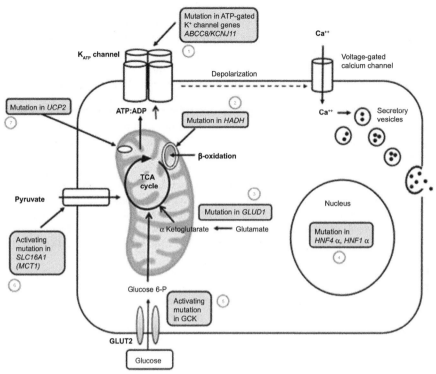

Fig. 1. Diagram of the β-cell showing the molecular mechanisms of unregulated insulin secretion in patients with congenital HH. (1) ATP-gated K^+ channel (K_{ATP}) encoded by *ABCC8* and *KCNJ11* genes, (2) L-3-hydroxyacyl-coenzyme A dehydrogenase (HADH) encoded by *HADH* gene, (3) GDH encoded by *GLUD1* gene, (4) hepatocyte nuclear factor 4α (HNF4α) encoded by *HNF4A* gene; (5) GCK encoded by the *GCK* gene, (6) the moncarboxylate transporter (MCT1) encoded by *SLC16A1* gene, and (7) uncoupling protein 2 (UCP2). TCA, tricarboxylic acid.

Defects in the K_{ATP} channel: mutations in the ABCC8 and KCNJ11 genes

Given the key role of the K_{ATP} channel in regulating insulin secretion, it is not surprising that defects in the genes *ABCC8* and *KCNJ11* are the major cause of severe congenital HH. These mutations involve defects in K_{ATP} channel biogenesis and turnover,[30] channel trafficking from the endoplasmic reticulum and Golgi apparatus[31,32] to the plasma membrane, and alterations of channels in response to nucleotide regulation and open-state frequency.[33] Inactivating mutations in these genes reduce or abolish the activity of the K_{ATP} channel, leading to unregulated release of insulin despite severe hypoglycemia.[34] In approximately 50% of the patients, germline mutations are found.[35]

Approximately 150 homozygous, compound heterozygous, and heterozygous inactivating mutations in *ABCC8* and about 24 *KCNJ11* mutations have been reported up to date.[35] Recessive mutations in these genes explain the most common causes of HH.[34,35] Recessive inactivating mutations in *ABCC8* and *KCNJ11* genes normally cause severe HH, which is unresponsive to medical treatment with diazoxide. Dominant inactivating mutations in *ABCC8* and *KCNJ11* usually cause a milder phenotype of HH,[36,37] but medically unresponsive forms have also been reported.[38]

Mutations in GLUD1

This gene encodes the mitochondrial matrix enzyme, GDH. Activating missense mutations in this gene are associated with the second most common form of HH known as hyperinsulinism/hyperammonemia syndrome (HI/HA).[39] GDH is expressed in the liver, kidney, brain, and pancreatic β-cells and catalyzes the reversible oxidative deamination of glutamate to α-ketoglutarate and ammonia using nicotinamide adenine dinucleotide (NAD) or NAD phosphate as cofactors. An increased GDH activity leads to inappropriate insulin secretion in pancreatic β-cells, as well as to excessive ammonia production (in the kidney)[40] and reduced urea synthesis in the liver.

Mutations in GLUD1 result in a gain of enzyme function by reducing its sensitivity to allosteric inhibition by the high-energy phosphates, such as GTP and ATP, and allowing activation by the amino acid leucine.[6] Patients manifest with recurrent symptomatic postprandial hypoglycemia after protein-rich meals (leucine-sensitive hypoglycemia) and fasting hypoglycemia accompanied by asymptomatic elevations of plasma ammonia.[41] There is a rare subgroup of patients with leucine hypersensitivity but with normal serum ammonia concentrations[42] who could perhaps be mosaic for GDH enzyme activity (normal GDH activity in the liver but elevated activity in the pancreas).

HI/HA phenotype is considered to be milder than other forms of congenital HH, hence escaping recognition for the first few months of life.[42] These patients have more neurologic issues such as epilepsy and learning disabilities.[43] Nevertheless, in contrast to patients with hyperammonemia due to urea cycle disorders, patients with HI/HA syndrome do not experience lethargy or headaches and do not manifest central nervous system symptoms that might be expected for their degree of hyperammonemia and are resistant to ammonia-scavenging agents or protein restriction.

Mutations in 3-hydroxyacyl-coenzyme A dehydrogenase

HADH codes for the enzyme 3-hydroxyacyl-coenzyme A dehydrogenase (HADH) and catalyzes the penultimate reaction in the β-oxidation of fatty acids (NAD^+-dependent conversion of L-HADH to 3-ketoacyl-CoA). HADH is expressed in most tissues, although the enzyme is highly active in the β-cells.[44] The expression of HADH is regulated by transcription factors such as Foxa2, involved in β-cell differentiation.[45] Mutations in this gene (mapped to chromosome 4q22–26)[46] are a rare cause of HH[7] and can cause either severe neonatal HH or mild late-onset HH.[45,47]

The exact mechanism of dysregulated insulin secretion in patients with an HADH mutation is not understood but could involve an interaction between GDH and HADH.[48] Some patients have abnormal acylcarnitine metabolites (raised plasma hydroxybutyrylcarnitine and urinary 3-hydroxyglutarate levels), and some patients are protein sensitive.[49] Most reported patients so far have responded to diazoxide. Genetic analysis for HADH gene is recommended in patients with diazoxide-responsive HH from consanguineous families, who test negative for mutations in the K_{ATP} channel.[50]

Mutations in glucokinase

GCK is a glycolytic enzyme that also functions as a glucose sensor in the pancreatic β-cell and similarly in enteroendocrine cells, hepatocytes, and hypothalamic neurons.[51] In β-cells, it controls glucose-stimulated insulin secretion. Autosomal dominant heterozygous activating mutations of GCK lead to an increased affinity of the enzyme for glucose, resulting in an increase in the ATP:ADP ratio in the pancreatic β-cell, closure of K_{ATP} channel, and inappropriate insulin secretion.[8] The age of presentation ranges from infancy to adulthood,[52] and the severity of symptoms varies within and between families.[53] Hypoglycemia occurs while fasting; some patients respond well to diazoxide, whereas others require more aggressive management including administration of octreotide and even surgery.[54]

Mutations in HNF4A and HNF1A

Mutations in genes *HNF4A* and *HNF1A* can cause maturity-onset diabetes of the young type 1 and type 3, respectively, characterized by progressive β-cell dysfunction with failure of glucose-induced insulin secretion.[55] *HNF4A* gene encodes for the transcription factor hepatocyte nuclear factor 4α (HNF4α), which controls the expression of genes involved in glucose-stimulated insulin secretion.[56] Heterozygous mutations in the *HNF4A* gene have recently been reported to result in transient[57] or persistent HH.[58] The mechanism by which *HNF4A* mutations cause HH is not understood but could involve a reduction in expression of the potassium channel subunit Kir6.2[56] or reduction in the levels of peroxisome proliferator-activated receptor α (PPARα).[59] PPARα is a transcription factor involved in the regulation of fatty acid β-oxidation. HNF4α-deficient β-cells have lower levels of PPARα[56] and possibly a decrease in β-oxidation of fatty acids important for insulin secretion during fasting.[60] This fact has been proved in PPARα-null mice, which present with fasting HH.[59]

HNF1A is a transcription factor important for the development of the pancreas, and 2 cases with mutations in this gene have been reported in diazoxide-responsive HH.[55] Patients with mutations in *HNF4A* or *HNF1A* have macrosomia and present with neonatal HH that can be controlled through diet or can be more severe and persistent requiring diazoxide treatment.[61]

Mutations in solute carrier family 16, member 1

Mutations in *SLC16A1* (solute carrier family 16, member 1) gene can cause exercise-induced hyperinsulinism (EIHI). The gene *SLC16A1* encodes monocarboxylate transporter 1 (MCT1), which transports lactate and pyruvate into the β-cells. *SLC16A1* is usually not expressed in β-cells, so in normal physiologic conditions, lactate and pyruvate concentrations are low in β-cells and do not stimulate insulin secretion.[62] However, dominantly inherited promoter-activating mutations in *SLC16A1* lead to failure of β-cell-specific transcriptional silencing of this gene, therefore inducing the expression of MCT1 in β-cells with consequent pyruvate uptake and pyruvate-stimulated insulin release despite ensuing hypoglycemia.[63]

During strenuous anaerobic exercise or when on a pyruvate load, cells accumulate lactate and pyruvate, which then act as insulin secretagogues.[64] These patients develop hypoglycemia typically 30 to 45 minutes after an intense anaerobic exercise.[64] So far, 13 patients have been reported, 12 from 2 Finnish pedigrees and 1 unrelated case.[63]

Mutations in the uncoupling protein 2 gene

This gene encodes uncoupling protein 2 (UCP2), which is expressed in different tissues. This protein plays an important role in protection against oxidative stress, participating in fatty acid metabolism and in the negative regulation of β-cell insulin secretion.[65] Parentally inherited heterozygous *UCP2* variants were found in 2 unrelated children with HH.[66] However, the role of UCP2 in patients with congenital HH is still unclear.

Syndromes Associated with Hyperinsulinemic Hypoglycemia

Many different developmental syndromes can present with HH during the neonatal period or at a later age (eg, congenital central hypoventilation syndrome). **Table 1** summarizes the different developmental syndromes associated with HH. The

Table 1	
Summarizing the developmental syndromes associated with HH	
Prenatal and postnatal overgrowth syndromes	Beckwith-Wiedemann syndrome Sotos syndrome Simpson-Golabi-Behmel syndrome Perlman syndrome
Chromosomal abnormality syndromes	Trisomy 13 (Patau syndrome) Mosaic Turner syndrome
Postnatal growth failure syndromes	Kabuki syndrome Costello syndrome
Contiguous gene deletion affecting the *ABCC8* gene	Usher syndrome
Syndromes with abnormal calcium homeostasis	Timothy syndrome
Insulin receptor mutation	Insulin resistance syndrome (Leprechaunism)
Others	Congenital disorders of glycosylation types Ia, Ib, and Ic Congenital central hypoventilation syndrome (Ondine syndrome)

syndrome that is most commonly associated with HH is Beckwith-Wiedemann syndrome (BWS). HH is found in around 50% of these patients.[67] BWS is a prenatal and/or postnatal overgrowth syndrome with typical features being macroglossia, anterior abdominal wall defects, organomegaly, hemihypertrophy, ear lobe creases, helical pits, and renal tract abnormalities. In most patients with BWS, HH usually resolves spontaneously in a few days,[67] although in 5% of cases, HH persists and medical therapy or even near-total pancreatectomy might be required.

Postprandial Hyperinsulinemic Hypoglycemia

Postprandial hyperinsulinemic hypoglycemia (PPHH) develops within a few hours of food intake because of inappropriate secretion of insulin in response to the meal. The most common cause of this is dumping syndrome that appears in young children after a gastroesophageal (Nissen fundoplication) surgery.[68] Rapid emptying of hyperosmolar carbohydrate-containing solutions into the small bowel results in rapid glucose absorption, hyperglycemia, and reactive hypoglycemia. Secretion of glucagon-like peptide-1 (GLP-1) in children who have undergone Nissen fundoplication and who develop PPHH is exaggerated, which could contribute to a high insulin surge and consequent hypoglycemia.[69]

The oral glucose tolerance test (OGTT) and the mixed-meal provocation test are the 2 tests used to diagnose dumping syndrome. A difference of more than 6 mmol/L between peak and nadir blood glucose levels during OGTT has been used as a diagnostic criterion for dumping syndrome,[70] the other indicators being biochemical evidence of endogenous hyperinsulinemia and symptoms of neuroglycopenia during a hypoglycemic episode.

Insulinoma

Insulinoma should be considered in HH with onset in childhood or adolescence.[71] Insulinoma may be part of multiple endocrine neoplasia syndrome type 1, and therefore a positive family history may shed light in the familial cases.

Munchausen Syndrome by Proxy

Exogenous administration of insulin or antidiabetic drugs such as sulfonylureas can lead to factitious HH. Some cases have led to misdiagnosis and resulting pancreatectomy.[72]

Histological Forms

There are 3 major histologic forms of congenital HH: diffuse, focal, and atypical.[73] The diffuse form affects all the β-cells of the islets of Langerhans but with variable involvement and preservation of the pancreatic architecture. The β-cells throughout the pancreas are enlarged/hypertrophied (very abundant cytoplasm) and are distinctly hyperfunctioning (nuclei are 3–4 times the size of acinar nuclei).[73] The most common genetic causes of diffuse HH are recessive and dominant mutations in *ABCC8* and *KCNJ11* genes.

The focal form usually affects a small and poorly delimited area of the pancreas (usually 2–10 mm in diameter), which is composed of islets that contain a heterogeneous population of endocrine cells of various sizes. This form consists of nodular adenomatous hyperplasia of islet-like cell clusters, including ductuloinsular complexes and giant β-cell nuclei, surrounded by a histologically and functionally normal pancreatic tissue, therefore with an abnormal pancreatic architecture.[74] The focal lesion may have tentacles or satellites in the nearby pancreas, which necessitates intraoperative margin analysis to ensure complete excision and avoid recurrence.

The inheritance of the focal form is sporadic, although a familial case has been reported in the literature.[75] The genetic mechanism in focal disease involves 2 independent events: the first is the inheritance of a paternal *ABCC8* or *KCNJ11* gene mutation[76] and the second is the somatic loss of the maternal 11p allele (11p15.1–11p15.5) involving the *ABCC8* and *KCNJ11* region within the focal lesion.[76] The maternal 11p loss leads to paternal uniparental disomy unmasking the paternally inherited K_{ATP} channel mutation and leading to abnormal expression of imprinted genes contained in this area, such as the maternally expressed tumor suppressor genes *H19* and *CDKN1C* and the paternally expressed growth factor insulin-like growth factor 2. The altered expression of these may very likely increase the proliferation of β-cells evolving into a focal adenomatous hyperplasia.[29]

In the past years, new atypical focal histologic forms of congenital HH have been characterized by morphologic mosaicism.[77] In these atypical forms, the pancreas has a normal architecture and contains 2 types of islets that coexist: large islets with cytoplasm-rich β-cells and occasional enlarged nuclei and shrunken islets with β-cells showing little cytoplasm and small nuclei.[78] The large hyperactive islets are mostly confined to one or few lobules. This form can potentially be cured with partial pancreatectomy and hence the relevance of its recognition by pathologists on intraoperative frozen sections.[78] In vitro studies on islets isolated from these patients showed increased insulin secretion at a low glucose threshold and immunohistochemistry revealed overexpression of hexokinase-I in the hyperfunctional islets and a somatic activating mutation of GCK in 1 patient.[79]

CLINICAL CHARACTERISTICS

Congenital HH most commonly presents in the newborn, but it can also present during infancy and childhood, in which cases it is usually a milder form. Hypoglycemic symptoms vary from nonspecific, such as poor feeding, lethargy, and irritability, to severe, such as apnea, seizures, or coma. In the clinical history, perinatal risk factors for HH such as gestational diabetes, type of delivery (fetal distress, birth asphyxia), intrapartum glucose infusions, and birth weight (especially if IUGR or macrosomia)[80] should be sought.

In the family history, certain aspects should be looked for such as consanguinity as well as diabetes mellitus and its age of onset. Undiagnosed hypoglycemia in other family members may be suggested by a history of neonatal and infantile seizures and unexplained infant deaths.[80] The relationship of the hypoglycemic episode to the most recent meal can be diagnostically important. Hypoglycemia that occurs after a short fast is highly suggestive of HH. Postprandial hypoglycemia may appear in dumping syndrome or in patients with insulin receptor gene mutations.[80] In some patients, hypoglycemia only manifests after protein ingestion or exercise.[81]

On physical examination, it should be noted if the patient had IUGR or macrosomia because these are more commonly associated with transient HH. Distinctive phenotypic signs may suggest the possibility of a developmental syndrome (such as BWS). Hepatomegaly should always be looked for, as it is associated with excessive glycogen deposition in infants with HH.[1] Hepatomegaly and hypertrophic cardiomyopathy might be related to the effect of fetal hyperinsulinemia.[1]

BIOCHEMICAL FEATURES

Making a prompt diagnosis of HH is important to avoid hypoglycemic brain injury, and therefore physicians should have a low threshold for recognizing these patients. HH is the only condition in which hypoglycemia can persist even with continuous intravenous administration of glucose. A glucose requirement greater than 8 mg/kg/min (normal 4–6 mg/kg/min) is virtually diagnostic of HH.[1]

An inappropriately raised/detectable level of insulin and/or C-peptide at the time of hypoglycemia (spontaneous or controlled diagnostic fast) is pathologic and concordant with HH. Also, low/suppressed plasma free fatty acid (<1.5 mmol/L)[82] and 3-β-hydroxybutyrate (<2 mmol/L) levels[82] and the absence of ketonuria during the hypoglycemic state are highly suggestive of HH.[1] There is no correlation between the serum insulin concentration and the severity of the hypoglycemia.[1] When the diagnosis is in doubt, measurement of C-peptide level (which has a longer half-life and reflects the endogenous insulin production) can be diagnostically more helpful than measurement of insulin levels (short half-life). **Table 2** summarizes the diagnostic criteria for HH.

Provocation tests are a helpful tool to confirm HH and its different causes in some patients. A positive glycemic response of greater than 1.5 mmol/L (27 mg/dL) to an injection of glucagon (0.5–1 mg dose) at the time of hypoglycemia also aids in the diagnosis of HH.[83] Glucagon stimulates the release of stored hepatic glycogen and causes a rapid increase in the blood glucose level in HH. Other tests that provide evidence of HH are improvement of hypoglycemia after a subcutaneous dose of octreotide and the finding of decreased serum concentrations of insulin-like growth factor binding protein 1 (IGFBP-1) because insulin suppresses the transcription of the *IGFBP-1* gene.[84]

An elevated serum ammonia concentration (between 2 and 5 times the upper limit of normal)[85] in a patient with HH suggests HI/HA syndrome,[40] although normal ammonia concentrations do not necessarily exclude it. In patients with HI/HA syndrome, fasting and protein/leucine load test precipitate hypoglycemia.[42] Increased levels of plasma hydroxylbutyrylcarnitine and urinary 3-hydroxyglutarate might indicate HADH deficiency.[46] Patients with EIHI require a formal exercise test and/or a pyruvate load to demonstrate hypoglycemia.[63]

The patient with a history that suggests PPHH should undergo a mixed-meal tolerance test,[22] which seems to be superior to an OGTT to exclude this particular diagnosis. Levels of insulin antibodies should be measured to rule out insulin autoimmune syndrome.

Table 2
Diagnostic criteria for HH

Hormone/Metabolite Measured	Result	HH Type
Glucose infusion rate	>8 mg/kg/min	All forms of hyperinsulinemic hypoglycemia
Laboratory blood glucose level	<3 mmol/L	
Levels of serum insulin/C-peptide	Detectable or elevated	
Levels of serum ketone bodies	Suppressed/low	
Levels of serum fatty acids	Suppressed/low	
Serum ammonia level	Elevated in HI/HA syndrome	HI/HA syndrome
Plasma hydroxyl-butyrylcarnitine level	Raised in HADH deficiency	HADH deficiency
Urinary 3-hydroxyglutarate level	Raised in HADH deficiency	
Supportive evidence (when diagnosis is in doubt or difficult):		
Administration of intramuscular/intravenous glucagon	Positive glycemic (>1.5 mmol/L) response	All forms of hyperinsulinemic hypoglycemia
Administration of subcutaneous/intravenous dose of octreotide	Positive glycemic response	
Serum levels of IGFBP1	Low (insulin negatively regulates the expression of IGFBP1)	
Branched-chain amino acids (leucine, isoleucine, and valine)	Suppressed	
Provocation tests (leucine loading and exercise testing)	Hypoglycemic hyperinsulinemic response	HI/HA and EIHI, respectively

Abbreviations: HADH, L-3-hydroxyacyl-coenzyme A dehydrogenase; IGFBP1, insulin growth factor binding protein 1.

IMPORTANCE OF GENETIC TESTING FOR CONGENITAL HYPERINSULINEMIC HYPOGLYCEMIA

Patients who are not responsive to first-line treatment with diazoxide need further investigations. It is important to distinguish focal from diffuse disease because the surgical approaches are completely different. A genetic cause for HH is found in about 80% to 90% of diazoxide-unresponsive cases, as opposed to only 22% to 47% of diazoxide-responsive patients. Genetic analysis for mutations in *ABCC8* and *KCNJ11* genes identifies most patients with medically unresponsive diffuse disease (homozygous or compound heterozygous mutations in *ABCC8* and *KCNJ11*).[28] Patients with a paternal mutation in *ABCC8* and *KCNJ11* (or those with no mutations in these genes) potentially have a focal disease and thus require further imaging.[28]

ROLE OF THE 18F-L-3,4-DIHYDROXYPHENYLALANINE-PET/COMPUTED TOMOGRAPHY IN THE MANAGEMENT OF CONGENITAL HYPERINSULINEMIC HYPOGLYCEMIA

In medically unresponsive HH with paternally inherited, de novo, or no identified mutation in K_{ATP} channel genes, the histologic subtypes (focal, diffuse, and atypical) need to be differentiated before planning surgery, because the surgical approaches for each of these are completely different. Diffuse disease is diagnosed in patients homozygous or compound heterozygous for K_{ATP} channel genes. The 18F-DOPA-PET/CT scan is the current gold standard technique for correctly localizing focal forms of congenital HH.[78] However, such imaging should be performed only in centers with the necessary expertise and the images should be interpreted only by experts in the field of combined PET and contrast-enhanced CT imaging.

This imaging technique is based on the fact that pancreatic islets take up L-DOPA and convert it into dopamine using the enzyme DOPA decarboxylase, which is expressed in islet cells.[28] The compound 18F-DOPA is an analog of DOPA, and thus the positron-emitting compound is useful for tracking the uptake of this dopamine precursor. Diffuse, focal, and atypical forms of congenital HH show a high DOPA decarboxylase activity.

A meta-analysis reported that the pooled sensitivity and specificity of 18F-DOPA-PET/CT in differentiating between focal and diffuse HH was 89% (95% confidence interval [CI], 81%–95%) and 98% (95% CI, 89%–100%), respectively.[86] The pooled accuracy in localizing focal HH was 80% (95% CI, 71%–88%).[86] **Fig. 2** depicts the algorithm for the management of patients with congenital HH.

TREATMENT

It is vital that blood glucose concentrations are maintained greater than 3.5 mmol/L in patients with HH[12] because there are no alternative energy substrates for the brain to use at the time of hypoglycemia. Should the child remain hypoglycemic despite increase in volume/frequency of feeds, then an intravenous bolus of 10% dextrose (1–2 mL/kg) can be administered and always be followed by a continuous infusion. Ideally, no more than 2 boluses should be administered, because repeated boluses may stimulate inappropriate insulin secretion. Typically, these patients require greater than 8 mg/kg/min of intravenous glucose infusion to maintain normoglycemia, and this is delivered by increasing the glucose concentration after the insertion of a secure central venous access.

Some children with congenital HH have major feeding issues (such as disturbed feeding pattern, feed refusal behavior, and gastroesophageal reflux),[1] so oral feeding can be a real challenge in these patients. However, enteral feeds should be encouraged to try and maintain orality. In some children, the feeding issues are so severe that they require a gastrostomy insertion and possibly a Nissen fundoplication for controlling the severe gastroesophageal reflux. Feeding may need to be frequent, enriched in carbohydrate content, or supplemented by raw corn starch (from the age of 1 year). If the clinical and biochemical investigations support the diagnosis of HH, the treatments discussed in the following sections may be introduced:

Diazoxide

Diazoxide is the first-line treatment of choice in HH.[1] Diazoxide keeps the K_{ATP} channels in the β-cells open and hence prevents the release of insulin. Diazoxide causes hypertrichosis and can also lead to fluid overload (especially during the neonatal period), hyperuricemia, tachycardia, and leukopenia. In the neonatal period, its use requires fluid restriction and conjunction with a diuretic such as chlorothiazide (7–10 mg/kg/d, given orally in 2 divided doses). The starting dose of diazoxide is 5 mg/kg/d, given orally in 3 divided doses, although in patients with less-severe HH, for example, those related to perinatal stress or IUGR, smaller initial doses (2–3 mg/kg/d) may be

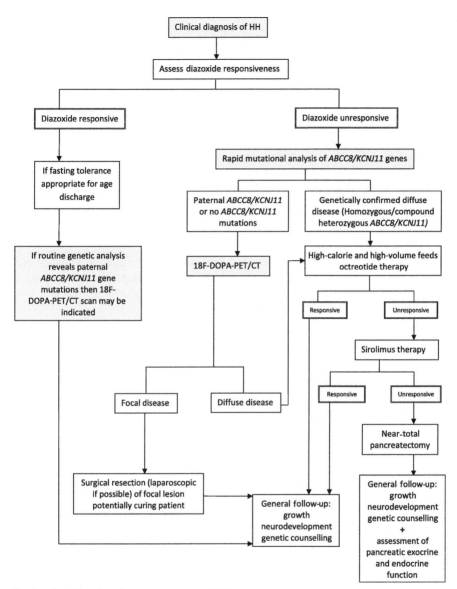

Fig. 2. Algorithm for the management of HH.

effective and safe. Diazoxide responsiveness is defined by (1) normal frequency and volume feeds, (2) ability to fast adequately for age and maintain normal blood glucose levels, (3) low or undetectable serum insulin concentration at the end of the fast, and (4) appropriate increase in serum fatty acids and ketone bodies at the end of the fast.[87] Should the patient show no response after 4 days of treatment, then the dose of diazoxide may be increased by increments of 5 mg/kg/d every 4 days. Patients unresponsive to maximum doses of diazoxide (15–20 mg/kg/d) need urgent genetic analysis. Inactivating mutations in *ABCC8* and *KCNJ11* genes linked to diffuse disease and those with focal congenital HH are less likely to respond to diazoxide.

Somatostatin Analogs

Somatostatin analogs, such as octreotide, are the second-line treatment for diazoxide-insensitive cases. Octreotide stabilizes the K_{ATP} channel in the β-cell, inhibits exocytosis of insulin granules, and reduces the entry of calcium into the β-cell. Octreotide is given subcutaneously at a starting dose of 5 μg/kg/d by continuous infusion (alternatively, 6–8 hourly subcutaneous injections) and may be used along with glucagon or diazoxide in those infants who are not responsive to diazoxide. The criteria for effectiveness are the same as those for diazoxide.[87] The dose may be modified in increments of 5 μg/kg/d every 3 to 4 days until a maximum of 35 μg/kg/d. A new long-acting formulation called lanreotide/LAR-octreotide[88] aids in long-term therapy for diazoxide-unresponsive patients, combined with frequent oral feeds during the day and in some cases, continuous enteral feeds overnight. Necrotizing entercolitis has been described in patients with other risk factors who are receiving octreotide therapy.[89] Octreotide use has been associated with cholelithiasis and tachyphylaxis.[89]

Glucagon

To help stabilize blood glucose levels before a more definitive treatment, glucagon can be given as a 0.5 to 1mg intravenous or intramuscular bolus or at 1 to 10 μg/kg/h continuous infusion. Glucagon acts by releasing hepatic glycogen stores and also stimulates gluconeogenesis, ketogenesis, and lipolysis.[90]

Calcium Channel Blockers

Nifedipine is a Ca^{2+} channel antagonist that inhibits the β-cell membrane depolarization required for insulin exocytosis and release. There have been limited reports of its use in congenital HH.[91] Nifedipine is given orally, and the starting dose is 0.25 mg/kg/d. If after 3 days there is no evidence of response, the dose may be increased to 0.5 mg/kg/d and so on, up to a maximum dose of 2.5 mg/kg/d.

Glucagon-Like Peptide-1 Receptor Antagonist

GLP-1 induces glucose-dependent stimulation of insulin secretion, which is why the GLP-1 receptor may be a new therapeutic target in the future for children with K_{ATP} HH. In both mice[92] and humans (adults only so far) with K_{ATP} HH,[93] exendin-(9–39) (GLP-1 receptor antagonist) has been shown to elevate fasting blood glucose levels. cAMP may have a role in K_{ATP} HH because cAMP content in SUR1 –/– was reduced by exendin-(9–39) both basally and when stimulated by amino acids. Further investigations regarding effectiveness, safety, and pharmacokinetics are needed before its use in children with congenital HH.

Mammalian Target of Rapamycin Inhibitors

Another novel medical therapy in the management of diffuse congenital HH is the mTOR inhibitor, sirolimus (formerly rapamycin). Senniappan and colleagues[94] reported the use of sirolimus in 4 infants with severe congenital HH who were unresponsive to maximal doses of diazoxide and octreotide. mTOR inhibitors had previously been described as successful agents in the treatment of malignant insulinomas.[95] A possible mechanism of hyperinsulinism and β-cell hyperplasia in diffuse HH involves the constitutive activation of the mTOR pathway,[96] implicated in the cellular response to nutrients and growth factor signaling.[97] The effect of sirolimus on β-cell mass is probably achieved through inhibition of the mTOR complex 1 (mTORC1) pathway, although the precise mechanism is not yet clear. The chronic insulin resistance induced by sirolimus is thought to be mediated through the subsequent disassembly and inactivation of mTORC2 and the downregulation of the prosurvival protein kinase B, leading to decreased function and viability of the existing β-cells.[96] Given its recent use for HH and its immunosuppressant nature, further studies are needed to understand the molecular mechanisms of sirolimus action in patients with congenital HH.

The Role of Surgery for Congenital Hyperinsulinemic Hypoglycemia

Identification of diffuse or focal congenital HH is of paramount importance because the management differs entirely. The focal form of the disease can be cured by surgical removal of the lesion, whereas diffuse disease that is completely medically unresponsive requires a near-total (95%–98% removal) pancreatectomy.[98] The latter is associated with a high incidence of diabetes mellitus and pancreatic exocrine insufficiency. Some patients require additional postoperative therapy with diazoxide, octreotide, and/or frequent feedings to maintain normoglycemia. A laparoscopic approach reduces the operative trauma and offers a faster recovery. Histopathologic liaison is of major relevance, because intraoperative histology determines when the margins of the frozen section of biopsies are clear from disease.

SUMMARY

HH is a complex challenging disorder that requires early diagnosis to prevent brain injury. The molecular basis of congenital HH involves defects in key genes that regulate insulin secretion. Rapid genetic analysis, imaging with 18F-DOPA-PET/CT, and new surgical techniques have changed the clinical approach to these patients. Newer treatment modalities are on the horizon for patients with severe diffuse disease.

REFERENCES

1. Aynsley Green A, Hussain K, Hall J, et al. Practical management of hyperinsulinism in infancy. Arch Dis Child Fetal Neonatal Ed 2000;82:F98–107.
2. Hussain K, Hindmarsh P, Aynsley-Green A. Neonates with symptomatic hyperinsulinemic hypoglycemia generate inappropriately low serum cortisol counter regulatory hormonal responses. J Clin Endocrinol Metab 2003;88(9):4342–7.
3. Hussain K, Bryan J, Christesen HT, et al. Serum glucagon counter regulatory hormonal response to hypoglycemia is blunted in congenital hyperinsulinism. Diabetes 2005;54(10):2946–51.
4. Thomas PM, Cote GJ, Wohllk N, et al. Mutations in the sulfonylurea receptor gene in familial persistent hyperinsulinemic hypoglycemia of infancy. Science 1995; 268:426–9.
5. Thomas P, Ye Y, Lightner E. Mutation of the pancreatic islet inward rectifier Kir6.2 also leads to familial persistent hyperinsulinemic hypoglycemia of infancy. Hum Mol Genet 1996;5:1809–12.
6. Stanley CA, Lieu YK, Hsu BY, et al. Hyperinsulinism and hyperammonemia in infants with regulatory mutations of the glutamate dehydrogenase gene. N Engl J Med 1998;338:1352–7.
7. Clayton PT, Eaton S, Aynsley Green A, et al. Hyperinsulinism in short chain L-3-hydroxyacyl-CoA dehydrogenase deficiency reveals the importance of beta-oxidation in insulin secretion. J Clin Invest 2001;108:457–65.
8. Glaser B, Kesavan P, Heyman M, et al. Familial hyperinsulinism caused by an activating glucokinase mutation. N Engl J Med 1998;338:226–30.

9. Cornblath M, Hawdon JM, Williams AF, et al. Controversies regarding definition of neonatal hypoglycemia: Suggested operational thresholds. Pediatrics 2000;105: 1141–5.

10. Williams AF. Hypoglycaemia of the newborn: a review. Bull World Health Organ 1997;75(3):261–90.

11. Koh TH, Aynsley-Green A, Tarbit M, et al. Neural dysfunction during hypoglycaemia. Arch Dis Child 1988;63:1353–8.

12. Hussain K, Blankenstein O, De Lonlay P, et al. Hyperinsulinaemic hypoglycaemia: biochemical basis and the importance of maintaining normoglycaemia during management. Arch Dis Child 2007;92:568–70.

13. Screening guidelines for newborns at risk for low blood glucose (Canadian Paediatric Society). Paediatr Child Health 2004;9(10):723–9.

14. Hawdon JM, Ward Platt MP, Aynsley-Green A. Patterns of metabolic adaptation for preterm and term infants in the first neonatal week. Arch Dis Child 1992; 67(4):357–65.

15. Aynsley-Green A, Lucas A, Bloom SR. The control of the adaptation of the human neonate to postnatal nutrition. Acta Chir Scand Suppl 1981;507:269–81.

16. Hussain K. Congenital hyperinsulinism and neonatal diabetes mellitus. Rev Endocr Metab Disord 2010;11:155–6.

17. Cook DL, Hales CN. Intracellular ATP directly blocks K+ channels in pancreatic B-cells. Nature 1984;311:271–3.

18. Ashcroft FM, Harrison DE, Ashcroft SJ. Glucose induces closure of single potassium channels in isolated rat pancreatic beta-cells. Nature 1984;312:446–8.

19. Inagaki N, Gonoi T, Clement JP 4th, et al. Reconstitution of IKATP: an inward rectifier subunit plus the sulfonylurea receptor. Science 1995;270:1166–70.

20. Tucker SJ, Gribble FM, Proks P, et al. Molecular determinants of KATP channel inhibition by ATP. EMBO J 1998;17:3290–6.

21. Matschinsky FM. Banting Lecture 1995. A lesson in metabolic regulation inspired by the glucokinase glucose sensor paradigm. Diabetes 1996;45:223–41.

22. Cryer PE, Axelrod L, Grossman AB, et al. Evaluation and management of adult hypoglycemic disorders: an Endocrine Society Clinical Practice Guideline. J Clin Endocrinol Metab 2009;94:709–28.

23. Cryer PE. Glucose counterregulation: prevention and correction of hypoglycemia in humans. Am J Physiol 1993;264:149–55.

24. Straub SG, Cosgrove KE, Ammala C, et al. Hyperinsulinism of infancy: the regulated release of insulin by KATP channel-independent pathways. Diabetes 2001; 50:329–39.

25. Gembal M, Detimary P, Gilon P, et al. Mechanisms by which glucose can control insulin release independently from its action on adenosine triphosphate-sensitive K + channels in mouse B cells. J Clin Invest 1993;91:871–80.

26. Aizawa T, Sato Y, Ishihara F, et al. ATP-sensitive K + channel-independent glucose action in rat pancreatic beta-cell. Am J Physiol 1994;266:622–7.

27. Ammala C, Eliasson L, Bokvist K, et al. Activation of protein kinases and inhibition of protein phosphatases play a central role in the regulation of exocytosis in mouse pancreatic beta cells. Proc Natl Acad Sci U S A 1994;91:4343–7.

28. Senniappan S, Shanti B, James C, et al. Hyperinsulinaemic hypoglycaemia: genetic mechanisms, diagnosis and management. J Inherit Metab Dis 2012;35: 589–601.

29. Fafoula O, Alkhayyat H, Hussain K. Prolonged hyperinsulinaemic hypoglycaemia in newborns with intrauterine growth retardation. Arch Dis Child Fetal Neonatal Ed 2006;91:F467.

30. Crane A, Aguilar-Bryan L. Assembly, maturation, and turnover of K (ATP) channel subunits. J Biol Chem 2004;279:9080–90.
31. Cartier EA, Conti LR, Vandenberg CA, et al. Defective trafficking and function of KATP channels caused by a sulfonylurea receptor 1 mutation associated with persistent hyperinsulinemic hypoglycemia of infancy. Proc Natl Acad Sci U S A 2001;98:2882–7.
32. Yan FF, Lin YW, MacMullen C, et al. Congenital hyperinsulinism associated ABCC8 mutations that cause defective trafficking of ATP-sensitive K+ channels: identification and rescue. Diabetes 2007;56:2339–48.
33. Lin YW, MacMullen C, Ganguly A, et al. A novel KCNJ11 mutation associated with congenital hyperinsulinism reduces the intrinsic open probability of beta-cell ATP-sensitive potassium channels. J Biol Chem 2006;281:3006–12.
34. Kane C, Shepherd RM, Squires PE, et al. Loss of functional KATP channels in pancreatic beta-cells causes persistent hyperinsulinemic hypoglycemia of infancy. Nat Med 1996;2:1344–7.
35. Flanagan SE, Clauin S, Bellanné-Chantelot C, et al. Update of mutations in the genes encoding the pancreatic beta-cell K (ATP) channel subunits Kir6.2 (KCNJ11) and sulfonylurea receptor 1 (ABCC8) in diabetes mellitus and hyperinsulinism. Hum Mutat 2009;30:170–80.
36. Huopio H, Reimann F, Ashfield R, et al. Dominantly inherited hyperinsulinism caused by a mutation in the sulfonylurea receptor type 1. J Clin Invest 2000;106:897–906.
37. Pinney SE, MacMullen C, Becker S, et al. Clinical characteristics and biochemical mechanisms of congenital hyperinsulinism associated with dominant KATP channel mutations. J Clin Invest 2008;118:2877–86.
38. Flanagan SE, Kapoor RR, Banerjee I, et al. Dominantly acting ABCC8 mutations in patients with medically unresponsive hyperinsulinaemic hypoglycaemia. Clin Genet 2011;79:582–7.
39. Senniappan S, Arya VB, Hussain K. The molecular mechanisms, diagnosis and management of congenital hyperinsulinism. Indian J Endocrinol Metab 2013;17(1):19–30.
40. Treberg JR, Clow KA, Greene KA, et al. Systemic activation of glutamate dehydrogenase increases renal ammoniagenesis: Implications for the hyperinsulinism/hyperammonemia syndrome. Am J Physiol Endocrinol Metab 2010;298:E1219–25.
41. Hsu BY, Kelly A, Thornton PS, et al. Protein-sensitive and fasting hypoglycemia in children with the hyperinsulinism/hyperammonemia syndrome. J Pediatr 2001;138:383–9.
42. Kapoor RR, Flanagan SE, Fulton P, et al. Hyperinsulinism-hyperammonaemia syndrome: Novel mutations in the GLUD1 gene and genotype-phenotype correlations. Eur J Endocrinol 2009;161:731–5.
43. Bahi-Buisson N, Roze E, Dionisi C, et al. Neurological aspects of hyperinsulinism-hyperammonaemia syndrome. Dev Med Child Neurol 2008;50:945–9.
44. Hardy OT, Hohmeier HE, Becker TC, et al. Functional genomics of the beta-cell: Short-chain 3-hydroxyacyl-coenzyme A dehydrogenase regulates insulin secretion independent of K+ currents. Mol Endocrinol 2007;21:765–73.
45. Molven A, Matre GE, Duran M, et al. Familial hyperinsulinemic hypoglycemia caused by a defect in the SCHAD enzyme of mitochondrial fatty acid oxidation. Diabetes 2004;53:221–7.
46. Vredendaal PJ, Van den Berg IE, Malingré HE, et al. Human short-chain L-3-hydroxyacyl-CoA dehydrogenase: Cloning and characterization of the coding sequence. Biochem Biophys Res Commun 1996;223:718–23.

47. Martins E, Cardoso ML, Rodrigues E, et al. Short-chain 3-hydroxyacyl-CoA dehydrogenase deficiency: The clinical relevance of an early diagnosis and report of four new cases. J Inherit Metab Dis 2011;34:835–42.

48. Li C, Chen P, Palladino A, et al. Mechanism of hyperinsulinism in short-chain 3-hydroxyacyl-CoA dehydrogenase deficiency involves activation of glutamate dehydrogenase. J Biol Chem 2010;285:31806–18.

49. Kapoor RR, James C, Flanagan SE, et al. 3-Hydroxyacyl-coenzyme A dehydrogenase deficiency and hyperinsulinemic hypoglycemia: characterization of a novel mutation and severe dietary protein sensitivity. J Clin Endocrinol Metab 2009;94:2221–5.

50. Flanagan SE, Patch AM, Locke JM, et al. Genome wide homozygosity analysis reveals HADH mutations as a common cause of diazoxide responsive hyperinsulinemic hypoglycemia in consanguineous pedigrees. J Clin Endocrinol Metab 2011;96:498–502.

51. Matschinsky FM. Regulation of pancreatic beta-cell glucokinase: from basics to therapeutics. Diabetes 2002;51(3):394–404.

52. Christesen HB, Jacobsen BB, Odili S, et al. The second activating glucokinase mutation (A456V): Implications for glucose homeostasis and diabetes therapy. Diabetes 2002;51:1240–6.

53. Wabitsch M, Lahr G, Van de Bunt M, et al. Heterogeneity in disease severity in a family with a novel G68V GCK activating mutation causing persistent hyperinsulinaemic hypoglycaemia of infancy. Diabet Med 2007;24:1393–9.

54. Cuesta-Muñoz AL, Huopio H, Otonkoski T, et al. Severe persistent hyperinsulinemic hypoglycemia due to a de novo glucokinase mutation. Diabetes 2004;53: 2164–8.

55. Abdulhadi-Atwan M, Bushman J, Tornovsky-Babaey S, et al. Novel de novo mutation in sulfonylurea receptor 1 presenting as hyperinsulinism in infancy followed by overt diabetes in early adolescence. Diabetes 2008;57(7):1935–40.

56. Gupta RK, Vatamaniuk MZ, Lee CS, et al. The MODY1 gene HNF-4alpha regulates selected genes involved in insulin secretion. J Clin Invest 2005;115: 1006–15.

57. Pearson ER, Boj SF, Steele AM, et al. Macrosomia and hyperinsulinaemic hypoglycaemia in patients with heterozygous mutations in the HNF4A gene. PLoS Med 2007;4:118.

58. Kapoor RR, Locke J, Colclough K, et al. Persistent hyperinsulinemic hypoglycemia and maturity onset diabetes of the young due to heterozygous HNF4A mutations. Diabetes 2008;57:1659–63.

59. Gremlich S, Nolan C, Roduit R, et al. Pancreatic islet adaptation to fasting is dependent on peroxisome proliferator activated receptor alpha transcriptional up-regulation of fatty acid oxidation. Endocrinology 2005;146:375–82.

60. Prentki M, Joly E, El-Assaad W, et al. Malonyl-CoA signaling, lipid partitioning, and glucolipotoxicity: Role in beta-cell adaptation and failure in the etiology of diabetes. Diabetes 2002;51(3):405–13.

61. Flanagan SE, Kapoor RR, Mali G, et al. Diazoxide responsive hyperinsulinemic hypoglycemia caused by HNF4A gene mutations. Eur J Endocrinol 2010;162:987–92.

62. Zhao C, Wilson MC, Schuit F, et al. Expression and distribution of lactate/monocarboxylate transporter isoforms in pancreatic islets and the exocrine pancreas. Diabetes 2001;50:361–6.

63. Otonkoski T, Jiao H, Kaminen-Ahola N, et al. Physical exercise induced hypoglycemia caused by failed silencing of monocarboxylate transporter 1 in pancreatic beta cells. Am J Hum Genet 2007;81:467–74.

64. Meissner T, Friedmann B, Okun JG, et al. Massive insulin secretion in response to anaerobic exercise in exercise induced hyperinsulinism. Horm Metab Res 2005; 37:690–4.

65. Chan CB, De Leo D, Joseph JW, et al. Increased uncoupling protein 2 levels in beta-cells are associated with impaired glucose stimulated insulin secretion: mechanism of action. Diabetes 2001;50:1302–10.

66. Gonzalez-Barroso MM, Giurgea I, Bouillaud F, et al. Mutations in UCP2 in congenital hyperinsulinism reveal a role for regulation of insulin secretion. PLoS One 2008;3:3850.

67. Munns CF, Batch JA. Hyperinsulinism and Beckwith-Wiedemann syndrome. Arch Dis Child Fetal Neonatal Ed 2001;84:67–9.

68. Bufler P, Ehringhaus C, Koletzko S. Dumping syndrome: a common problem following Nissen's fundoplication in young children. Pediatr Surg Int 2001;17:351–5.

69. Palladino AA, Sayed S, Levitt Katz LE, et al. Increased glucagon-like peptide-1 secretion and postprandial hypoglycemia in children after Nissen's fundoplication. J Clin Endocrinol Metab 2009;94:39–44.

70. Kneepkens CM, Fernandes J, Vonk RJ. Dumping syndrome in children. Diagnosis and effect of glucomannan on glucose tolerance and absorption. Acta Paediatr Scand 1988;77:279–86.

71. Shin JJ, Gorden P, Libutti SK. Insulinoma: pathophysiology, localization and management. Future Oncol 2010;6:229–37.

72. Giurgea I, Ulinski T, Touati G, et al. Factitious hyperinsulinism leading to pancreatectomy: severe forms of Munchausen syndrome by proxy. Pediatrics 2005;116: 145–8.

73. Rahier J, Guiot Y, Sempoux C. Morphologic analysis of focal and diffuse forms of congenital hyperinsulinism. Semin Pediatr Surg 2011;20(1):3–12.

74. Sempoux C, Guiot Y, Jaubert F, et al. Focal and diffuse forms of congenital hyperinsulinism: the keys for differential diagnosis. Endocr Pathol 2004;15:241–6.

75. Ismail D, Smith VV, de Lonlay P, et al. Familial focal congenital hyperinsulinism. J Clin Endocrinol Metab 2011;96:24–8.

76. Fournet JC, Mayaud C, de Lonlay P, et al. Unbalanced expression of 11p15 imprinted genes in focal forms of congenital hyperinsulinism: Association with a reduction to homozygosity of a mutation in ABCC8 or KCNJ11. Am J Pathol 2001;158:2177–84.

77. Sempoux C, Capito C, Bellanne-Chantelot C, et al. Morphological mosaicism of the pancreatic islets: a novel anatomopathological form of persistent hyperinsulinemic hypoglycemia of infancy. J Clin Endocrinol Metab 2011;96:3785–93.

78. Hardy OT, Hernandez-Pampaloni M, Saffer JR, et al. Diagnosis and localization of focal congenital hyperinsulinism by 18F-fluorodopa PET scan. J Pediatr 2007; 150:140–5.

79. Henquin JC, Sempoux C, Marchandise J, et al. Congenital hyperinsulinism caused by hexokinase I expression or glucokinase-activating mutation in a subset of beta-cells. Diabetes 2013;62:1689–96.

80. Hussain K. Investigations for neonatal hypoglycaemia. Clin Biochem 2011;44: 465–6.

81. Arya VB, Senniappan S, Guemes M, et al. Neonatal hypoglycaemia. Indian J Pediatr 2014;81(1):58–65.

82. Dekelbab BH, Sperling MA. Recent advances in hyperinsulinemic hypoglycemia of infancy. Acta Paediatr 2006;95:1157–64.

83. Finegold DN, Stanley CA, Baker L. Glycemic response to glucagon during fasting hypoglycemia: An aid in the diagnosis of hyperinsulinism. J Pediatr 1980;96:257–9.

84. Levitt Katz LE, Satin Smith MS, Collett Solberg P, et al. Insulin like growth factor binding protein 1 levels in the diagnosis of hypoglycemia caused by hyperinsulinism. J Pediatr 1997;131:193–9.

85. Palladino AA, Stanley CA. The hyperinsulinism/hyperammonemia syndrome. Rev Endocr Metab Disord 2010;11:171–8.

86. Treglia G, Mirk P, Rufini V. Diagnostic performance of fluorine-18-dihydroxyphenylalanine positron emission tomography in diagnosing and localizing the focal form of congenital hyperinsulinism. Pediatr Radiol 2012;42(11):1372–9.

87. Arnoux J-B, Saint-Martin C, Montravers F, et al. An update on congenital hyperinsulinism: advances in diagnosis and management. Expert Opin Orphan Drugs 2014;2(8):1–17.

88. Le Quan Sang KH, Arnoux JB, Mamoune A, et al. Successful treatment of congenital hyperinsulinism with long acting release octreotide. Eur J Endocrinol 2012;166:333–9.

89. Thornton PS, Alter CA, Katz LE, et al. Short and long-term use of octreotide in the treatment of congenital hyperinsulinism. J Pediatr 1993;123:637–43.

90. Deshpande S, Ward Platt M. The investigation and management of neonatal hypoglycaemia. Semin Fetal Neonatal Med 2005;10:351–61.

91. Muller D, Zimmering M, Roehr CC. Should nifedipine be used to counter low blood sugar levels in children with persistent hyperinsulinaemic hypoglycaemia? Arch Dis Child 2004;89:83–5.

92. De Leon DD, Li C, Delson MI, et al. Exendin-(9-39) corrects fasting hypoglycemia in SUR-1-/- mice by lowering cAMP in pancreatic beta-cells and inhibiting insulin secretion. J Biol Chem 2008;283:25786–93.

93. Calabria AC, Li C, Gallagher PR, et al. GLP-1 receptor antagonist exendin-(9-39) elevates fasting blood glucose levels in congenital hyperinsulinism owing to inactivating mutations in the ATP-sensitive K + channel. Diabetes 2012;61:2585–91.

94. Senniappan S, Alexandrescu S, Tatevian N, et al. Sirolimus therapy in infants with severe hyperinsulinemic hypoglycemia. N Engl J Med 2014;370(12):1131–7.

95. Kulke MH, Bergsland EK, Yao JC. Glycemic control in patients with insulinoma treated with everolimus. N Engl J Med 2009;360:195–7.

96. Alexandrescu S, Tatevian N, Olutoye O, et al. Persistent hyperinsulinemic hypoglycemia of infancy: constitutive activation of the mTOR pathway with associated exocrine-islet transdifferentiation and therapeutic implications. Int J Clin Exp Pathol 2010;3:691–705.

97. Kwon G, Marshall CA, Pappan KL, et al. Signaling elements involved in the metabolic regulation of mTOR by nutrients, incretins, and growth factors in islets. Diabetes 2004;53(3):225–S232.

98. Fékété CN, de Lonlay P, Jaubert F, et al. The surgical management of congenital hyperinsulinemic hypoglycemia in infancy. J Pediatr Surg 2004;39:267–9.

Genome, Exome, and Targeted Next-Generation Sequencing in Neonatal Diabetes

Elisa De Franco, PhD, Sian Ellard, PhD, FRCPath*

KEYWORDS

- Next-generation sequencing • Gene discovery • Genetic testing • Neonatal diabetes

KEY POINTS

- Next-generation sequencing has revolutionized the approach to genetic testing and research.
- The 3 main applications of next-generation sequencing technology are targeted gene panels and exome and genome sequencing.
- Neonatal diabetes is a genetically and clinically heterogeneous disease, which means that genetic testing and research of new causes of the disease are challenging.
- A targeted gene panel has been developed to test all the known causes of neonatal diabetes in a single test. Early comprehensive testing has changed the way patients with neonatal diabetes are managed.
- Exome sequencing is a powerful tool to identify novel disease genes. In neonatal diabetes, it has led to the identification of 2 novel causes: mutations in *GATA6* and *STAT3*.
- Genome sequencing is the most comprehensive test available, and it was used to identify mutations in a novel enhancer that cause pancreatic agenesis.

INTRODUCTION TO NEONATAL DIABETES

Neonatal diabetes diagnosed before 6 months is a rare disease (approximate incidence of 1:100,000 live births[1]) that reflects severe β-cell dysfunction (**Fig. 1**). Two separate studies[2,3] have shown that diabetes diagnosed before 6 months of age is most likely to have a monogenic cause rather than being caused by autoimmunity.

The authors declare no conflicts of interest. S. Ellard is a Wellcome Trust Senior Investigator.
Institute of Biomedical and Clinical Science, University of Exeter Medical School, Barrack Road, Exeter EX2 5DW, UK
* Corresponding author. University of Exeter Medical School, RILD level 3, Royal Devon & Exeter Hospital, Barrack Road, Exeter EX2 5DW, UK.
E-mail address: sian.ellard@nhs.net

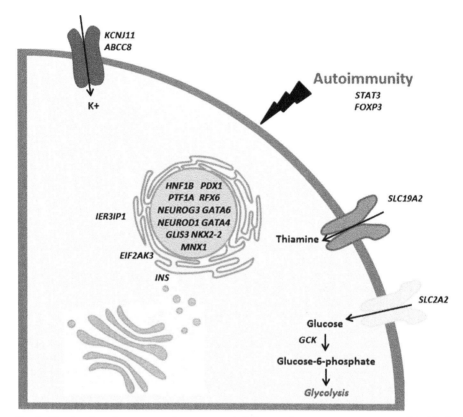

Fig. 1. The β cell and genes causing neonatal diabetes. Gene names are reported in black font. KCNJ11, ABCC8, SLC19A2, and SLC2A2 are transmembrane channels. FOXP3 and STAT3 are involved in the immune response. HNF1B, PDX1, PTF1A, RFX6, NEUROG3, GATA6, NEUROD1, GATA4, GLIS3, NKX2-2, and MNX1 are transcription factors that regulate genes in the nucleus. EIF2AK3 and IER3IP1 regulate protein trafficking in the endoplasmic reticulum. Mutations in the *INS* gene cause neonatal diabetes either by resulting in absence of insulin or by producing a defective insulin protein that accumulates in the endoplasmic reticulum and is not secreted in the blood stream. For genes encoding proteins acting within the β cell, the position of the gene name indicates the intracellular location of the protein. Substrates and transported molecules are indicated in blue. Biological processes are indicated in red.

Neonatal diabetes is a clinically and genetically heterogeneous disease. To date there are 23 different genetic causes of neonatal diabetes that identify different clinical subtypes of the disease (De Franco and colleagues, *submitted for publication* and[4]) (see **Fig. 1, Table 1**).

The most common causes of neonatal diabetes are mutations in the genes encoding the subunits of the voltage-dependent potassium channel *ABCC8* and *KCNJ11*.[8,9,27] Correct function of the potassium channel is necessary for secretion of insulin in response to glucose levels. Approximately 40% of patients with neonatal diabetes have a potassium channel gene mutation.[27,50] Patients with mutations in these two genes are sensitive to sulfonylurea treatment, and their glycemic control can be greatly improved switching from insulin to sulfonylurea therapy.[51,52] This finding has led to international guidelines suggesting immediate referral for genetic testing after a clinical diagnosis of neonatal diabetes.[53] Mutations in *KCNJ11* and *ABCC8* can cause transient neonatal diabetes, permanent neonatal diabetes, or DEND (developmental delay, epilepsy, and neonatal diabetes) syndrome.[8,9,27,28,54]

Clinically neonatal diabetes can be divided into 3 broad categories:

- Transient neonatal diabetes (The diabetes remits and eventually relapses later in life.)
- Permanent neonatal diabetes (The diabetes does not remit.)
- Syndromic neonatal diabetes (Neonatal diabetes is one of the clinical features characterizing a syndrome.)

The most common causes of transient neonatal diabetes are methylation abnormalities resulting in overexpression of paternally expressed genes at the 6q24 locus[5–7] and mutations in *ABCC8* or *KCNJ11* (see **Table 1**).[28,54] Patients with a transient form of neonatal diabetes are diagnosed with hyperglycemia in the first 6 months of life; the diabetes then remits, and in most cases it relapses later in life.

Isolated insulin-requiring permanent neonatal diabetes is caused by mutations in the *INS* and *GCK* genes.[17,25,26] Mutations in 18 genes are known to cause syndromic neonatal diabetes (see **Table 1**), in which neonatal diabetes is just one of the features of the clinical spectrum that defines a particular condition. Because neonatal diabetes is diagnosed in the first 6 months of life, in most cases it is the presenting feature of the syndrome; additional clinical features will sequentially appear later in life. For this reason, a differential clinical diagnosis in the first 6 months of life is often difficult and can only be achieved months or even years after the first presentation with neonatal diabetes.

INTRODUCTION TO NEXT-GENERATION SEQUENCING

The term *next-generation sequencing* collectively refers to the high throughput DNA sequencing technologies that are able to sequence many DNA sequences in a single reaction (ie, in parallel). The advent of next-generation sequencing enables DNA sequencing at several orders of magnitude greater than was possible using the Sanger method developed in the 1970s. The Sanger methodology permits sequencing of a maximum of a few hundred nucleotides in a single reaction with each nucleotide being sequenced (or read by the instrument) just once. In contrast, next-generation sequencing allows entire exomes or genomes to be sequenced in a single test with each nucleotide being independently read multiple times (**Fig. 2**).

The introduction of next-generation sequencing technologies on the market in 2005[55] has resulted in the possibility to sequence entire exomes and genomes much more quickly and at a much lower cost. A widely quoted example is the first human genome sequence that took 13 years and cost nearly £2 billion, compared with the current cost of approaching £1000 for a genome sequence obtained in just 2 days. Next-generation sequencing technologies are now extensively used both for new disease gene discovery and for improving diagnostic genetic tests for known diseases.

Preparation of samples for next-generation sequencing usually includes fragmentation of DNA, ligation of adapters, and, in most cases, amplification via polymerase chain reaction. Several kits for library preparation are commercially available that allow for automation of the process and preparation of multiple samples in parallel.

The most widely used applications of next-generation sequencing are targeted analysis of a panel of genes and exome sequencing with genome sequencing

Table 1
Genetic causes of neonatal diabetes

Gene	Mode of Inheritance	Neonatal Diabetes Phenotype	Additional Features	Frequency in NDM Patients (De Franco et al, *Submitted*) (%)	References
6q24	—	Transient	Intrauterine growth retardation, macroglossia, umbilical hernia, neurologic features (rare)	11.1	Gardner et al,[5] Temple et al,[6] Temple & Shield[7]
ABCC8	Dominant/recessive	Transient, permanent	Developmental delay with/without epilepsy	14.7	Babenko et al,[8] Proks et al[9]
EIF2AK3	Recessive	Permanent	Skeletal dysplasia, liver dysfunction	7.5	Delepine et al,[10] Rubio-Cabezas et al[11]
FOXP3	X-linked	Permanent	Eczema, enteropathy, other autoimmune features	1.4	Chatila et al[12]
GATA4	Dominant	Transient, permanent	Exocrine insufficiency, congenital heart malformations	0.4	D'Amato et al,[13] Shaw-Smith et al[14]
GATA6	Dominant	Transient, permanent	Exocrine insufficiency, congenital heart malformation, neurologic defects, hypothyroidism, gut and hepatobiliary malformations	2.8	Lango Allen et al,[15] De Franco et al[16]
GCK	Recessive	Permanent	—	2.9	Njolstad et al,[17] Barbetti et al[18]
GLIS3	Recessive	Permanent	Hypothyroidism	0.9	Dimitri et al,[19] Senee et al[20]
HNF1B	Dominant	Transient	Exocrine insufficiency, renal cysts	0.2	Edghill et al,[21] Yorifuji et al[22]
IER3IP1	Recessive	Permanent	Microcephaly, epilepsy	0.1	Abdel-Salam et al,[23] Poulton et al[24]
INS	Dominant/recessive	Transient, permanent	—	10.8	Garin et al,[25] Stoy et al[26]

Gene	Inheritance	Transient, permanent	Features	%	References
KCNJ11	Dominant	Transient, permanent	Developmental delay with/without epilepsy	23.5	Gloyn et al,[27] Gloyn et al[28]
MNX1	Recessive	Permanent	Sacral agenesis, neurologic defects	0.1	Flanagan et al[29]
NEUROD1	Recessive	Permanent	Cerebellar hypoplasia, sensorineural deafness, visual impairment	0.3	Rubio-Cabezas et al[30]
NEUROG3	Recessive	Permanent	Congenital malabsorptive diarrhea	0.2	Rubio-Cabezas et al[31]
NKX2-2	Recessive	Permanent	Corpus callosum agenesis	0.2	Flanagan et al[29]
PDX1	Recessive	Permanent	Exocrine insufficiency	0.6	Schwitzgebel et al,[32] Stoffers et al,[33] Thomas et al,[34] De Franco et al,[35] Nicolino et al[36]
PTF1A	Recessive	Permanent	Exocrine insufficiency, cerebellar agenesis (only for coding mutations)	2.2	Al-Shammari et al,[37] Sellick et al,[38] Tutak et al,[39] Weeden et al[40]
RFX6	Recessive	Permanent	Intestinal atresia and/or malrotation, gall bladder agenesis	0.1	Smith et al,[41] Spiegel et al[42]
SLC19A2	Recessive	Permanent	Thiamine-responsive megaloblastic anemia, sensorineural deafness	0.7	Bay et al,[43] Bergmann et al,[44] Mandel et al,[45] Shaw-Smith et al[46]
SLC2A2	Recessive	Transient	Hepatorenal glycogen accumulation, renal dysfunction, impaired utilization of glucose and galactose	0.6	Sansbury et al[47]
STAT3	Dominant	Permanent	Autoimmune enteropathy, thyroid dysfunction, pulmonary disease, juvenile-onset arthritis	0.4	Flanagan et al[4]
ZFP57	Recessive	Transient	Intrauterine growth retardation	1.2	Mackay et al,[48] Mackay & Temple[49]

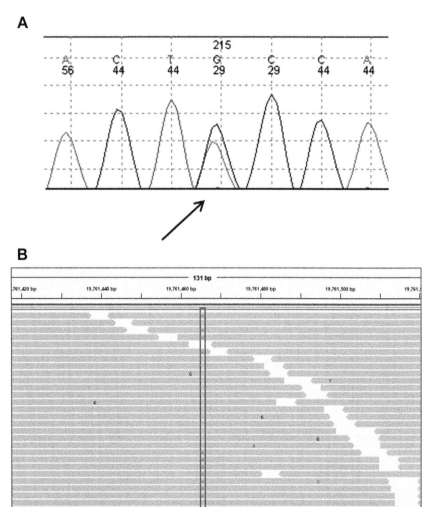

Fig. 2. With Sanger sequencing each nucleotide is sequenced (or read by the instrument) once. With next-generation sequencing entire exomes or genomes can be sequenced in a single test, and each position is covered by multiple reads. (*A*) Sanger sequencing trace of a mutation in *GATA6*. (*B*) The same mutation is detected by multiple reads with a next-generation sequencing assay. Black arrows indicate the mutation.

becoming more popular as prices decrease. Details on these technologies and their applications in neonatal diabetes are discussed in the following sections.

TARGETED NEXT-GENERATION SEQUENCING
Method

Next-generation sequencing technologies provide the potential for simultaneous analysis of all the genes known to cause a disease in a single assay at a similar cost to testing a few genes by Sanger sequencing. A widely used application is targeted next-generation sequencing of a given set of genes. Various methods have been successfully used to target specific genomic regions, currently the most commonly used is hybridization capture.[56–58] With this approach, several marked oligonucleotides (or baits) with sequences complementary to the targeted regions are used to capture the genes in the panel.

The error rate for next-generation sequencing is estimated at 1%[59]; therefore, multiple reads are required to obtain equivalent sensitivity to Sanger sequencing. The minimum depth of coverage needed (number of reads per base) will depend on the reason for testing (eg, clinical diagnostic vs prescreen before exome analysis). For clinical diagnostic testing the minimum read depth required is 30 reads, which enables reliable detection of heterozygous single nucleotide variants. Detection of small (<30 base pairs) insertions and deletions has proven more difficult, and optimization of the process is still ongoing. Various specific methods for detection of larger deletions and duplications have been developed (reviewed in[60,61]).

The use of targeted next-generation sequencing gene panels has become very common for genetic testing of genetically heterogeneous diseases, such as breast cancer,[62] polycystic kidney disease,[63] Bardet-Biedl/Alström syndrome,[58] and retinal disease.[57]

Targeted Next-Generation Sequencing in Neonatal Diabetes

To date mutations in 22 genes are known to cause neonatal diabetes (see **Fig. 1**, **Table 1**) (De Franco and colleagues, *submitted for publication*, and[4]). Three targeted next-generation sequencing assays have been developed for testing of monogenic forms of diabetes, including one developed by the authors.[64–66]

The targeted panel test developed in Exeter, United Kingdom uses a capture-in-solution system with baits for 48 genes known to cause monogenic forms of diabetes (eg, maturity-onset diabetes of youth, lipodystrophy), including the 22 known neonatal diabetes genes. This test can detect single nucleotide mutations and small deletions/insertions as well as large deletions and duplications.[65]

Because approximately 40% of patients diagnosed with neonatal diabetes have a mutation in a potassium channel gene (De Franco and colleagues, *submitted for publication*) and can be successfully treated with sulfonylurea tablets instead of insulin,[51,52] early comprehensive genetic testing in neonatal diabetes is of the utmost importance for patients' clinical management.

A recent study has evaluated the impact of early comprehensive genetic testing in a large cohort of patients with neonatal diabetes (De Franco and colleagues, *submitted for publication*). Comprehensive genetic analysis, including targeted next-generation sequencing and a methylation assay to detect 6q24 methylation abnormalities (**Fig. 3**), was performed on 1020 patients diagnosed with neonatal diabetes before 6 months of age and referred from 79 countries over 14 years.

De Franco and colleagues showed that a genetic diagnosis could be identified in more than 80% of patients with neonatal diabetes. As expected, the genetic causes of neonatal diabetes were very different in patients born to nonconsanguineous and

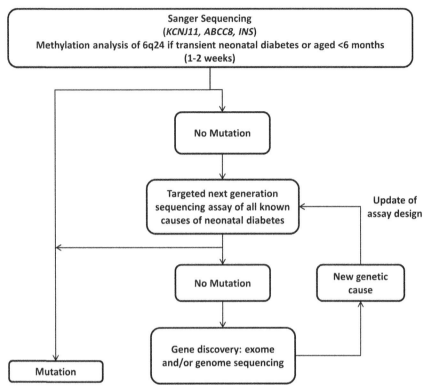

Fig. 3. Current genetic testing pipeline for neonatal diabetes referrals in the Exeter Genetics laboratory.

consanguineous parents. Mutations in *KCNJ11* and *ABCC8* were common in the non-consanguineous cohort, accounting for 46% of cases, but were present in only 12% of the patients in the consanguineous group.

The authors also reported that the median time from diagnosis of neonatal diabetes to referral for genetic testing has decreased from more than 5 years in 2000 to less than 3 months in 2012, indicating that now patients are more likely to be referred for genetic testing when neonatal diabetes is the only clinical feature present, before development of other clinical characteristics suggestive of their specific neonatal diabetes subtypes. This change means that comprehensive testing of all the known causes of neonatal diabetes results in these patients receiving a genetic diagnosis before development of the full clinical spectrum.

This has important implications for the patients with one of the neonatal diabetes subtypes for which an alternative treatment is available (potassium channel,[51,52] Thiamine-responsive megaloblastic anemia[67]) and for patients with syndromic forms of neonatal diabetes for whom clinicians will be aware of the likely development of specific additional features before these present. The authors conclude that the availability of a comprehensive genetic test has resulted in a paradigm shift in genetic testing for neonatal diabetes: although traditionally genetic testing was used only to confirm a diagnosis made by a set of clinical features, now genetic testing is a first-line investigation that makes the diagnosis and guides decisions for clinical care of patients.

EXOME SEQUENCING
Method

Exome sequencing allows simultaneous investigation of the less than 2% of the human genome (the exons) that encodes for proteins. About 80% of the disease-causing mutations are predicted to be located in a protein-coding part of the genome, thus making exome sequencing an attractive strategy to investigate the genetic basis of Mendelian diseases.

The exonic sequences are generally selected from genomic DNA by hybridization capture. Multiple capture systems are available, and the number of targeted exons is approximately 200,000, representing approximately 95% of known genes (**Table 2**).

Selection of the coding regions of the genome for sequencing is at the same time the main advantage and main disadvantage for exome sequencing when compared with whole-genome sequencing. In fact selection of the exonic sequences means that exome sequencing is currently cheaper and produces far less data to analyze than whole-genome sequencing. At the same time, the target selection process is subjected to different efficiency depending on the genomic region (for example, GC rich regions are captured far less efficiently than other parts of the genome); this results in uneven coverage (different number of reads) of the different targets, affecting the ability to detect variants in some parts of the genome.

Typically, between 20,000 and 50,000 variants are identified per exome sequenced.[68] Filtering and prioritizing strategies are needed to reduce this number to a small subset of variants that are most likely to be pathogenic. The filtering steps applied to exome sequencing data account for qualitative requirements, predicted effect of the variant on the protein, and whether the variant has been previously identified. Generally, these steps leave 150 to 500 nonsynonymous or splice-site variants to be considered as potentially pathogenic.[69] This number is generally too large to allow follow-up of all the variants, and additional prioritization strategies are needed. These strategies are generally based on the likely inheritance pattern of the disease (eg, looking for recessive mutations in linkage interval or de novo mutations in apparently sporadic disease).

Exome Sequencing in Neonatal Diabetes

More than 100 genes causing Mendelian disorders have been identified using exome sequencing,[70] including 2 novel causes of syndromic neonatal diabetes: *GATA6*[15] and *STAT3*.[4]

Identification of mutations in GATA6 as the most common cause of pancreatic agenesis

Neonatal diabetes caused by pancreatic agenesis is an extremely rare condition characterized by insulin-dependent diabetes and pancreatic exocrine insufficiency requiring enzyme supplementation therapy.[15] Before the identification of mutations in *GATA6*, only recessive mutations in 2 pancreatic developmental factors, *PDX1* and *PTF1A*, were known to cause pancreatic agenesis in humans. Mutations in

Table 2
Comparison between exome and genome sequencing

Technology	Amount of Data	Number of Variants	Cost ($)
Exome sequencing	50 Mb	~25,000	500
Genome sequencing	200 Gb	~3,000,000	5000

PDX1 had been described in 4 cases with isolated agenesis of the pancreas.[32–34] Mutations in *PTF1A* had been reported in 4 families in which affected individuals had both pancreatic and cerebellar agenesis.[37–39]

Lango Allen and colleagues[15] investigated a cohort of 27 patients with pancreatic agenesis and noticed that most patients with syndromic pancreatic agenesis were born to unaffected, unrelated parents. This finding suggested that the mutation causing the condition was most likely sporadic. To investigate this hypothesis, the investigators performed exome sequencing of 2 probands with pancreatic agenesis and a congenital heart malformation and their unaffected, unrelated parents with the objective of identifying de novo mutations (present in the patients but not inherited from either parent). After exclusion of common variants and variants that were unlikely to be pathogenic (eg, synonymous variants that do not lead to changes in the amino acid sequence), a single de novo variant was confirmed in each patient. Both variants, a missense mutation and a frameshift deletion, affected the coding region of the developmental transcription factor gene *GATA6*.

GATA6 is a transcription factor involved in early embryonic development of multiple organs, including the pancreas.[71] Traditionally, identification of novel causes of neonatal diabetes was guided by a candidate gene approach, based on the phenotype of mouse models. These studies were not suggestive of a role of Gata6 in pancreatic development in rodents,[71,72] and for this reason investigation of *GATA6* in patients with neonatal diabetes had not been considered before. In this case exome sequencing led to the identification of a novel disease gene and gave unexpected insights into human pancreatic development.

Lango Allen and colleagues[15] then sequenced *GATA6* in 25 additional patients with pancreatic agenesis and identified mutations in 13 additional cases. The investigators concluded that heterozygous mutations in *GATA6* are the most common cause of pancreatic agenesis.

A subsequent study[16] looked at the contribution of *GATA6* mutations in patients with neonatal diabetes but no reported exocrine insufficiency. The results showed that mutations in this gene cause a broad phenotypic spectrum of diabetes, from complete pancreatic agenesis to adult-onset diabetes without exocrine pancreatic insufficiency.

Identification of activating STAT3 mutations as a cause of early onset multiorgan autoimmune disease

In some cases diabetes diagnosed before 6 months can be caused by mutations in a single gene causing a polyendocrinopathy syndrome characterized by severe early autoimmunity leading to β-cell destruction. The most common of these conditions is IPEX syndrome (immune dysregulation, polyendocrinopathy, enteropathy, X-linked), which is caused by mutations in the *FOXP3* gene.[12] Identification of the genes causing these conditions is crucial to understand the mechanisms involved in the pathogenesis of more common autoimmune diseases.

In order to identify the gene causing early onset poly-autoimmunity, Flanagan and colleagues[4] performed exome sequencing of a proband/parents trio for a patient diagnosed with diabetes at 2 weeks and early onset additional autoimmune conditions (autoimmune hypothyroidism diagnosed at 3 years and celiac disease diagnosed at 17 months). A single de novo mutation in the transcription factor gene *STAT3* was identified. Sequencing of *STAT3* in 63 additional patients (24 with early onset autoimmune disease and 39 with neonatal diabetes) identified mutations in 4 further individuals.

Functional studies on the mutated STAT3 protein showed that the changes identified in patients with the early onset poly-autoimmunity phenotype were all activating mutations, whereas mutations resulting in decreased activity of the STAT3 protein have been previously described as a cause of hyper immunoglobulin E syndrome.[73] The investigators proposed a mechanism in which *STAT3* activating mutations lead to early autoimmunity by impairing the development of regulatory T cells.[4]

In this study the use of exome sequencing lead to the identification of a novel cause of neonatal diabetes and gave important insights into the complex mechanisms leading to autoimmunity. This knowledge can be exploited to better understand the basis of more common autoimmune diseases, such as type 1 diabetes.

GENOME SEQUENCING
Method

Genome sequencing allows the analysis of approximately the entire genomic sequence ($\sim$98%[74]), without prior selection of specific regions. Each genome sequenced produces about 200 Gb of data with 3 to 4 million single nucleotide variants expected to be detected in each individual (see **Table 2**).

Genome sequencing is considered the most comprehensive test currently available[75] and presents some technical advantages compared with whole-exome sequencing: It is more sensitive and accurate for detecting structural variation (such as insertions, deletions, and translocations) because it does not rely on capture of a subset of regions and it allows a more even coverage throughout the genome. Another advantage of genome sequencing is the possibility to investigate nonexonic regulatory regions that are missed by exome sequencing. The main obstacles to the use of whole-genome sequencing for diagnostics have been the relatively high cost (which is rapidly falling) and the enormous amount of data produced, resulting in challenging data analysis (see **Table 2**). Most of the studies reporting the use of whole-genome sequencing so far have limited the initial variants analysis to the part of the genome encoding for proteins and have proceeded to the investigation of the noncoding variants just when a causing mutation could not be identified in the exome.

Genome Sequencing in Neonatal Diabetes

The use of genome sequencing in patients with isolated pancreatic agenesis recently led to the identification of mutations in a previously unrecognized regulatory element of the *PTF1A* gene.[40]

Biallelic mutations affecting the gene encoding for the transcription factor *PTF1A* are a known cause of pancreatic and cerebellar agenesis, with 4 families reported so far.[37–39] Weedon and colleagues[40] used whole-genome sequencing to identify the genetic cause of isolated pancreatic agenesis. The investigators studied 3 consanguineous pedigrees, which included multiple affected individuals, suggesting a recessive pattern of inheritance. Linkage analysis in the 3 families highlighted a single shared region on chromosome 10, including the *PTF1A* gene. No coding mutation segregating with the disease was identified.

Genome sequencing was subsequently performed in 2 probands; analysis was performed prioritizing coding variants for the initial analysis, but no likely cause was found. The investigators then concentrated on molecular changes affecting genomic regions regulating early pancreatic development. A single shared homozygous variant located in a highly conserved region approximately 25 kb from the *PTF1A* locus was identified. Sequencing analysis of the putative regulatory element in 19 additional patients with pancreatic agenesis identified a mutation in 8 of them.

Functional studies showed that the regulatory element is indeed a previously unrecognized *PTF1A* enhancer (a genomic element enhancing gene transcription), which is selectively active during pancreatic development.[40] These results probably explain why patients with mutations in the *PTF1A* distal enhancer do not present the severe cerebellar phenotype associated with mutations affecting the *PTF1A* gene.[37–39]

In this study the application of genome sequencing has been crucial to identify the genetic cause of pancreatic agenesis in 10 families and uncover the role of a previously unsuspected regulatory element necessary for normal pancreatic development in humans.

CONCLUDING REMARKS

Next-generation sequencing applications are now widely used both for diagnostic genetic testing and for identification of novel causes of genetic conditions. Neonatal diabetes, being a genetically heterogeneous Mendelian disorder, has greatly benefitted from the application of next-generation sequencing technologies both in diagnostic and research settings.

Impact of Next-Generation Sequencing in Diagnosis of Neonatal Diabetes

There are 23 known causes of neonatal diabetes that identify different clinical subtypes of the disease (De Franco and colleagues, *submitted for publication*, and[4]), including isolated permanent neonatal diabetes, transient neonatal diabetes, and complex syndromes whereby neonatal diabetes is often the presenting feature (eg, Wolcott-Rallison syndrome). Traditional genetic testing for neonatal diabetes requires accurate clinical information regarding the patients' phenotype to allow selection of a small number of genes to test. Because patients are now referred soon after diagnosis with neonatal diabetes, this approach is limited by the clinical features present at the moment of genetic testing.

Targeted next-generation sequencing allows comprehensive analysis of all the genes known to cause neonatal diabetes in a single test. A genetic diagnosis can be identified in more than 80% of patients (De Franco and colleagues, *submitted for publication*), including approximately 40% of patients who have the genetic subtypes (mutations in *KCNJ11* and *ABCC8*) treatable with high-dose sulfonylurea instead of insulin.

For patients with syndromic forms of neonatal diabetes, hyperglycemia in the first 6 months of life is often the presenting feature of the disease. The other phenotypic features characterizing the disease can often present months or years after the initial diagnosis of neonatal diabetes. The most common of these conditions is Wolcott-Rallison syndrome, a recessive disease characterized by neonatal diabetes, skeletal dysplasia, and liver dysfunction.[13,14] For these patients an early genetic diagnosis predicts the future development of additional clinical features and raises awareness of the potential life-threatening complications (De Franco and colleagues, *submitted for publication*).

In the context of neonatal diabetes, next-generation sequencing allowed a shift in the paradigm of genetic testing: the genetic investigation is not merely confirmatory anymore, but it makes the diagnosis and guides clinical management of the patients.

Impact of Next-Generation Sequencing for Identification of Novel Causes of Neonatal Diabetes

Applications of next-generation sequencing technologies, exome sequencing in particular, have led to the identification of many novel causes of different genetic conditions.

Before the introduction of next-generation sequencing, identification of disease-causing genes was focused on analysis of candidate genes, selected by observations coming from animal model experiments, and linkage studies that are possible only when multiple affected individuals are available. Strategies based on exome sequencing are not biased by the prior knowledge on biological function suggested by experiments on animal models. For this reason discoveries of novel causes of disease by next-generation sequencing can sometimes highlight previously unrecognized roles for known genes. This circumstance is the case for the identification of mutations in *GATA6* as the most common cause of pancreatic agenesis in humans by exome sequencing.[15] Mutations in *GATA6* account for approximately 50% of pancreatic agenesis cases, but experiments looking at the development of the pancreas in mouse models had not suggested a role of this gene in pancreatic development.[71,72]

Identification of a genetic defect causing extreme phenotypes, such as early onset multiorgan autoimmunity, has important implications in the study of complex diseases, such as type 1 diabetes. The use of exome sequencing recently led to the identification of activating mutations in *STAT3* as a cause of early onset poly-autoimmunity, highlighting a fundamental role of this transcription factor in immune system regulation.[4]

Genome sequencing is considered the most comprehensive of the genetic tests currently available[75] as it allows investigation of complex genomic rearrangements, copy number variation, and variants in intronic and regulatory regions as well as in the coding parts of the genome. A combination of linkage studies and whole-genome sequencing in 2 consanguineous families with isolated pancreatic agenesis led to the identification of mutations in a previously unknown enhancer regulating expression of *PTF1A* during development of the pancreas.[40]

The introduction of next-generation sequencing has greatly expanded the potential of the strategies used to identify novel causes of genetic diseases. The research of novel causes of neonatal diabetes is a perfect example of how applications of next-generation sequencing technologies, coupled with appropriate analysis strategies, are powerful tools to successfully identify novel disease-causing genes.

ACKNOWLEDGMENTS

The authors thank all their colleagues in Exeter for their contributions in developing of the next-generation sequencing capacity for monogenic diabetes.

REFERENCES

1. Iafusco D, Massa O, Pasquino B, et al. Minimal incidence of neonatal/infancy onset diabetes in Italy is 1:90,000 live births. Acta Diabetol 2012;49(5):405–8.
2. Edghill EL, Dix RJ, Flanagan SE, et al. HLA genotyping supports a nonautoimmune etiology in patients diagnosed with diabetes under the age of 6 months. Diabetes 2006;55(6):1895–8.
3. Iafusco D, Stazi MA, Cotichini R, et al. Permanent diabetes mellitus in the first year of life. Diabetologia 2002;45(6):798–804.
4. Flanagan SE, Haapaniemi E, Russell MA, et al. Activating germline mutations in STAT3 cause early-onset multi-organ autoimmune disease. Nat Genet 2014; 46(8):812–4.
5. Gardner RJ, Mackay DJ, Mungall AJ, et al. An imprinted locus associated with transient neonatal diabetes mellitus. Hum Mol Genet 2000;9(4):589–96.

6. Temple IK, Gardner RJ, Robinson DO, et al. Further evidence for an imprinted gene for neonatal diabetes localised to chromosome 6q22-q23. Hum Mol Genet 1996;5(8):1117–21.
7. Temple IK, Shield JP. Transient neonatal diabetes, a disorder of imprinting. J Med Genet 2002;39(12):872–5.
8. Babenko AP, Polak M, Cave H, et al. Activating mutations in the ABCC8 gene in neonatal diabetes mellitus. N Engl J Med 2006;355(5):456–66.
9. Proks P, Arnold AL, Bruining J, et al. A heterozygous activating mutation in the sulphonylurea receptor SUR1 (ABCC8) causes neonatal diabetes. Hum Mol Genet 2006;15(11):1793–800.
10. Delepine M, Nicolino M, Barrett T, et al. EIF2AK3, encoding translation initiation factor 2-alpha kinase 3, is mutated in patients with Wolcott-Rallison syndrome. Nat Genet 2000;25(4):406–9.
11. Rubio-Cabezas O, Patch AM, Minton JA, et al. Wolcott-Rallison syndrome is the most common genetic cause of permanent neonatal diabetes in consanguineous families. J Clin Endocrinol Metab 2009;94(11):4162–70.
12. Chatila TA, Blaeser F, Ho N, et al. JM2, encoding a fork head-related protein, is mutated in X-linked autoimmunity-allergic disregulation syndrome. J Clin Invest 2000;106(12):R75–81.
13. D'Amato E, Giacopelli F, Giannattasio A, et al. Genetic investigation in an Italian child with an unusual association of atrial septal defect, attributable to a new familial GATA4 gene mutation, and neonatal diabetes due to pancreatic agenesis. Diabet Med 2010;27(10):1195–200.
14. Shaw-Smith C, De Franco E, Allen HL, et al. GATA4 mutations are a cause of neonatal and childhood-onset diabetes. Diabetes 2014;63(8):2888–94.
15. Lango Allen H, Flanagan SE, Shaw-Smith C, et al. GATA6 haploinsufficiency causes pancreatic agenesis in humans. Nat Genet 2012;44(1):20–2.
16. De Franco E, Shaw-Smith C, Flanagan SE, et al. GATA6 mutations cause a broad phenotypic spectrum of diabetes from pancreatic agenesis to adult-onset diabetes without exocrine insufficiency. Diabetes 2013;62(3):993–7.
17. Njolstad PR, Sovik O, Cuesta-Munoz A, et al. Neonatal diabetes mellitus due to complete glucokinase deficiency. N Engl J Med 2001;344(21):1588–92.
18. Barbetti F, Cobo-Vuilleumier N, Dionisi-Vici C, et al. Opposite clinical phenotypes of glucokinase disease: description of a novel activating mutation and contiguous inactivating mutations in human glucokinase (GCK) gene. Mol Endocrinol 2009; 23(12):1983–9.
19. Dimitri P, Warner JT, Minton JA, et al. Novel GLIS3 mutations demonstrate an extended multisystem phenotype. Eur J Endocrinol 2011;164(3):437–43.
20. Senee V, Chelala C, Duchatelet S, et al. Mutations in GLIS3 are responsible for a rare syndrome with neonatal diabetes mellitus and congenital hypothyroidism. Nat Genet 2006;38(6):682–7.
21. Edghill EL, Bingham C, Ellard S, et al. Mutations in hepatocyte nuclear factor-1beta and their related phenotypes. J Med Genet 2006;43(1):84–90.
22. Yorifuji T, Kurokawa K, Mamada M, et al. Neonatal diabetes mellitus and neonatal polycystic, dysplastic kidneys: phenotypically discordant recurrence of a mutation in the hepatocyte nuclear factor-1beta gene due to germline mosaicism. J Clin Endocrinol Metab 2004;89(6):2905–8.
23. Abdel-Salam GM, Schaffer AE, Zaki MS, et al. A homozygous IER3IP1 mutation causes microcephaly with simplified gyral pattern, epilepsy, and permanent neonatal diabetes syndrome (MEDS). Am J Med Genet A 2012;158A(11): 2788–96.

24. Poulton CJ, Schot R, Kia SK, et al. Microcephaly with simplified gyration, epilepsy, and infantile diabetes linked to inappropriate apoptosis of neural progenitors. Am J Hum Genet 2011;89(2):265–76.
25. Garin I, Edghill EL, Akerman I, et al. Recessive mutations in the INS gene result in neonatal diabetes through reduced insulin biosynthesis. Proc Natl Acad Sci U S A 2010;107(7):3105–10.
26. Stoy J, Edghill EL, Flanagan SE, et al. Insulin gene mutations as a cause of permanent neonatal diabetes. Proc Natl Acad Sci U S A 2007;104(38):15040–4.
27. Gloyn AL, Pearson ER, Antcliff JF, et al. Activating mutations in the gene encoding the ATP-sensitive potassium-channel subunit Kir6.2 and permanent neonatal diabetes. N Engl J Med 2004;350(18):1838–49.
28. Gloyn AL, Reimann F, Girard C, et al. Relapsing diabetes can result from moderately activating mutations in KCNJ11. Hum Mol Genet 2005;14(7):925–34.
29. Flanagan SE, De Franco E, Lango Allen H, et al. Analysis of transcription factors key for mouse pancreatic development establishes NKX2-2 and MNX1 mutations as causes of neonatal diabetes in man. Cell Metab 2014;19(1):146–54.
30. Rubio-Cabezas O, Minton JA, Kantor I, et al. Homozygous mutations in NEUROD1 are responsible for a novel syndrome of permanent neonatal diabetes and neurological abnormalities. Diabetes 2010;59(9):2326–31.
31. Rubio-Cabezas O, Jensen JN, Hodgson MI, et al. Permanent neonatal diabetes and enteric anendocrinosis associated with biallelic mutations in NEUROG3. Diabetes 2011;60(4):1349–53.
32. Schwitzgebel VM, Mamin A, Brun T, et al. Agenesis of human pancreas due to decreased half-life of insulin promoter factor 1. J Clin Endocrinol Metab 2003; 88(9):4398–406.
33. Stoffers DA, Zinkin NT, Stanojevic V, et al. Pancreatic agenesis attributable to a single nucleotide deletion in the human IPF1 gene coding sequence. Nat Genet 1997;15(1):106–10.
34. Thomas IH, Saini NK, Adhikari A, et al. Neonatal diabetes mellitus with pancreatic agenesis in an infant with homozygous IPF-1 Pro63fsX60 mutation. Pediatr Diabetes 2009;10(7):492–6.
35. De Franco E, Shaw-Smith C, Flanagan SE, et al. Biallelic PDX1 (insulin promoter factor 1) mutations causing neonatal diabetes without exocrine pancreatic insufficiency. Diabet Med 2013;30(5):e197–200.
36. Nicolino M, Claiborn KC, Senee V, et al. A novel hypomorphic PDX1 mutation responsible for permanent neonatal diabetes with subclinical exocrine deficiency. Diabetes 2010;59(3):733–40.
37. Al-Shammari M, Al-Husain M, Al-Kharfy T, et al. A novel PTF1A mutation in a patient with severe pancreatic and cerebellar involvement. Clin Genet 2011;80(2):196–8.
38. Sellick GS, Barker KT, Stolte-Dijkstra I, et al. Mutations in PTF1A cause pancreatic and cerebellar agenesis. Nat Genet 2004;36(12):1301–5.
39. Tutak E, Satar M, Yapicioglu H, et al. A Turkish newborn infant with cerebellar agenesis/neonatal diabetes mellitus and PTF1A mutation. Genet Couns 2009; 20(2):147–52.
40. Weedon MN, Cebola I, Patch AM, et al. Recessive mutations in a distal PTF1A enhancer cause isolated pancreatic agenesis. Nat Genet 2014;46(1):61–4.
41. Smith SB, Qu HQ, Taleb N, et al. Rfx6 directs islet formation and insulin production in mice and humans. Nature 2010;463(7282):775–80.
42. Spiegel R, Dobbie A, Hartman C, et al. Clinical characterization of a newly described neonatal diabetes syndrome caused by RFX6 mutations. Am J Med Genet 2011;155A(11):2821–5.

43. Bay A, Keskin M, Hizli S, et al. Thiamine-responsive megaloblastic anemia syndrome. Int J Hematol 2010;92(3):524–6.
44. Bergmann AK, Sahai I, Falcone JF, et al. Thiamine-responsive megaloblastic anemia: identification of novel compound heterozygotes and mutation update. J Pediatr 2009;155(6):888–92.e1.
45. Mandel H, Berant M, Hazani A, et al. Thiamine-dependent beriberi in the "thiamine-responsive anemia syndrome". N Engl J Med 1984;311(13):836–8.
46. Shaw-Smith C, Flanagan SE, Patch AM, et al. Recessive SLC19A2 mutations are a cause of neonatal diabetes mellitus in thiamine-responsive megaloblastic anaemia. Pediatr Diabetes 2012;13(4):314–21.
47. Sansbury FH, Flanagan SE, Houghton JA, et al. SLC2A2 mutations can cause neonatal diabetes, suggesting GLUT2 may have a role in human insulin secretion. Diabetologia 2012;55(9):2381–5.
48. Mackay DJ, Callaway JL, Marks SM, et al. Hypomethylation of multiple imprinted loci in individuals with transient neonatal diabetes is associated with mutations in ZFP57. Nat Genet 2008;40(8):949–51.
49. Mackay DJ, Temple IK. Transient neonatal diabetes mellitus type 1. Am J Med Genet C Semin Med Genet 2010;154C(3):335–42.
50. Ellard S, Flanagan SE, Girard CA, et al. Permanent neonatal diabetes caused by dominant, recessive, or compound heterozygous SUR1 mutations with opposite functional effects. Am J Hum Genet 2007;81(2):375–82.
51. Codner E, Flanagan S, Ellard S, et al. High-dose glibenclamide can replace insulin therapy despite transitory diarrhea in early-onset diabetes caused by a novel R201L Kir6.2 mutation. Diabetes Care 2005;28(3):758–9.
52. Pearson ER, Flechtner I, Njolstad PR, et al. Switching from insulin to oral sulfonylureas in patients with diabetes due to Kir6.2 mutations. N Engl J Med 2006; 355(5):467–77.
53. Hattersley A, Bruining J, Shield J, et al. ISPAD clinical practice consensus guidelines 2006-2007. The diagnosis and management of monogenic diabetes in children. Pediatr Diabetes 2006;7(6):352–60.
54. Flanagan SE, Patch AM, Mackay DJ, et al. Mutations in ATP-sensitive K+ channel genes cause transient neonatal diabetes and permanent diabetes in childhood or adulthood. Diabetes 2007;56(7):1930–7.
55. Margulies M, Egholm M, Altman WE, et al. Genome sequencing in microfabricated high-density picolitre reactors. Nature 2005;437(7057):376–80.
56. Johansson H, Isaksson M, Sorqvist EF, et al. Targeted resequencing of candidate genes using selector probes. Nucleic Acids Res 2011;39(2):e8.
57. O'Sullivan J, Mullaney BG, Bhaskar SS, et al. A paradigm shift in the delivery of services for diagnosis of inherited retinal disease. J Med Genet 2012;49(5):322–6.
58. Redin C, Le Gras S, Mhamdi O, et al. Targeted high-throughput sequencing for diagnosis of genetically heterogeneous diseases: efficient mutation detection in Bardet-Biedl and Alstrom syndromes. J Med Genet 2012;49(8):502–12.
59. Shendure J, Ji H. Next-generation DNA sequencing. Nat Biotechnol 2008;26(10): 1135–45.
60. Duan J, Zhang JG, Deng HW, et al. Comparative studies of copy number variation detection methods for next-generation sequencing technologies. PloS One 2013;8(3):e59128.
61. Wang H, Nettleton D, Ying K. Copy number variation detection using next generation sequencing read counts. BMC Bioinformatics 2014;15:109.
62. Morgan JE, Carr IM, Sheridan E, et al. Genetic diagnosis of familial breast cancer using clonal sequencing. Hum Mutat 2010;31(4):484–91.

63. Rossetti S, Hopp K, Sikkink RA, et al. Identification of gene mutations in autosomal dominant polycystic kidney disease through targeted resequencing. J Am Soc Nephrol 2012;23(5):915–33.
64. Bonnefond A, Philippe J, Durand E, et al. Highly sensitive diagnosis of 43 monogenic forms of diabetes or obesity through one-step PCR-based enrichment in combination with next-generation sequencing. Diabetes Care 2014;37(2):460–7.
65. Ellard S, Lango Allen H, De Franco E, et al. Improved genetic testing for monogenic diabetes using targeted next-generation sequencing. Diabetologia 2013; 56(9):1958–63.
66. Gao R, Liu Y, Gjesing AP, et al. Evaluation of a target region capture sequencing platform using monogenic diabetes as a study-model. BMC Genet 2014;15(1):13.
67. Neufeld EJ, Fleming JC, Tartaglini E, et al. Thiamine-responsive megaloblastic anemia syndrome: a disorder of high-affinity thiamine transport. Blood Cells Mol Dis 2001;27(1):135–8.
68. Gilissen C, Hoischen A, Brunner HG, et al. Disease gene identification strategies for exome sequencing. Eur J Hum Genet 2012;20(5):490–7.
69. Vissers LE, de Ligt J, Gilissen C, et al. A de novo paradigm for mental retardation. Nat Genet 2010;42(12):1109–12.
70. Rabbani B, Mahdieh N, Hosomichi K, et al. Next-generation sequencing: impact of exome sequencing in characterizing Mendelian disorders. J Hum Genet 2012; 57(10):621–32.
71. Morrisey EE, Tang Z, Sigrist K, et al. GATA6 regulates HNF4 and is required for differentiation of visceral endoderm in the mouse embryo. Genes Dev 1998; 12(22):3579–90.
72. Watt AJ, Zhao R, Li J, et al. Development of the mammalian liver and ventral pancreas is dependent on GATA4. BMC Dev Biol 2007;7:37.
73. Holland SM, DeLeo FR, Elloumi HZ, et al. STAT3 mutations in the hyper-IgE syndrome. N Engl J Med 2007;357(16):1608–19.
74. Gilissen C, Hehir-Kwa JY, Thung DT, et al. Genome sequencing identifies major causes of severe intellectual disability. Nature 2014;511(7509):344–7.
75. Lupski JR, Reid JG, Gonzaga-Jauregui C, et al. Whole-genome sequencing in a patient with Charcot-Marie-Tooth neuropathy. N Engl J Med 2010;362(13): 1181–91.

Index

Note: Page numbers of article titles are in **boldface** type.

A

ABC gene, 1021, 1025, 1027, 1029, 1038, 1040, 1044, 1048
Acanthosis nigricans, 825
Acidosis, in diabetes mellitus. *See* Ketoacidosis, diabetic.
Activities of daily living, short stature and, 970
Adaptation, to short stature, 966–968
Adenomas, thyroid, 934–935
Adrenal inefficiency, 992
Affirmed gender, definition of, 1002
Age factors, in diabetic ketoacidosis, 860
Alkaline phosphatase, measurement of, 846
Amenorrhea, 945, 948, 951–954
American Academy of Pediatrics, weight management guidelines of, 5 As of
    Obesity Management, 826
Aminocaproic acid, for abnormal uterine bleeding, 946, 951
Amiodarone, thyroid dysfunction from, 935
Ammonia, in hyperinsulinemic hypoglycemia, 1026
Anatomic sex, 1002
Androgens
    deficiency of, in disorders of sex evelopment, 986, 991–992, 994
    excess of, in disorders of sex development, 986
Androstenedione, deficiency of, in disorders of sex development, 991–992, 994
Anxiety
    in diabetes mellitus, 913–914
    in obesity, 825
Artificial pancreas (closed-loop delivery system), 881–882
Aspart, 875–876, 878
Attention, diabetes mellitus effects on, 901–902, 913
Autonomic neuropathy, diabetic, 893, 898

B

Background diabetic retinopathy, 892, 895, 897
Bariatric surgery, for obesity, 829–833
Barker hypothesis, of short stature, 968–969, 971
Beckwith-Wiedemann syndrome, 1024
Behavioral approach, for obesity, 831
Behavioral issues, in diabetes mellitus, 892
Beta cells, insulin secretion from, 1020
3β-Hydroxysteroid dehydrogenase deficiency, 994
Biological sex, 1002
Biopsy, bone, 851

Pediatr Clin N Am 62 (2015) 1055–1069
http://dx.doi.org/10.1016/S0031-3955(15)00101-7
0031-3955/15/$ – see front matter © 2015 Elsevier Inc. All rights reserved.

pediatric.theclinics.com

Moving?

Make sure your subscription moves with you!

To notify us of your new address, find your **Clinics Account Number** (located on your mailing label above your name), and contact customer service at:

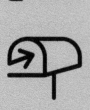

Email: journalscustomerservice-usa@elsevier.com

800-654-2452 (subscribers in the U.S. & Canada)
314-447-8871 (subscribers outside of the U.S. & Canada)

Fax number: 314-447-8029

Elsevier Health Sciences Division
Subscription Customer Service
3251 Riverport Lane
Maryland Heights, MO 63043

*To ensure uninterrupted delivery of your subscription, please notify us at least 4 weeks in advance of move.

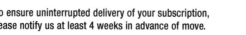

Printed and bound by CPI Group (UK) Ltd, Croydon, CR0 4YY

03/10/2024

01040489-0007